SOURCE BOOK OF GERIATRIC ASSESSMENT

Vol. 1

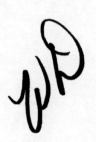

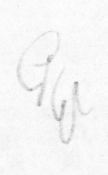

Liliane Israël

Djordje Kozarević

Norman Sartorius

SOURCE BOOK OF GERIATRIC ASSESSMENT

Preface to the English Edition by Anne Gilmore

Produced with the collaboration
of the World Health Organization

Vol. 1

Evaluations in Gerontology

The English edition of this book has been produced with the technical collaboration of

R. LYLE

Department of General Psychology, Southmead District General Hospital, Westbury-on-Trim, Bristol

L. WAINTRAUB   B. LEFEVRE

G. Israël, M. Bucci, M. Israël

Centre Régional de Gériatrie, Service Hospitalo-Universitaire de Gérontologie Clinique, Grenoble

S. KUNIJEVIĆ   Lj. KOZAREVIĆ

G. Milisavljević, M. Bosković, S. Petrović

Institute of Chronic Diseases and Gerontology, Belgrade

D. MASSARI

M. Vaccari, L. Chiaruttini

Fidia Data Centre for Clinical Research, Abano Terme

G. FILLENBAUM

Center for Study of Aging and Human
Development, Duke University, Durham

R. TAYLOR

Medical Research Council
Medical Sociology Unit, Aberdeen

S. Karger · Basel · München · Paris · London · New York · Tokyo · Sydney · 1984

National Library of Medicine, Cataloging in Publication
Israël, Liliane
Source book of geriatric assessment
Liliane Israël, Djordje Kozarević, Norman Sartorius, with the collaboration of the World Health Organization WHO.
Basel; New York: Karger, 1984
2 v.
Contents: v. 1. Evaluations in gerontology. v. 2. Review of analysed instruments. Includes bibliographies and index.
1. Geriatric Psychiatry 2. Mental Processes - in old age 3. Psychological Tests - instrumentation 4. Psychiatric Status Rating Scales
I. Kozarević, Djordje II. Sartorius, N. III. World Health Organization IV. Title
WT 150 I85s
ISBN 3-8055-3832-4 (set)
ISBN 3-8055-3830-8 (v.1)

CONTENTS

Foreword by T.A. Lambo
Preface to the English Edition by Anne Gilmore

I GUIDING PRINCIPLES AND CLASSIFICATION CRITERIA

II DESCRIPTIVE FORMS

Section 1: Uni-dimensional Instruments

(*) Translated title

(*) Translated title

Section 3: Three-Dimensional Instruments

(*) Translated title

III COMPLEMENTARY INSTRUMENTS

IV INDEX

V BIBLIOGRAPHIES

(*) Translated title

ACKNOWLEDGEMENTS

The authors wish to offer their special appreciation to all those who contributed to the preparation of the book. They would like to thank in particular:

The authors of the instruments who gave their authorization for reproduction and also actively participated in the preparation of the descriptive forms.

The collaborative institutions whose contribution was essential:

THE "SERVICE DE GERIATRIE DU CENTRE HOSPITALIER REGIONAL ET UNIVERSITAIRE DE GRENOBLE", directed by Prof. R. Hugonot and the "Association pour le Developpement des Recherches" (A.D.R.) in Grenoble, France.
THE INSTITUTE OF CHRONIC DISEASES AND GERONTOLOGY, (I.C.D.G.), Belgrade, Yugoslavia.
THE CENTER FOR MULTIDISCIPLINARY STUDIES of the University of Belgrade, Yugoslavia, directed by Prof. R. Andjus.
THE INSTITUTIONS DE GERIATRIE of Geneva directed by Prof. J.P. Junod, with the assistance of Dr. Th. Hovaguimian, Consultant, Division of Mental Health, W.H.O., Geneva, Switzerland.

The technical collaborators for their excellent support:
Dr. **D. McGee**
    Senior Statistician, Center for Disease Control, Atlanta, Ga U.S.A.
Dr. **R. Dimitrijević**
    Resident in Psychiatry, Institute of Chronic Diseases and Gerontology, Belgrade, Yugoslavia.
Dr. **R. Krunić**
    Resident in Rehabilitation Medicine, Service of Prof. Congić, Belgrade, Yugoslavia.
Dr. **V. Trifković**
    Resident in Gerontology, Institute of Chronic Diseases and Gerontology, Belgrade, Yugoslavia.
Dr. **L. Waintraub**
    Resident in Psychiatry, Service du Prof. Pichot, Clinique des Maladies Mentales et de l'Encéphale, Faculté Médecine Cochin Port-Royal, Paris, France.

Their final thanks to Prof. **L. Bolis**, World Health Organization, Geneva, for her cooperation in the realization of the book, Dr. **H. Hermanova**, World Health Organization, Regional Office for Europe, Copenhagen, for her encouragements, and to **Prof. R. Hugonot**, who arranged support for the French edition and without whose help this book could not have been published.

Ai miei nonni Armando ed Elena, a mio padre
Giuseppe e a mia madre Evelina dalla cui
convivenza è nato il rispetto e l'amore per
gli anziani.

Liliane

Tout le monde se servait d'une même langue
et des mêmes mots.....

Et Yahvé dit: "Voici que tous font un seul
peuple et parlent une seule langue, et tel est
le début de leurs entreprises!

Maintenant, aucun dessein ne sera
irréalisable pour eux."

Genèse, 11, 6

FOREWORD

The large number of instruments presented in this book demonstrates better than any volume of words that at present there is no single instrument that would satisfy all users and be appropriate for all purposes. Perhaps to envisage such an instrument is utopian. The needs of clinical research and training are many, and the preferences – whether theoretical or practical – of investigators are even more numerous.

As a result, confusion reigns in the assessment of mental functioning. The mental health programme of the World Health Organization, among whose tasks it is to support international and national research, has for many years worked actively on the development of standardized instruments and on the creation of a common language which will allow examinations to be made in a reliable and comparable way and the results to be expressed in terms that will be understood by all concerned. The availability of such a common language will enable resources to be pooled and knowledge shared in a way that is at present impossible.

A number of instruments have been developed by WHO either from scratch or by adapting existing instruments which have been used with remarkable success. These instruments were mainly concerned with the assessment of the mental state of an adult suffering from a mental disorder. In the assessment of the elderly, relatively little has been done by the World Health Organization and it is only during the last few years, when the problems of the elderly have acquired a new urgency, that there has been the development of a global programme on aging, mental health being an important component. Here, as in any programme that aims at developing on an international scale, the availability of a common language is essential.

The first steps in such a programme are to review the instruments that have been developed and tested, to examine evidence of their reliability and validity and other metric characteristics, and to offer this material to researchers, clinicians and health services. The purpose of this book therefore is to provide a means of access to the most frequently used instruments and to give concise information on their characteristics. This will facilitate the selection of an instrument likely to be suitable or requiring adaptation to specific clinical work or, when the work in question requires a new approach, facilitate the examination of existing knowledge and experience.

Care of the elderly – healthy or ill – is a complex undertaking calling for compassion, understanding, and the participation of many groups and services ranging from the family to Ministries of Health and of Social Welfare. However, the contribution which the elderly person is able to make is perhaps the most important factor in determining the quality of care and the quality of life. Measurement of the state of health and ability seen in this context is only one of the technical requirements in the care of the elderly, but an essential one since a real need exists. It is therefore encouraging to see this book come into print.

The authors of this book have received strong support from a large number of investigators who responded to an invitation from WHO to participate in this work, but its publication would not have been possible without the intensive and creative efforts of the three authors who have produced a work of reference of direct use to those who seek to improve the care of the elderly and to research workers in the fields of medicine, behavioural sciences and epidemiology.

T.A. LAMBO
World Health Organization
Geneva

PREFACE

The major demographic change in age structure experienced in most countries this century has been accompanied by an unprecedented but now wholly necessary interest in both the physical and psychosocial capabilities of the elderly population.

This interest has arisen largely because of the demand that large numbers of elderly people are liable to make on every type of support service available to the community and with such a demand greatly increased if these elderly people are in some way incapacitated.

The rise of gerontology as a specialised area of academic work and the advent of geriatric medicine and psychogeriatrics in many countries, together with the awakening of interest in these disciplines in others, has encouraged investigation into such problems of ageing. It is generally acknowledged that although, most probably, continuing progress in medical discovery will contribute to the slight prolongation of the lifespan and assist a greater number of people to reach 75 years and beyond, it will not necessarily be able to prolong total physical or mental independence. It is therefore predictable that there will be an increase in the number of people of advanced age, incapable of total self-care, who will depend on constant medical, nursing or social support.

Such predictions serve to underline the great need which exists already for scientific observation and evaluation by sustained, systematic and accurate means of the disabilities of ageing and of the aged themselves. Often the assessment of the individuals and the organization of their therapy or care is dependent on a treatment plan in which mental state is one of the most important determinant as to whether or not the complaint can be treated or has to be managed and relieved rather than cured.

Assessing the affective mood or level of cognition of the impaired aged individual presents a considerable problem, much more so than rating the ambulatory and clearly functioning person, since with progressive mental disability the patient becomes less able to co-operate and self-assessment may be impossible.

Often there is a requirement for health professionals other than the highly specialised to present to others information about a patient's mental state and behaviour, and it is important and in the best interest of the patient that the report of this information should be as objective and authentic as possible.

Mere descriptions by lay persons are hard to compare because oral or written reportage varies even when the observers are highly trained and intelligent. Thus it is important to transform such information into a standard form to convey it accurately in order to permit formal analysis and perhaps even scientific comparison.

Further, in order to answer any scientific question it is essential to have available the precise instrument to measure the particular parameter which has attracted interest. For example, the physician in his estimation of blood pressure requires a sphygmomanometer and for the cardiac sounds a stethoscope or echocardiograph machine. So what and which instrument is required if memory or cognition have to be examined in the elderly patient? Fortunately there is a multiplicity of tests and instruments available but less fortunately outside the traditional clinical interview there is a "free for all" use of these instruments. Certainly even specialist health professionals may be unfamiliar with the minutiae of psychometrics and will meet with some difficulties when required to document in some form the cognitive state of their elderly patients. Bearing in mind that inconsistent and unreliable data has invalidated much otherwise excellent research, there is a need, therefore, for an evaluation, in detail, of such tests in use today.

The present work is the result of a unique partnership between psychologist, epidemiologist, and psychiatrist. Dr. Lilian Israel, a clinical psychologist previously working in Neurology, and lecturer in Psychology at the University of Social Science in Grenoble, France, who since 1973 has devoted her works to Gerontology; Prof. Djordje Kozarević, Director of the Institute of Chronic Diseases and Gerontology and professor of biomedical population survey methods, University of Belgrade, working for many years in epidemiology and public health; Dr. Norman Sartorius, psychiatrist and psychologist, Director of the Division of Mental Health, WHO headquarters, Geneva.

It is fortunate that the authors using their expertise in psychology, epidemiology, public health and psychiatry have been able to produce a classification and have assembled a large number of assessment instruments, indicating their use with the elderly. This work of reference will prove invaluable to all who are attempting to work creatively in the field of investigation and will contribute ultimately to the greater understanding and better care of the elderly.

ANNE GILMORE M.D.
University of Glasgow and
The Prince and Princess of Wales Hospice
Glasgow

I - GUIDING PRINCIPLES AND CLASSIFICATION CRITERIA

"Pour connaitre la rose, quelqu'un
emploie la géométrie, et un autre
emploie le papillon."

Paul CLAUDEL

I - GUIDING PRINCIPLES AND CLASSIFICATION CRITERIA

1. INTRODUCTION

This source book, in two volumes, is the result of a broad documentary research study conceived with the practical aim of identifying, collecting and classifying evaluative instruments for the elderly, details of which were previously dispersed throughout the literature of many disciplines. The contents concern the multidimensional assessment of the elderly, particularly in the field of mental health. The principle has been to start with the reality of the situation and not with some theoretical concept.

This book is an analysis and synthesis of information aimed at defining and determining the possible applications of each instrument, thus offering the reader a wide range of tools for use in gerontology. The instruments here described and analysed are of different types: questionnaires, check-lists, rating scales and tests. This review was completed from bibliographical and institutional sources; information provided directly by authors was also incorporated. The source book enables the user to select quickly the best tools suited for his purpose. The range of instruments is presented in a standardized way which allows comparisons to be made. The detailed analysis and tabulation has been designed with the purpose of presenting the user with a fixed frame of references which allows him to determine the type of information needed to identify each instrument.

The *"frame of reference"* responds to the necessity of defining axes applicable to all types of instruments. It has been constructed with the view to consider the following questions: *Which are the common characteristics shared by these instruments which allow us to differentiate them? Which aspects are of particular interest to different disciplines?* We were also concerned with the goal, adequacy, reliability and validity of each instrument: *for which purpose has it been designed and how? What does it measure? By whom is it scored or rated? What are its limitations and restrictions? What are its uses? For whom may it be applicable?*

Therefore, with this frame we can answer two types of questions. The first are those we ask ourselves as authors before designing an instrument. *What should be measured? How? Why? On whom? By whom?* Then there are those questions concerning standardization and appropriateness which arise if a specific field of research is contemplated. In order to answer these questions and to solve some of the inherent problems we have attempted to devise a method of presentation which can be readily understood.

Our overall aim has been to provide a common language and to facilitate multidisciplinary communication.

2. CLASSIFICATION CRITERIA

A preliminary review of published work enabled us to distinguish the aspects most frequently assessed and group them into the *three principal dimensions* of physical, mental and social aspects of *functioning* of an individual in his relationship to himself or to his surroundings (Fig. 1).

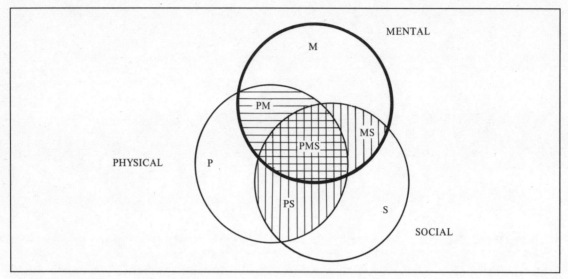

Figure 1: Schematic illustration of interaction between the three principal dimensions.

· ***The physical field*** concerns functional aspects which are the essential components of self-care and activities of daily living.

· ***The mental field*** concerns psychological factors influencing the individual's behavior, and includes cognitive potential, emotional and behavioral elements.

· ***The social field*** concerns the individual's approach to his surrounding, his relationships with others, his interaction with his environment and life events, and his attitudes, adaptability and sociability.

Number of categories assessed

The three main dimensions can be regarded separately or combined in different proportion into seven exclusive groups ranging from specific to global (Fig. 2).

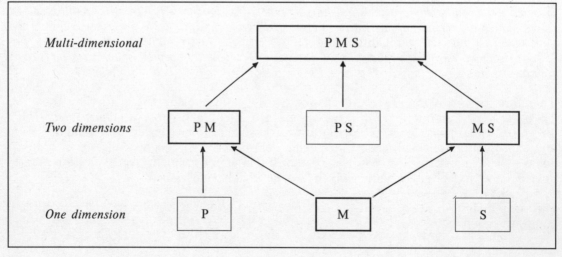

Figure 2: The seven categories discussed in the text showing classification according to evaluated parameters: physical, mental and social.

The specific *uni-dimensional* instruments can assess physical aspects (P), mental aspects (M) or social aspects (S). The principle applied was that when over 80% of the instrument dealt with only one aspect of the three, it should be classified as unidimensional. For example, if a rating scale consisting of 20 items had 16 items measuring aspects of mental health and 4 measuring physical or social activities, the instrument was classified as M and not as PMS.

Two-dimensional instruments were grouped accordingly as being either physical-mental (PM), mental-social (MS) or physical-social (PS).

Three-dimensional instruments deal with the *three dimensions* of health consisting of physical, mental and social elements (PMS). It was required that the instrument should deal with all of the aspects to a similar extent in order to qualify for this category.

The number of aspects dealt with and their combinations formed the basis of first classification criterion. This volume focuses on the four categories dealing with mental health, these being: Physical-Mental-Social (PMS), Physical-Mental (PM), Mental-Social (MS) and Mental (M) (Fig. 3).

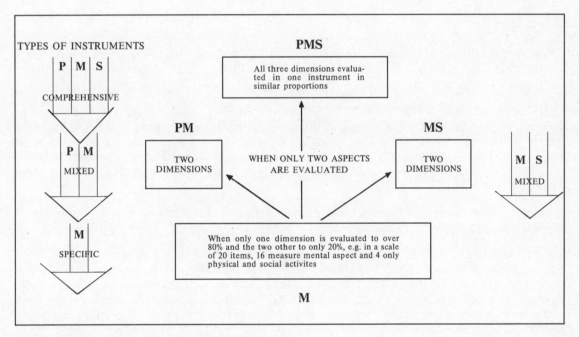

Figure 3. Schematic representation of fields investigated.

The apparent division into different categories should be considered as a device to re-group different instruments into exclusive classes with common inclusion criteria. As ageing progresses the individual's health status becomes more and more susceptible to changes in physical and mental status, as does his capacity for interaction and communication with his habitual environment. However, the different aspects of health (physical, mental and social), should be considered as *perspectives of functioning* rather than as *fields of independent activity,* since in reality they interact and are not separable. One has to deal with the whole person. When planning any intervention, these aspects must be jointly considered, although here they have been subject to separate analysis.

Content of instruments

Within the instruments specific to the mental dimension three main modes can be found: (a) *mood,* (b) *cognition,* and (c) *behavior.* These modes are also present in the other sections in association with physical or social aspects. However, this further subdivision is presented only for those instruments which contain a mental component. In the case of multidimensional instruments (MS, PM and PMS) classification into the categories of mood, cognition and behavior is also indicated in the Index by the letters (a), (b), (c).

Division into three such modes had no preconceived theoretical basis but was a division already inherent in the literature. However, the reader may refer to the index for a classification by author, type of instrument, variable, study population, rater, application, country of origin and language availability.

3. INCLUSION AND EXCLUSION CRITERIA

In order to be included in this source book, the instrument had first to satisfy certain standards. Content, specificity, date of publication and validity were all considered carefully.

· *Content.* The instrument had to have a mental evaluation component, i.e. to refer essentially to psychological functioning. Instruments without a mental component and concerned only with physical or social aspects (P or S), or combined (PS), have been excluded.

· *Specificity.* Although the degree of specificity for that purpose might vary, only instruments applicable to the elderly, i.e. designed for and used in the study of the elderly have been included.

· *Date of publication.* It was the authors intention to review all such tests over the period of the last fifteen years, i.e. from 1965, but it was found possible to review some one hundred instruments which were in operation prior to this data and also to include some recent work covering the period 1980-1982. Details of the one hundred older instruments are included in a complementary bibliography, and their analyses have been presented in descriptive tables, p. 374 - 385.

· *Validity.* The instrument had to yield a quantitative or qualitative score and assessment criteria must have been mentioned.

Some instruments are still in an experimental phase and complete validation has not yet been established, while others have been validated to a greater or lesser extent. All of these have been included. The authors consider that lack of validation need not necessarily negate the potential value of an instrument. Validation is never completely finished and this should be a continuing process. No judgement has, therefore, been made regarding the quality or adequacy of validation studies, although information concerning these aspects is given in detail in the following chapters so that the reader may form his own opinion of the scientific value of the instrument.

In this manner the authors have tried to inform the reader without influencing him. The fact that an instrument has been the subject of numerous validation studies and has been used more, need not necessarily imply that it is better than another. The aim was to provide the user with sufficient information to enable him to choose the tool best adapted to his intended purpose.

4. STAGES IN THE DEVELOPMENT OF THE BOOK

This book was prepared in five stages:

1. *Documentation.* The bibliographic survey used data from different sources.

Standard references in the relevant fields: former works on this theme served as a starting point.
Medlars the data bank of the "National Library of Medicine" provided information.*
Postal enquiries were sent to a great number of institutions identified by the W.H.O. on all five continents.

2. *Correspondence with authors.* It was necessary to classify the instruments identified according to the type of instrument: questionnaire, check-list, rating scale or psychometric test. A specially constructed questionnaire (see appendix vol. 2) was therefore sent to the authors. Most authors (90%) answered during the period of three months. Some completed the questionnaire entirely while others answered only some of the questions. A few sent documentation with the request for us to complete the questionnaire on that basis. Only 3% of the letters in the postal survey were returned undelivered. In some cases English-speaking authors edited the report of the DESCRIPTIVE FORM of their own work. This is indicated by a sign on the left top of the page: (A).

3. *Content analyses and final selection.* A team of three independent experts analysed the instruments after reading the main reference and its related literature. Information was collected and analysed, and the instrument was thereby classified into its appropriate category according to the format described earlier.

4. *Preparation and drafting of Descriptive Forms.* Information available for the content analyses was compared with the responses of the authors to the questionnaire. In preparing the DESCRIPTIVE FORMS attention was paid mainly to these responses. Final synthesis was done by presenting this data in conjunction with relevant bibliography.

5. *Construction of indices.* From the computerised data bank it was possible to derive INDICES according to the elements contained in the descriptive form. These elements were next incorporated into new categories. All necessary instructions for understanding these INDICES can be found in the introduction to the fourth part of this book.

5. GENERAL PRESENTATION

The DESCRIPTIVE FORMS are presented in the *second part* of this volume and they are grouped into three sections corresponding to the number of dimensions included.
Each descriptive form in followed by its corresponding bibliography which is presented in a standardized way.

    Section one : Uni-dimensional instruments.
    Section two : Two-dimensional instruments.
    Section three: Three-dimensional instruments.

Summary tables by category and sub-categories of different sections are presented after the DESCRIPTIVE FORMS for the 145 instruments included in this book. They contain the key words detailing principal areas and the validation studies relating to each of them.

The third part of volume one contains a list of titles and information of one hundred complementary instruments which did not satisfy the selection criteria. A short and condensed analysis of these instruments is presented on the basis of the same model as for the instruments which were included.

(*) INSERM Documentation Center, Hopital de Bicêtre, 78 rue du Général Leclerc, 94270 Le Kremlin Bicêtre, France.

In the *fourth part* the INDICES are presented under the following headings which are author, type of instrument, category of classification, subject and area of application, year of publication, country, specificity, study population and raters.

Bibliographies are presented in the *fifth part*. They include references for the two hundred and forty-five instruments, together with a general bibliography for the book.

VOLUME TWO presents the actual instruments for which we have obtained full authorisation for reproduction from those concerned.

These volumes are therefore intended to meet many different demands and are addressed to all those in the various professions concerned with the elderly, i.e. medical and nursing personnel and other practitioners, research workers and teachers in the field of geriatrics and gerontology.

II - DESCRIPTIVE FORMS

"..... L'homme se découvre quand il se mesure avec l'obstacle. Mais pour l'atteindre, il lui faut un outil."

Antoine de Saint-Exupery

II – DESCRIPTIVE FORMS

This part of VOLUME ONE is a collection of one hundred and forty-five DESCRIPTIVE FORMS and provides specific data for each instrument arranged according to the three dimensions previously outlined. These data are presented after the title as: Identifying information, analysis of content and references.

· *Identifying information* includes the author, the title of the principal reference, title of review, year of publication, language and translations available, the addresses of author or editor.

· *Analysis of content* is derived from several convergent sources of information: correspondence with the authors, analyses of the content of principal references and of complementary instruments prepared by different experts. Each DESCRIPTIVE FORM has its own particular reference system which appears immediately after the information has been given for the instrument.

· *The references* are of two kinds:

The first is related to the *content* of the DESCRIPTIVE FORM and is arranged under three headings:

      Origin of the Instrument
      Validation Studies
      Other works (cited by author)

The second type is also related to the content and appears in a bibliography which has been indicated by the author, or extracted from the principal references. These additional references may be of use to those interested more specifically in a given instrument.

1 – FRAME OF REFERENCE AND VALIDATION

FRAME OF REFERENCE

Our assessment of these instruments is provided in the DESCRIPTIVE FORMS under eleven headings.

1. *Specificity.*

   The material for different degrees of specificity has been graded in the following manner:

   *** : Developed *particularly for the elderly population* and used in connection with them.

   ** : Not particularly developed for, *but already used with the elderly.*

   * : Neither developed nor used for the elderly, but according to the authors *applicable with some restrictions or reservations.*

2. *Type of instrument*

   Several different measuring techniques have been identified in these instruments.

   Test. May be *projective, psychometric, verbal* or *non-verbal.*

   Questionnaire. Includes the semi-structured interview and the open-ended questionnaire.

   Check-list. This is an inventory in which the rater's choice is between one of two possible answers, e.g. yes-no, correct-incorrect, present-absent.

   Scale. Such an instrument allows for gradation of response. The scale itself can vary in type: nominal, ordinal, or interval.

   > *The nominal* type of scale records membership or non-membership of a class, e.g. types of disabilities.
   >
   > *The ordinal* scale has the same characteristics as the nominal, but the classes in addition to being different can be internally ordered or ranked, e.g. the grade of severity of disability.
   >
   > *The interval scale* in addition to the idea of rank, has equal intervals between scale points.

   Whilst the first two scales relate solely to qualitative aspects, the last one is, in addition, concerned with quantity.

3. *Origin.*

   Details are given of the source references which have provided the starting point for the development of the instrument in question. If the instrument is original, this is also stated.

4. *Purpose.*

   This gives the authors' reasons for the creation of the instrument.

5. *Population involved.*

The suitability of the instrument for work with various groups and types of patients. Information is also given with due regard to place of residence and specific diagnostic category.

6. *Administration.*

Concerns the method of implementing the instrument and more particularly an attempt is made to answer the question *"By whom and how is it to be scored?"*

Rater is the term applied to the person in charge of the collection and assessment of the data. Raters may be any of the following: physician, psychologist, nurse, nurse's aide, social worker. In some cases there may be self-evaluation by the patient with or without assistance.

Time required. This information is of practical value and permits the division of instruments into categories of different duration.

Training. Whether or not training is necessary for the rater: its duration and intensity.

Scoring. According to the kind of instrument, detailed information is provided on the type of scoring whether quantitative or qualitative, the number of items and the score obtained.

7. *Description.*

Under this heading will be found more precise details of the psychometric tests.

8. *Variables.*

The actual content of the instrument, and the various dimensions evaluated are described, thus providing information on what the instrument measures.

9. *Validation.*

This is presented in the following manner. The population observed, together with corresponding references, type of validity, reliability and sensitivity, other norms and scaling.

10. *Other works cited by the author.*

Past or current circumstances under which the instrument was used are described; this information does not appear in every case and is mentioned only when produced by the author himself or when available in the bibliography.

11. *Application.*

This covers many possible areas, *Research or clinical:* diagnostic, prognostic, screening, care planning, drug trials, epidemiological studies, teaching, training, planning and management. Those instruments concerned with diagnosis are fusther categorised into medical of functional.

The value of an instrument depends on its psychometric qualities. Work concerning validation testifies that value. Such work covers three main aspects: validity, reliability and sensitivity.

VALIDITY

Is the capacity of the instrument to evaluate, to a greater or lesser extent, those characteristics for which it was originally developed. A review of the literature in French and English permits differentiation of five types of validity.

Face validity evaluates the correspondence of content with actual situations or attitudes appearing in everyday life.

Construct validity evaluates the adequacy of the content of an instrument in relation to the hypothesis or theoretical concept under consideration. This is frequently measured using factor analytic techniques.

Concurrent validity is the degree of correlation obtained between two instruments, one of which has already been validated.

External validity describes the greater or lesser correspondence between the results of the measurement and clinical assessment.

Predictive validity is the ability of an instrument to predict outcome. This is a most important capacity of an instrument since case-management may depend on the results obtained by it.

RELIABILITY

A reliable test is one which gives comparable results in comparable situations. Different forms of reliability exist depending on whether reference is to an individual, to the time, or to the instrument.

Inter-rater reliability expresses the correlation between results obtained by two or more different observers assessing the same individual at the same time and using the same instrument. It is evaluated by a *"concordance coefficient"* ranging from 0-1.

Test-retest reliability refers to agreement between two or more assessments of the same individual undertaken under the same experimental conditions on different occasions. Test-retest reliability is usually calculated by using a correlation or a constancy coefficient calculated on the basis of the results of two applications of the test. (The Bravais Pearson "r" is used for numerical values, while the Spearman "rho" is used for ranked data).

Internal consistency, parallel forms and *split-half* method provide more details on the psychometric properties of the instrument.

We speak of this internal consistency as the degree to which the various items of the instrument are all measuring the same concept. This is assessed by the degree of correlation among the individual items in addition to the correlation between the individual items and the total score.

The method of parallel forms examines the correlation between different versions of the same instrument which are similar with respect to the number of items, the order of their difficulty, but are different in regard to their contents. The index of equivalence is the *correlation coefficient* between the scores of the two forms.

The correlation between the two halves of an instrument or between the total scores obtained using the odd and even items separately, is called the "split-half correlation". It is relatively economical to calculate this form of reliability as it requires only one application of the instrument. It is expressed by the *homogeneity coefficient*.

SENSITIVITY

An instrument is sensitive when it discriminates maximally between individuals of different types. A distinction can be made between:

Inter-individual sensitivity which is the capacity of a scale to distinguish between different individuals to a greater or lesser degree.

Intra-individual sensitivity, which consists of the detection of differences in one and the same individual at different points in time.

The sensitivity of an instrument tends to be related to the number of items and the sensitivity of the scoring system. The degree of sensitivity can be increased by a system of weighting which stresses differences.

•

• •

These DESCRIPTIVE FORMS are now presented in three different sections, at the beginning of which a list of the instruments is provided:

Section 1 groups **uni-dimensional** instruments. These instruments cover three aspects:

Mood	Cognitive functions	Behavior
(a)	(b)	(c)

For example on page 25 the Identification Boxes at the upper right hand corner of the DESCRIPTIVE FORM read: M (Mental), Ia (Section I-a=mood), 1 (Instrument No 1).

Section 2 groups **two-dimensional** instruments where the mental component is present but is associated with either social or physical parameters, e.g.

Mental-Social	Physical-Mental
(MS)	(PM)

For example on page 211 the Identification Boxes at the upper right hand corner of the DESCRIPTIVE FORM read: MS Instrument No 1 of Mental Social.

Section 3 groups **three-dimensional** instruments, i.e.;

Physical – Mental – Social
(PMS)

For example on page 273 the Identification Boxes at the upper right hand corner of the DESCRIPTIVE FORM read: PMS 1 Instrument No 1 of Physical Mental Social.

SUMMARY TABLES are provided at the end of the DESCRIPTIVE FORM section which list the instruments in chronological order and give: title, year, author country, specificity, type of instrument, language, origin, population, rater, number of items and grades, duration, training, application and variables included.

2 - DESCRIPTIVE FORMS

Section 1
UNI-DIMENSIONAL INSTRUMENTS

MOOD

DEPRESSION ADJECTIVE CHECK-LIST (D.A.C.L.)

SPECIFICITY

* *

TYPE OF INSTRUMENT

7 Check-lists
of 32 items

REFERENCE	**Lubin (B.)** · – Adjective check-lists for measurement of depression. *Archives of General Psychiatry,* 1965, 12, 57-62.

Language: Original version published in English. Translated into Spanish, Dutch, Hebrew and Chinese.
U.S.A.

Location: See ref. biblio n° 18

For all information concerning the instrument and the translations, write to the author or the publisher at the following addresses:

Bernard Lubin,
Department of Psychology,
University of Missouri-Kansas City
5319 Holmes Street
Kansas City, Missouri 64110, U.S.A.

Educational and Industrial Testing
Service
Inc., P.O. Box 7234
San Diego, CA 92107, U.S.A.

ORIGIN   A list of 171 different adjectives depicting the tone of mood has been established by the author. The application to two groups of normal and depressed females made it possible to retain 128 adjectives of higher discriminating potential that have been compiled according to precise criteria into four lists (A.B.C.D.). The same procedure applied to two groups of males made it possible to make other three lists (E.F.G.) (ref. 18).

PURPOSE   The instrument is designed for clinical, experimental and epidemiological use, conceived to measure depressive mood in a simple and viable way without taking into account the patient's clinical history.

POPULATION   Any person capable of reading and understanding the items.

ADMINISTRATION   *Rater:* Self-administration.

Time required: 2 minutes.

Training: Consists of supervising application and scoring of at least 20 respondents.

Scoring: In the list A, B, C, D there are 22 "positive" adjectives (qualifying depressive mood) and 10 "negative" adjectives (relating to normal mood). The list E, F, G comprises 22 positive and 12 negative items.

VARIABLES   Depressive mood.

VALIDATION   With several groups of both sexes differing in state of mood, the validation consisted of (ref. 18):
Cross validation with intercorrelation of lists particularly with regard to sex.
Concurrent validity with measurement of depression by MMPI (ref. 11) and Depression Inventory by Beck (ref. 1).
Reliability of each list: split-half study of internal consistency, parallel form.

OTHER WORKS
cited by author
· Geriatric studies (U.S.A. - Israel)
· Translation and validation in Spanish and Hebrew with the help of a specialist translator (ref. 31, 34).
· Composition of a similar instrument for evaluation by observer (ref. 30).

APPLICATION   **Clinical:** diagnostic, screening.
Research: drug trials, epidemiological studies.
The instrument is useful whenever self-reported depressive mood needs to be measured.

Ia.1

1 Beck (A.T.), Ward (C.H.), Mendelson (M.), Mock (J.), Erbaugh (J.): An inventory for measuring depression. *Archives of General Psychiatry*, 1961, 4, 561-571.

2 Byerly (F.C.): Comparison between inpatients, outpatients, and normals on three self-report depression inventories. Unpublished doctoral dissertation. Western Michigan University, 1979.

3 Christenfeld (R.), Lubin (B.), Satin (M.): Concurrent validity of the depression adjective check-list. *American Journal of Psychiatry*, 1978, 135, 582.

4 Constantino (R.E.B.): Nursing care of widows in grief and mourning through bereavement crisis intervention. Unpublished doctoral dissertation. University of Pittsburgh, 1979.

5 Dunnette (M.D.): Self-description adjective check-list as indicator of behavioral modalities. Paper read before the American Psychological Association Convention, Chicago, September 1960.

6 Durham (R.C.): Lewinsohn's behavioral measures of social skill: their stability and relationship to mood level and depression among college students. *Journal of Clinical Psychology*, 1979, 33, 599-604.

7 Fogel (M.L.), Curtis (G.C.), Kordasz (F.), Smith (W.G.): Judges ratings, self-ratings, and checklist report of affect. *Psychological Reports*, 1966, 19, 299.

8 Giambra (L.M.): Independent dimensions of depression: factor-analysis of three self-report depression measures. *Journal of Clinical Psychology*, 1977, 33, 928-935.

9 Giambra (L.M.): Depression and day-dreaming: analysis based on self-ratings. *Journal of Clinical Psychology*, 1978, 34, 14-25.

10 Gough (H.G.): Adjective check-list as personality assessment research technique. *Psychological Reports*, 1960, 6, 107-122.

11 Hathaway (S.R.), Mc Kinley (J.C.): Minnesota Multiphasic Personality Inventory: manual. New York: Psychological Corporation, 1951.

12 Heilbrun (A.B. Jr.): Validation of need scaling technique for adjective checklist. *J. Consult. Psychol.*, 1959, 23, 347-351.

13 La Forge (R.), Suczek (R.): Interpersonal dimensions of personality. III: Interpersonal check list. *J. Personality*, 1955, 24, 94-112.

14 Levitt (E.E.), Lubin (B.): Depression: concepts, controversies and some new facts. New York: Springer, 1975.

15 Lewinsohn (P.M.), Bary (M.): Pleasant activities and depression. *Journal of Consulting and Clinical Psychology*, 1973, 41, 261.

16 Lomranz (J.), Lubin (B.), Eyal (N.), Medini (G.): A hebrew version of the depression adjective check lists. *Journal of Personality Assessment*, 1981, vol. 45, n° 4, 380-384.

17 Lomranz (J.), Lubin (B.), Eyal (N.), Medini (G.): Norms for the revised form of the hebrew depression adjective check list. *Journal of Clinical Psychology*, April 1981, vol. 37, n° 2, 318-319.

18 Lubin (B.): Adjective check-lists for measurement of depression. *Archives of General Psychiatry*, 1965, 12, 57-62.

19 Lubin (B.): Fourteen brief lists for the measurement of depression. *Archives of General Psychiatry*, 1966, 15, 205-208.

20 Lubin (B.): Depression adjective check-lists: manual. San Diego, CA: Educational and Industrial Testing Service, 1967.

21 Lubin (B.): Bibliography for the depression adjective check-lists. San Diego, CA: Edits, 1977.

22 Lubin (B.): Research on the instrument itself. In: Symposium: Recent research with the depression adjective check-lists. Western Psychological Association, 1980.

23 Lubin (B.), Caplan (M.E.), Collins (J.F.): Additional evidence for the comparability of set 2 (E, F, and G) of the depression adjective check-lists. *Psychological Reports*, 1980, 46, 849-850.

24 Lubin (B.), Dupre (V.A.), Lubin (A.W.): Comparability and sensitivity of set 2 (Lists E, F, and G) of the depression adjective check-lists. *Psychological Reports*, 1967, 20, 756-758.

25 Lubin (B.), Gardiner (S.H.), Roth (A.): Mood and somatic symptoms during pregnancy. *Psychosomatic Medicine*, 1975, 37, 136-146.

26 Lubin (B.), Himelstein (P.): Reliability of the depression adjective check-lists. *Perceptual and Motor Skills*, 1976, 43, 1037-1038.

27 Lubin (B.), Hornstra (R.K.), Dean (L.M.): Concurrent validity of the depression adjective chek-list in a psychiatric population. *Journal of Community Psychology*, 1978, 6, 157-162.

28 Lubin (B.), Hornstra (R.K.), Love (A.): Course of depressive mood in a psychiatric population upon application for service and at three month and twelve month reinterview. *Psychological Reports*, 1974, 34, 424.

29 Lubin (B.), Levitt (E.E.): Norms for depression adjective check list: age group and sex. *Journal of Consulting and Clinical Psychology*, 1979, 47, 192.

30 Lubin (B.), Marone (J.G.), Nathan (R.G.): Comparison of self-administered and examiner-administered depression adjective check-lists. *Journal of Consulting and Clinical Psychology*, 1978, vol. 46, n° 3, 584-585.

31 Lubin (B.), Millham (J.), Paredes (F.): Spanish language versions of the depression adjective check lists. *Hispanic Journal of Behavioral Sciences*, 1980, vol. 2, n° 1, 51-57.

32 Lubin (B.), Nathan (M.M.), Nathan (R.G.): Comparison of response formats for the depression adjective check-lists. *Journal of Clinical Psychology*, 1981, 37, 1, 172-175.

33 Lubin (B.), Roth (A.V.), Dean (L.M.), Hornstra (R.K.): Correlates of depressive mood among normals. *Journal of Clinical Psychology*, 1978, 34, 650-653.

34 Lubin (B.), Schoenfeld (L.S.), Rinck (C.), Millham (J.): Reliability and validity of the spanish depression adjective check-lists: psychiatric patients and normals. *Interamerican Journal of Psychology*, 1980, 14, 1, 53-55.

35 Marone (J.), Lubin (B.): Relationship between set 2 of the depression adjective check-lists (DACL) and the Zung self-rating depression scale (SDS). *Psychological Reports*, 1968, 22, 333-334.

SELF RATING DEPRESSION SCALE

SPECIFICITY

* *

TYPE OF INSTRUMENT

Ordinal rating scale.
20 items, 4 grades

REFERENCE	**Zung (W.W.K.)** · – A self rating depression scale. *Archives of General Psychiatry,* 1965, 12, 63-70.
	Language: Original version published in English. Translated into 30 languages. **U.S.A.**
	Location: Enclosed in volume two page 95 See ref. biblio nº 16
	For all information concerning the instrument or translations, write to the author at the following address:
	William Zung, Department of Psychiatry Duke University Medical Center, Veterans Administration Hospital, Durham, North Carolina 27705, U.S.A.

ORIGIN

The instrument results from a census of diagnostic criteria on depression and an analysis of tape recorded interviews with depressed patients aimed to formulate and refine the items. It was inspired by studies carried out by **Grinker** (ref. 5), **Overall** (ref. 12) and **Friedman** concerned with the symptomatology of mood (ref. 4).

PURPOSE

The scale was made to measure depression conceived as a clinical entity by self-evaluation, brief and easy to use, providing both quantitative and qualitative data.

POPULATION

All depressed patients.

ADMINISTRATION

Rater: Self-administration.

Time required: 3 minutes.

Training: Some instructions to the patients on the method of responding are necessary.

Scoring: Items deal with respondent's condition during past week. There are 10 positive and 10 negative items, assessed according to a frequency scale containing 4 grades from 4-1 or from 1-4, so that global score becomes higher if the syndrome is intense. The crude total score divided by the score maximum total of 80 is converted to a percentage, yielding an index of depression. However, morbidity scores in aged persons are not the same as in adult young persons.

VARIABLES

According to factor analysis: 7 factors:
1. Feeling of emptiness
2. Mood disorders
3. General somatic symptoms
4. Specific somatic symptoms
5. Psycho-motor symptoms
6. Suicidal ideas
7. Irritability-indecisiveness

VALIDATION

Carried out with depressed hospitalized or ambulatory patients suffering from psychiatric or organic diseases (ref. 16), it consists of:
External validity with regard to clinical diagnosis and factor analysis.
Concurrent validity with other instruments, scale of Hamilton, Beck, Lubin "Depression status Inventory", Zung and M.M.P.I.
Sensitivity between depressed and non-depressed patients, before and after treatment; between groups differing in age, sex, race, education, social and financial status.
Several **factor analyses** and comparison of results.
Reliability. Split-half
Norms differentiating stages of depression severity as a function of total score.

OTHER WORKS
cited by author

Application of scale in geriatrics.
Studies of non-depressed psychiatric patients, alcoholics, hospitalized children following suicidal attempts, drug addicts, normal persons, somatic patients (cardiac surgery, chronic pain).
Transcultural studies (USA, Australia, Canada, Czechoslovakia, Great Britain, Germany, India, Japan, Korea, Holland).
Construction of a similar inventory for completion by one observer: "Depression Status Inventory" (ref. 17).

APPLICATION

Clinical: Contribution to diagnostic and clinical studies of depression. Screening.
Research: Drug trials

1 Beck (A.T.), Ward (C.H.), Mendelson (M.), Mock (J.), Erbaugh (J.): An inventory for measuring depression. *Arch. Gen. Psychiat.*, 1961, 4, 561-571.

2 Clyde (D.J.): Construction and validation of emotional association test. Unpublished PhD Thesis. Pennsylvania State College, Philadelphia, 1950.

3 Fleminger (J.J.), Groden (B.): Clinical features of depression and response to imipramine ("Tofranil"). *J. Ment. Sci.*, 1962, 108, 101-104.

4 Friedman (A.S.), et al.: Syndromes and themes of psychotic depression. *Arch. Gen. Psychiat.*, 1963, 9, 504-509.

5 Grinker (R.R.), et al: Phenomena of depressions. New York: Paul B. Hoeber, Inc. Medical Book Department of Harper and Row Publishers, Inc, 1961.

6 Hamilton (M.): Development of a rating scale for primary depressive illness. *Brit. Journ. Soc. Clin. Psychol.*, 1967, 6, 278-296.

7 Hathaway (S.), Mc Kinley (C.): Minnesota Multiphasic Personality Inventory. New York: The Phychological Corporation, 1951.

8 Hedlund (J.L.), Vieweg (B.W.): The Zung self-rating depression scale: a comprehensive review. *Journal of Operational Psychiatry,* 1979, vol. 10, n° 1, 51-64.

9 Hildreth (H.M.): Battery of feeling and attitude scales for clinical use. *J. Clin. Psychol.*, 1946, 2, 214-221.

10 Hutchinson (J.T.), Smedberg (D): Phenelzine ("Nardil") in treatment of endogenous depression. *J. Ment. Sci.*, 1960, 106, 704-710.

11 Lubin (B): Adjective checklists for measurement of depression. *Arch. Gen. Psychiat.*, 1965, 12, 37-62.

12 Overall (J.E.): Dimensions of manifest depression. *Psychiat. Res.*, 1962, 1, 239-245.

13 Steuer (J.), Bank (L.), Olsen (E.J.), Jarvik (L.F.): Depression, physical health and somatic complaints in the elderly: a study of the Zung self-rating depression scale. *Journal of Gerontology*, 1980, vol. 35, n°. 5, 683-688.

14 Wechsler (H.), Grosser (G.), Busfield (B.): Depression rating scale. *Arch. Gen. Psychiat.*, 1963, 9, 334-343.

15 Wessman (A.E.), Ricks (D.), Tyl (M.): Characteristics and concomitants of mood fluctuation in college women. *J. Abnorm. Soc. Psychol.*, 1960, 60, 117-126.

16 Zung (W.W.K.): A self-rating depression scale. *Arch. Gen. Psychiat.*, 1965, 12, 63-70.

17 Zung (W.W.K.): The depression status inventory: an adjunct to the self-rating depression scale. *Journ. Clin. Psychol.*, 1972, 28, 539-543.

18 Zung (W.W.K.): How normal is depression? Upjohn Company, 1981. (Current Concepts).

19 Zung (W.W.K.), Wilson (W.P.), Dodson (W.E.): Effect of depressive disorders on sleep EEG responses. *Arch. Gen. Psychiat.*, 1964, 10, 439-445.

HAMILTON RATING SCALE FOR DEPRESSION

SPECIFICITY

TYPE OF INSTRUMENT

* *

Ordinal rating scale, 17 items of 3-5 grades + 4 items

REFERENCE	**Hamilton (M.)** · – Development of a rating scale for primary depressive illness. *British Journal of Social and Clinical Psychology,* 1967, 6, 278-296.
	Language: Original version published in English. Translations in all European languages, Japanese and Korean **Great Britain**
	Location: Enclosed in volume two page 96 See ref. biblio nº 5
	For all information concerning the instrument or translations, write to the author at the following address:
	Max Hamilton, The School of Medicine Psychiatry Annexe The University of Leeds 30 Clarendon Road Leeds LS2, 9NZ, Great Britain

ORIGIN	The author was inspired from general psychiatric and psychometric texts.
PURPOSE	The instrument was conceived to measure the severity of depression for clinical and experimental purposes.
POPULATION	Adult persons of all ages suffering from depression.
ADMINISTRATION	*Rater:* Psychiatrist and any person adequately trained. It is useful to have two raters. *Time required:* 20 to 30 minutes. *Training:* Background knowledge of psychiatry and experience with about ten patients are necessary. *Scoring:* 9 items are scored from 0-4. The six items scored from 0-2, represent variables which cannot be expressed quantitatively. An individual not suffering from depression would have a total score of 0. The maximum total score of 52 corresponds to the greatest intensity of depressive syndrome. The last four items do not measure the intensity of depression.
VARIABLES	Symptoms of melancholia (depression).
VALIDATION	Was done with groups of melancholic patients and covered a reduced scale of the first 17 items, the last 4 define clinical type of depression or correspond to rare symptoms. **Factors analyses** (ref. 6, 12) of principal components and varimax rotation was done separately for a group of male and female patients. Three factors were identified: the first "general factor of depression", the second "anxious depression", the third factor is an index of instability (ref. 5). **Concurrent validity** with other scales from 1960 onwards. Study of **inter-rater reliability.**
OTHER WORKS cited by author	Too numerous to mention here. See "Science Citation Index".
APPLICATION	Therapeutic trials Other applications are possible on different clinical categories subject to an appropriate validation.

1 Cattell (R.B.): The basis of recognition and interpretation factors. *Educ. Psychol. Measur.*, 1962, 22, 667-697.

2 Eysenck (H.J.): The questionnaire measurement of neuroticism and extraversion. *Riv. Psicol. Norm. Patol. Appl.*, 1955, 1, 3-17.

3 Hallworth (H.J.): Programs for correlations and factor analysis. *Br. J. Math. Stat. Psychol.*, 1965, 18, 142-143.

4 Hamilton (M.): A rating scale for depression. *J. Neurol. Neurosurg. Psychiat.*, 1960, 23, 56-62.

5 Hamilton (M.): Development of a rating scale for primary depressive illness. *Brit. J. Soc. Clin. Psychol.*, 1967, 6, 278-296.

6 Hamilton (M.): Comparison of factors by Ahmavaara's method. *Brit. J. Math. Stat. Psychol.*, may 1967, 20, 1, 107.

7 Hamilton (M.): Standardized assessment and recording of depressive symptoms. *Psychiat. Neurol. Neurochir.*, 1969, 72, 201-205.

8 Hamilton (M.), Mc Guire (R.J.), Goodman (M.J.): The P.L.U.S. system of programs: an integrated system of computer programs for biological data. *Br. J.Math.Stat.Psychol.*, 1965, 18, 265-266.

9 Hamilton (M.), White (J.M.): Clinical syndromes in depressive states. *J.Ment.Sci.*, 1959, 105, 985-998.

10 Harman (H.H.): Modern factor analysis. Univ.Chicago Press, 1960.

11 Jacobsen (M.): The use of rating scales in clinical research. *Brit.J.Psychiat.*, 1965, 111, 545-546.

12 Kaiser (H.F.): The Varimax criterion for analytic rotation in factor analysis. *Psychometrika*, 1958, 23, 187-200.

13 Kaiser (H.F.): Comments on communalities and the number of factors. Read at an informal conference "the communality problem in factor analysis". St. Louis: Washington University, 1960.

14 Kaiser (H.F.): Formulas for component scores. *Psychometrika*, 1962, 27, 83-87.

15 Kiloh (L.G.), Garside (R.F.): The independence of neurotic depression and endogenous depression. *Br.J.Psychiat.*, 1963, 109, 451-463.

16 Lorr (M.), Klett (C.J.), Mc Nair (D.M.): Syndromes of psychosis. Pergamon Press, 1963.

17 Pawlik (K.), Cattell (R.B.): Third-order factors in objective personality tests. *Br.J.Psychol.*, 1964, 55, 1-18.

18 Schwab (J.J.) et al.: Hamilton rating scale for depression and medical in-patients. *Brit.J.Psychiat.*, jan. 1967, 113, 83-88.

19 Wittenborn (J.R.): Symptom patterns in a group of mental hospital patients. *J.Consult.Psychol.*, 1951, 15, 290-302.

20 Wittenborn (J.R.): The dimensions of psychosis. *J.Nerv.Ment.Dis.*, 1962, 134, 117-128.

NEW PHYSICIAN'S RATING LIST

SPECIFICITY

* *

TYPE OF INSTRUMENT

Ordinal rating scale
19 items, 6 grades

REFERENCE	**Free (S.M. Jr.), Guthrie (M.B.)** · – A new rating scale for evaluating clinical response in the psychoneurotic outpatients. *Journal of Clinical Pharmacology,* 1969, 9, 187-194.

Language: Original version in English.
U.S.A.

Location: Enclosed in volume two page 97
See ref. biblio nº 6

For all information concerning the instrument write to the author at the following address:

Spencer Free,
Applebrook Research Center
Smithkline Animal Health Products
1600, Paoli Pike
West Chester, Pennsylvania 19380, U.S.A.

ORIGIN

The instrument was developed from factor analysis and studies of external validity of the "Physician's Rating List" (ref. 3). This ordinal scale with 18 items and 4 grades is original and was inspired by numerous works, such as: **Lorr's** "Inpatient Multidimensional Psychiatric Scale" (ref. 10) and **Overall's** "Brief Psychiatric Scale" (ref. 12).

PURPOSE

To allow an evaluation of syndromes of anxiety for psycho-pharmacological research.

POPULATION

Non-hospitalized patients whose symptomatology is either primarily anxious or depressive, or a mixture of the two.

ADMINISTRATION

Rater: Physician, not necessarily a psychiatrist.

Time required: Interview plus five minutes.

Training: Familiarization with items.

Scoring: Based on an interview with the patient. Each of the 19 items ranges from 0-5 according to the scale of intensity beginning with "absent" (0) to "disabling" (5). The total score ranging from 0-95, indicates "morbidity".

VARIABLES

Four factor scores in addition to the total morbidity score. In addition to the specific orientation to out-patients, a unique feature is the two symptom complexes associated with anxiety.
· Anxiety syndrome   · Depression factor
· Psychomotor activitation factor   · Somatization factor

VALIDATION

Was done on out-patients, presenting psychic and emotional symptomatology, subjected to an anxiolytic regime (ref. 7):
Factor analysis of principal components and by varimax rotation giving evidence of 4 factors.
Concurrent validity and sensitivity with other instruments used in therapeutic trials.
External validity through numerous trials of global score and factor scores.
Reliability: internal consistency of different factors.

OTHER WORKS
cited by author

Factor analysis resulted in an abridged scale "Brief Out-patient Psychopathology Scale" (ref. 7), by the author.

APPLICATION

Clinical: Contribution to diagnosis.
Research: Drug trials with out-patients.

1 Burdock (E.I.), Hakerem (G.), Hardesty (A.S.), Zubin (J.): A ward behavior rating scale for mental hospital patients. *J. Clin. Psychol.*, 1960, 16, 246.

2 Davidson (A.B.), Cook (L.): Effects of combined treatment with trifluoperazine HC1 and amobarbital on punished behavior in rats. *Psychopharmacologia*, 1969, 15, 159-168.

3 Free (S.M.Jr.): Experimental design considerations for outpatient studies. In: "Neuropharmacology". Proceedings of the V Congress of the Collegium Internationale Neuropsychopharmacologicum, Washington 28-31 March 1966. Amsterdam: Excerpta Medica, 1967, 72-78.

4 Free (S.M.Jr.): Factor analysis of outpatient clinical data. *J. Clin. Pharmacol.*, 1969, 9, 195.

5 Free (S.M. Jr.): Statistical problems in the measurement of change. In: "Neuropharmacology". Proceedings of the IX Congress of the Collegium Internationale Neuropsychopharmacologicum, Paris 7-12 July 1974. Amsterdam: Excerpta Medica, 1975, 223-228.

6 Free (S.M. Jr.), Guthrie (M.B.): A new rating scale for evaluating clinical response in psychoneurotic outpatients. *J. Clin. Pharmacology*, 1969, 9, 187-194.

7 Free (S.M. Jr.), Overall (J.E.): The Brief Outpatient Psychopathology Scale (BOPS). *Journal of Clin. Psychology*, 1977, vol. 33, n°. 3, 677-688.

8 Guthrie (M.B.), Free (S.M. Jr): Response to trifluoperazine-amobarbital in outpatients with anxiety. *Diseases of Nervous System*, 1969, 30, 195-200.

9 Honigfeld (G.), Klett (C.J.): The nurses'observation scale for inpatient evaluation: a new scale for measuring improvement in chronic schizophrenia. *J. Clin. Psychol.*, 1965, 21, 65.

10 Lorr (M.), Klett (C.J.), Mc Nair (D.M.), Lasky (J.J.): Inpatient multidimensional psychiatric scale. Manual. Palo Alto, Calif.: Consulting Psychologists Press, 1962.

11 Lorr (M.), O'Connor (J.P.), Stafford (J.W.): The psychotic reaction profile. *J. Clin. Psychol*, 1960, 16, 241.

12 Overall (J.E.), Gorham (D.R.): The brief psychiatric rating scale. *Psychol. Reports*, 1962, 10, 799.

13 Overall (J.E.), Hollister (L.E.), Dalal (S.N.): Psychiatric drug research: sample size requirements for one vs two raters. *Arch. Gen. Psychiat.*, 1967, 16, 152.

PSYCHOTIC INPATIENT PROFILE (P.I.P.)

SPECIFICITY

> ** *

TYPE OF INSTRUMENT

> Ordinal rating scale
> and check-list
> 96 items, 4-2 grades

REFERENCE	**Lorr (M.), Vestre (N.D.)** · – The psychotic inpatient profile: a nurse's observation scale. *Journal of Clinical Psychology,* 1969, 25, 137-140.

Language: Original version published in English.
                   U.S.A.

Location: Enclosed in volume two page 185
                   See ref. biblio nº 8

For all information concerning the instrument write to the author or the publisher at the following addresses.

Maurice Lorr,   Western Psychological Services
The Catholic University of America   12031 Wilshire Boulevard
Center for the Study of Youth Dpt   Los Angeles, California 90025,
Washington D.C. 20064, U.S.A.   U.S.A.

ORIGIN

Almost 40% of items were taken from "Psychotic Reaction Profile" (ref. 6), the others are original.

PURPOSE

The instrument is designed for clinical use by nurses and nurse's aides to evaluate a broad range of behaviors.

POPULATION

Inpatients of all ages and categories of diagnosis.

ADMINISTRATION

Rater: Nurse, nurse's aide in psychiatry or any person frequently seeing the patient.

Time required: 10 to 15 minutes.

Training: Familiarization with the items through discussion with physician or psychologist.

Scoring: Is based on three-day observation of the patient and is done according to a frequency scale of 4 grades for items 1-74, from 0 (never) to 3 (almost always). The others require a reply of the yes-no type, assessed respectively 3 and 0.

VARIABLES

Manifest symptomatology
· Excitement
· Hostile belligerence
· Paranoid projection
· Anxious depression
· Retardation
· Seclusiveness
· Need of care
· Psychotic disorganization

Observation data
· Grandiosity
· Perceptual disorganization
· Depressive mood
· Disorientation

VALIDATION

Was carried out with hospitalized psychiatric patients and included (ref. 8):
Factor analysis
Inter-rater and test-retest **reliability**
Sensitivity to effects of tranquillisers
Differentation between two groups of patients, from open and closed wards
Norms calculated for 4 groups of patients: male, female, under psychotropic treatment, and control group.

APPLICATION

Clinical: Contribution to diagnosis treatment choice and allocation to type of ward.
                    Prognosis.
Research: Drug trials.

1 Caffey (E.M.), Diamond (L.S.) et al. Discontinuation of chemotherapy in chronic schizophrenics. *J. Chronic Diseases*, 1964, 17, 347-350.

2 Lorr (M.): Ward behavior types. In: Lorr (M.) Ed.: «Explorations in typing psychotics». Oxford: Pergamon Press, 1966.

3 Lorr (M.), Cave (R.L.): The equivalence of psychotic syndromes across two media. *Multivariate Behavioral Research*, 1966, 1, 189-195.

4 Lorr (M.), Klett (C.J.), Mc Nair (D.M.): Ward-observable psychotic behavior syndromes. *Educ. Psychol. Meas.*, 1964, 24, 291-300.

5 Lorr (M.), O'Connor (J.P.): Psychotic symptom patterns in a behavior inventory. *Educ. Psychol. Meas.*, 1962, 22, 139-146.

6 Lorr (M.), O'Connor (J.P.), Stafford (J.W.): The psychotic reaction profile. *J. Clin. Psychol.*, 1960, 16, 241-245.

7 Lorr (M.), Vestre (N.D.): The psychotic inpatient profile: manual. Los Angeles: Western Psychological Services, 1968.

8 Lorr (M.), Vestre (N.D.): The psychotic inpatient profile: a nurse's observation scale. *J. Clin. Psychol.*, 1969, 25, 137-140.

9 Vestre (N.D.): Validity data on the psychotic reaction profile. *J. Consult. Psychol.*, 1966, 30, 84-85.

10 Vestre (N.D.), Zimmerman (R.): A validity study of the psychotic inpatient profile. Unpublished report.

11 Watson (C.G.), Klett (W.G.): A validation of the psychotic inpatient profile. *Journal of Clinical Psychol.*, 1972, 28, 102-109.

MEASUREMENT OF MORALE IN THE ELDERLY

SPECIFICITY

* * *

TYPE OF INSTRUMENT

Check-list, 45 items

REFERENCE	**Pierce (R.C.), Clark (M.M.)** · – Measurement of morale in the elderly. *International Journal of Aging and Human Development,* 1973, 4, 2, 83-101.

Language: Original version published in English.
U.S.A.

Location: Enclosed in volume two page 73 and 74
See ref. biblio nº 14

There is a more recent version (1978), with 35 items in the form of a five-point scale, also to be found in volume two. For all information concerning the instrument write to the author at the following address:

Robert Pierce,
99 Golden Hinde Blvd
San Rafael, CA 94903, U.S.A.

ORIGIN — The check-list is composed of original items and those taken from the scales by **Srole** (ref. 15) and **Thompson** et al. (ref. 16).

PURPOSE — It was designed to assess the level of morale amongst aged persons with mental disorders, in contrast to those who are mentally sound.

POPULATION — Elderly adults, out-patients, or those in long term care.

ADMINISTRATION — *Rater:* Psychologist, physician.

Time required: The questionnaire is embedded in a structured interview lasting from 2 to 4 hours.

Training: Knowledge of instrument and how to interview in a semi-direct way.

Scoring: Is dichotomous but can be extended on certain items. Factor scores can be calculated by adding up items belonging to the same factor.

VARIABLES — Eight identifiable factors resulted from factor analysis:
· Three refer to morale: depression-satisfaction, will-to-live, equanimity
· Three represent attitudes connected with morale: ageing thought of in a positive or negative sense, social alienation.
· Two others, physical health and sociability, belong to different spheres of morale, but are correlated with it.

VALIDATION — Discriminative validity of the instrument has been studied for each factor by comparing the results for 2 groups of aged subjects: hospitalized mental patients and normals (ref. 14).

APPLICATION — Designed for clinical use as well as for research allowing multidimensional evaluation of the morale of elderly persons, and hence differential studies, intra-individual, inter-individual or inter-group.

1 Clark (M.), Anderson (B.G.): Culture and aging. Springfield, Ill.: Charles C. Thomas, 1967.

2 Comrey (A.L.), Levonian (E.A.): A comparison of three-point coefficients in factor analyses of MMPI items. *Educational and Psychological Measurement*, 1958, 18, 739-755.

3 Cotton (J.W.), Campbell (D.T.), Malone (R.D.): The relationship between factorial composition of test items and measure of test reliability. *Psychometrika*, 1957, 22, 348-358.

4 Cumming (E.), Dean (L.R.), Newell (D.S.): What is "morale"? A case history of a validity problem. *Human Organization*, 1958, 17, 3-8.

5 Eysenck (H.J.): Personality and sexual behavior. *Journal of Psychosomatic Research*, 1972, 16, 141-152.

6 Fisher (J.), Pierce (R.C.): Dimensions of intellectual functioning in the aged. *Journal of Gerontology*, 1967, 22, 166-173.

7 Kutner (B.), Fanshel (D.), Togo (A.M.), Langner (T.S.): Five-hundred over sixty: a community survey on aging. New York: Russel Sage Foundation, 1956, 531.

8 Lawton (M.P.): The dimensions of morale. Paper presented to the Gerontological Society. New York, 1966.

9 Lowenthal (M.F.): Lives in distress. New York: Basic Books, 1964.

10 Lowenthal (M.F.), Berkman (P.L.) et al.: Aging and mental disorder in San Francisco. San Francisco: Jossey-Bass, 1967.

11 Lowenthal (M.F.), Boler (D.): Voluntary vs. involuntary social withdrawal. *Journal of Gerontology*, 1965, 20, 363-371.

12 Neugarten (P.L.), Havighurst (R.J.), Tobin (S.S.): The measurement of life satisfaction. *Journal of Gerontology*, 1961, 16, 134-143.

13 Palmore (E.), Luikart (C.): Health and social factors related to life satisfaction. *Journal of Health and Social Behavior,* 1972, 13, 68-80.

14 Pierce (R.C.), Clark (M.M.): Measurement of morale in the elderly. *Int'l. J. Aging and Human Development*, 1973, vol. 4, n°. 2, 83-101.

15 Srole (L.), Langner (T.S.), Michael (S.T.) Opler (M.K.), Rennie (T.A.C.): Mental health in the metropolis: the midtown Manhattan study. Vol. 1. New York: Mc Graw-Hill, 1962.

16 Thompson (W.E.), Streib (G.F.), Kosa (J.): The effect of retirement on personal adjustment: a panel analysis. *Journal of Gerontology*, 1960, 15, 165-169.

17 Tryon (R.C.), Bailey (D.E.): Cluster analysis. New York: Mc Graw-Hill, 1970.

BECK DEPRESSION INVENTORY (B.D.I.)

SPECIFICITY

* *

TYPE OF INSTRUMENT

Ordinal rating scale 21 items, 4 grades

REFERENCE	Beck (A.T.), Beamesderfer (A.) · – Assessment of depression: The depression inventory. In: Pichot (P.). Ed. "Psychological measurements in psychopharmacology. Modern problems in pharmacopsychiatry". Vol. 7. Basel, Switzerland: Karger, 1974, 151-169.
	Language: Original version published in English. Translated into Indian and Spanish, Polish, Hungarian, Japanese, Dutch, Finnish, German, French. **U.S.A.**
	Location: Enclosed in volume two page 98 See ref. biblio nº 7
	For translations write to the author at the following address:
	Aaron Beck, Center for Cognitive Therapy, Room 602 133 South 36th Street Philadelphia, PA 19104, U.S.A.
	For technical information write to:
	Evelyn Paley, School of Professional Psychology University of Denver University Park, Denver, Colorado, 80210, U.S.A.

ORIGIN — Original instrument inspired by clinical observation, particularly in analytical psychotherapy of depressed patients.

PURPOSE — Evaluation of severity of depression for clinical and experimental purposes.

POPULATION — All psychiatric patients.

ADMINISTRATION — *Rater:* Self-administration or evaluation by observer (psychologist, psychiatrist).

Time required: 5 minutes.

Training: Brief.

Scoring: Each item is rated on a 4 point severity scale, from 0 (absence of symptoms) to 3 (maximum intensity).

VARIABLES — Intensity of depression.

VALIDATION — Was done on psychiatric in and out-patients, at time of admission or first referral excluding subjects affected by cerebral organic syndromes or mental deficiency (ref. 7). External validity was tested with a clinical appreciation of severity of depression on a 4 point scale.
Predictive validity for outcome of syndrome.
Sensitivity to change in the severity of depressive syndrome.
Discriminative sensitivity between groups differing in severity of depressive syndrome.
Reliability: internal consistency, split-half.
Test-retest: Study of correlation between assessments at 2-6 weeks interval also by a psychiatrist observer.

OTHER WORKS cited by author — Studies of depressive syndromes in several types of patients (gastroduodenal ulcer, cancer, renal dialysis).
Translations and validations in foreign languages.
Studies of depression in children and adolescents.

APPLICATION — Screening of depression, diagnostic, outcome.

1 American Psychiatric Association: Diagnostic and statistical manual: mental disorders. Washington: Amer. Psychiat. Ass., 1952.

2 American Psychological Association: Technical recommendations for psychological tests and diagnostic techniques. *Psychol. Bull.*, 1954, 51 Suppl., 13-28.

3 Barraclough (B.M.), Nelson (B.), Sainsbury (P.): The diagnostic classification and psychiatric treatment of 25 suicides. Proc. 4 th Int. Conf. Suicide Prevention Center. Los Angeles: Delmar, 1968.

4 Beck (A.T.): A systematic investigation of depression. *Comprehens. Psychiat.*, 1961, 2, 162-170.

5 Beck (A.T.): Reliability of psychiatric diagnoses. I: a critique of systematic studies. *Amer. J. Psychiat.*, 1962, 119, 210-216.

6 Beck (A.T.): Depression: causes and treatment. Philadelphia: Univ. Pennsylvania Press, 1972.

7 Beck (A.T.): Beamesderfer (A.): Assessment of depression: the depression inventory. In: Pichot (P.) Ed.: "Psychological measurements in psychopharmacology. Mod. probl. pharmacopsychiat." Vol. 7. Basel: Karger, 1974, 151-169.

8 Beck (A.T.), Sethi (B.), Tuthill (R.): Childhood bereavement and adult depression. *Arch. Gen. Psychiat.*, 1963, 9, 295-302.

9 Beck (A.T.), Stein (D.): The self concept in depression. Unpublished study, 1960.

10 Beck (A.T.), Ward (C.H.): Dreams of depressed patients. Characteristic themes in manifest content. *Arch. Gen. Psychiat.*, 1961, 5, 462-467.

11 Beck (A.T.), Ward (C.H.), Mendelson (M.), Mock (J.E), Erbaugh (J.K.): An inventory for measuring depression. *Arch. Gen. Psychiat.*, 1961, 4, 561-571.

12 Beck (A.T.), Ward (C.H.), Mendelson (M.), Mock (J.E.), Erbaugh (J.K.): Reliability of psychiatric diagnoses. II: A study of consistency of clinical judgments and ratings. *Amer. J. Psychiat.*, 1962, 119, 351-357.

13 Blaser (R.), Low (D), Schaublin (A.): Die Messung der Depressionstiefe mit einem Fragebogen. *Psychiat. Clin.*, 1968, 1, 299-319.

14 Bloom (P.M.), Brady (J.P.): An ipsative validation of the multiple affect adjective check-list. *J. Clin. Psychol.*, 1968, 24, 45-46.

15 Brand (D.): Beyond the blues. *Wall Street J.*, april 7 1972, 1.

16 Clyde (D.J.): Clyde mood scale. Washington: George Washington University, 1961.

17 Comrey (A.L.): A factor analysis of items on the MMPI depression scale. *Educ. Psychol. Measur.*, 1957, 17, 578-585.

18 Cronbach (L.J.), Meehl (P.E.): Construct validity in psychological tests. *Psychol. Bull.* 1955, 52, 281-302.

19 Cropley (A.J.), Weckowicz (T.E.): The dimensionality of clinical depression. *Austr. J. Psychol.*, 1966, 18, 18-25.

20 Delay (J.), Pichot (P.), Lemperiere (T.), Mirouze (R.): La nosologie des états dépressifs. Rapports entre l'étiologie et la sémiologie. Il: Résultats du questionnaire de Beck. *Encéphale*, 1963, 52, 497-505.

21 Gottschalk (L.), Gleser (G.), Springer (K.): Three hostility scales applicable to verbal samples. *Arch. Gen. Psychiat.*, 1963, 9, 254-269.

22 Hamilton (M.): A rating scale for depression. *J. Neurol. Neurosurg. Psychiat.*, 1960, 23, 56-61.

23 Hathaway (W.R.), Mc Kinley (J.C.): A multiphasic personality schedule. III: The measurement of symptomatic depression. *J. Psychol.*, 1942, 10, 249-254.

24 Jasper (H.H.): A measurement of depression-elation and its relation to a measure of extraversion-intraversion. *J. Abnorm. Soc. Psychol.*, 1930, 25, 307-318.

25 Lehmann (H.E.): Epidemiology of depressive disorders. In: "Fieve depression in the 70'S". Amsterdam: Excerpta Medica, 1971.

26 Loeb (A.), Beck (A.T.), Diggory (J.C.): Differential effects of success and failure on depressed and non depressed patients. *J. Nerv. Ment. Dis.*, 1971, 152, 106-114.

27 Loeb (A.), Feshbach (S.), Beck (A.T.), Wolf (A.): Some effects of reward upon the social perception and motivation of psychiatric patients varying in depression. *J. Abnorm. Soc. Psychol.*, 1964, 68, 609-616.

28 May (A.E.), Urquhart (A.), Tarran (J.): Self-evaluation in various diagnostic and therapeutic groups. *Arch. Gen. Psychiat.*, 1969, 21, 191-194.

29 Mendels (J.), Hawkins (D.R.): Sleep and depression. *Arch. Gen. Psychiat.*, 1968, 19, 445-452.

30 Messick (M.): Response style and content measures from personality inventories. *Educ. Psychol. Measur.*, 1960, 22, 41-56.

31 Metcalfe (M.), Goldman (E.): Validation of an inventory for measuring depression. *Brit. J. Psychiat.*, 1965, 111, 240-242.

32 Nielsen (A.), Secunda (S.), Friedman (R.), Williams (T.): Prevalence and recognition of depression among ambulatory patients in a group medical practice. Proc. Meet. Amer. Psychiat. Ass., Dallas, 1972.

33 Nussbaum (K.), Michaux (W.W.): Response to humor in depression. A prediction and evaluation of patient change? *Psychiat. Quart.*, 1963, 37, 527-539.

34 Nussbaum (K.), Wittig (B.A.), Hanlon (T.E.), Kurland (A.A.): Intravenous nialamide in the treatment of depressed female patients. *Comprehens. Psychiat.*, 1963, 4, 105-116.

35 O'Connor (J.), Stefic (E.), Gresock (C.): Some patterns of depression. *J. Clin. Psychol.*, 1957, 13, 122-125.

36 Pichot (P.), Lemperiere (T.): Analyse factorielle d'un questionnaire d'autoévaluation des symptômes dépressifs. *Rev. Psychol. Appl.*, 1964, 14, 15-29.

37 Pichot (P.), Piret (J.), Clyde (D.J.): Analyse de la symptomatologie dépressive subjective. *Rev. Psychol. Appl.*, 1966, 16, 103-115.

38 Rawnsley (K.): The early diagnosis of depression. Office of Health Economics. Early diagnosis, paper 4, 1968.

39 Salkind (M.R.): Beck depression inventory in general practice. *J. Roy. Coll. Gen. Pratic,* 1969, 18, 267.

40 Schwab (J.J.), Bialow (M.), Brown (J.M.), Holzer (C.E.): Diagnosing depression in medical inpatients. *Ann. Intern. Med.*, 1967, 67, 695-707.

41 Schwab (J.J.), Bialow (M.), Holzer (C.E.): A comparison of two rating scales for depression. *J. Clin. Psychol.*, 1967, 23, 94-96.

42 Silver (M.), Bohnert (M.), Beck (A.T.), Marcus (D.): Relation of depression to attempted suicide and seriousness of intent. *Arch. Gen. Psychiat.*, 1971, 24, 495-500.

43 Spitzer (R.L.), Fleiss (J.L.), Endicott (J.), Cohen (J.): Mental status schedule. Properties of factor analytically derived scales. *Arch. Gen. Psychiat.*, 1967, 16, 479-493.

44 Stenback (A.), Rimon (R.), Turunen (M.): Validitet av Taylor manifest anxiety scale. *Nord. Psykiat. T.*, 1967, 21, 79-85.

45 Vinar (0.), Grof (P.): Die depressive Symptomatologie im Lichte des Beckschen Fragebogens. In: Hippius: "Das depressive Syndrom". Berlin: Publisher, 1968.

46 Ward (C.H.), Beck (A.T.), Mendelson (M.), Mock (J.E.), Erbaugh (J.K.): The psychiatric nomenclature. Reasons for diagnostic disagreement. *Arch. Gen. Psychiat.*, 1962, 7, 198-205.

47 Weckowicz (T.E.), Muir (W.), Cropley (A.J.): A factor analysis of the Beck inventory of depression. *J. Cons. Psychol.*, 1967, 31, 270-278.

48 Williams (J.G.), Barlow (D.H.), Agras (W.S.): Behavioral measurement of severe depression. *Arch. Gen. Psychiat.*, 1972, 27, 330-333.

49 Zuckerman (M.), Lubin (B.): Manual for the multiple affect adjective check list. San Diego: Educational and Industrial Testing Service, 1965.

50 Zung (W.W.K.): A self-rating depression scale. *Arch. Gen. Psychiat.*, 1965, 12, 63-70.

51 Zung (W.W.K.): A cross-cultural study of symptoms in depression. *Amer. J. Psychiat.*, 1969, 126, 154-159.

ÉCHELLE D'OBSERVATION CLINIQUE
CLINICAL OBSERVATION RATING SCALE

SPECIFICITY

TYPE OF INSTRUMENT

*

Ordinal rating scale 20 items, 6 grades

REFERENCE	**Crocq (L.), Fondarai (J.)** · – Exploitation par ordinateur des échelles d'appréciation psychiatrique. Extraits du compte rendu du congrès de psychiatrie et de neurologie de langue française. LXXIe session, Monaco, 2-7 juillet 1973. Paris, Masson 1974, 403-415.
	Language: Original version published in French. Translations in English, Spanish and Arabic. **France**
	Location: Enclosed in volume two page 99 See ref. biblio nº 3
	For all information concerning the instrument or translation write to the author at the following address:
	Louis Crocq, Ministère de la Défense Direction des Recherches, Etudes et Techniques (D.R.E.T.) Groupe 9 26, bd Victor 75996 Paris Armées, France

ORIGIN	Clinical scale B.P.R.S. type (ref. 10), inspired by **Hamilton's** studies (ref. 8), and **Wittenborn** (ref. 12).
PURPOSE	To enable a clinical analysis of depressive states, as well as monitoring of progress during treatment.
POPULATION	Adults of all ages suffering from non-psychotic depression.
ADMINISTRATION	*Rater:* Physician. *Time required:* 20 minutes. *Training:* Not necessary. *Scoring:* The total score of this scale varies from 0-100. Severity of depression increases with score.

VARIABLES	Clinical signs of neurotic or reactive depression:
	     Intellectual efficiency (3 items)
	     Behaviour (3 items)
	     Mood (3 items)
	     Neurotic symptoms (7 items)
	     Will (4 items)

OTHER WORKS cited by author	Drug trials (ref. 2). Studies concerning computer analysis of psychiatric evaluation scales (ref. 3, 5, 6, 7). Works in psychometric methodology (ref. 4).
APPLICATION	Drug trials.

1 Crocq (L.): L'homogénéisation des données cliniques dans les recherches coopératives. LXXVe Congrès de Psychiatrie et de Neurologie de Langue Française, Limoges, 1977.

2 Crocq (L.), Benoist (P.), Boule (J.), Carof (J.), Cron (M.), Digo (R.), Etchegaray (B.), Kulik (J.), Maleysson (M.), Pagot (R.): Essais cliniques multicentres contrôlés par l'Echelle d'Observation Clinique "E.O.C." *Psychologie Médicale*, 1978, tome 10, n°. 6, 1147-1162.

3 Crocq (L.), Fondarai (J.): Exploitation par ordinateur des échelles d'application psychiatrique. Congrès de Psychiatrie et de Neurologie de Langue Française. LXXIe session, Monaco, 2-7 juillet 1973. Paris: Masson, 1974, 403-415.

4 Crocq (L.), Fournier (A.), Martin de Lasalle (J.): Validation des critères de probabilité d'inadaptation neuro-psychique au milieu militaire et de leur application collective sous forme de questionnaire. *Société de Médecine Militaire Française*, mai 1965, tome 5, 281-291.

5 Crocq (L.), Longevialle (C.), Fondarai (J.): Bilan de santé individuel et santé de la population. Journées d'informatique médicale, Toulouse, mars 1973.

6 Fondarai (J.): L'informatique médicale – réalisations actuelles et perspectives d'avenir. *Marseille Médical*, 1967, 104, n°. 9, 763-771.

7 Fondarai (J.), Allain (P.), Etaix (J.), Longevialle (C.): Mise au point d'un système de triage et d'exploitation statistique pour la sélection de masse. Journées d'informatique médicale, Saint-Lary, 1-5 mars 1971, 361-365.

8 Hamilton (M.): Development of a rating scale for primary depressive illness. *Brit. J. Soc. Clin. Psychol.*, 1967, 6, 278-296.

9 Heaulme (M.de.), Amiel (A.), Leroy (C.): Bilan de santé mentale du centre de santé mentale de la Mutuelle de l'Education Nationale. Journées d'informatique médicale, Saint-Lary, 1-5 mars 1971.

10 Overall (J.E.), Gorham (D.R.): The brief psychiatric rating scale. *Psychological Reports*, 1962, 10, 799-812.

11 Pichot (P.), Debray (H.R.): Hospitalisation psychiatrique, statistique descriptive. Paris: Sandoz, 1971, 149 p.

12 Wittenborn (J.R.): Manual: Wittenborn psychiatric rating scales. New York: The Psychological Corporation, 1955.

PHILADELPHIA GERIATRIC CENTER MORALE SCALE

SPECIFICITY

* * *

TYPE OF INSTRUMENT

Check-list, 17 items

REFERENCE	**Lawton (M.P.)** · – The Philadelphia Geriatric Center Morale Scale: a revision. *Journal of Gerontology,* 1975, 30, 85-89.

Language: Original version published in English. Translated into Japanese by Maeda, Asano and Yaguchi (ref. 13).
U.S.A.

Location: Enclosed in volume two page 77
See ref. biblio n° 11

For all information concerning the instrument write to the author at the following address:

M. Powell Lawton,
Philadelphia Geriatric Center
5301 Old York Road
Philadelphia, Pennsylvania 19141, U.S.A.

ORIGIN
The instrument resulted from a factor analysis of "P.G.C. Morale Scale", with a validation study (ref. 10) of the 22 items, inspired by various works concerned with psychological determinants of ageing, degree of satisfaction and morale (ref. 15, 16).

PURPOSE
To enable evaluation of morale as a multi-dimensional concept adapted to very old people through a compact and reliable instrument that does not provoke fatigue or excessive inattention.

POPULATION
All aged persons, in or out-patients.

ADMINISTRATION
Rater: Self administration.

Time required: 10 minutes.

Training: Not necessary.

Scoring: Questions of the yes-no type are read to the respondent and not presented in writing.

VARIABLES
Psychological wellbeing.

VALIDATION
Factorial analysis by the author on aged persons whether out-patients or residents in institutions, average age 72, 6 resulted in 3 factors explaining 43% of the total variance (ref. 11):
  Agitation, anxiety,
  Attitude to own aging,
  Dissatisfaction, loneliness
Several other factor analyses have been performed on different versions of the instrument and the results compared, particularly that by Morris and Sherwood (ref. 14).
Reliability: internal consistency of factors (ref. 11).
The Japanese version has also been validated (ref. 13).

APPLICATION
Clinical and research in the progress of treatment aimed at improving the well-being of the elderly.

1   Adams (D.L.): Analysis of a life satisfaction index. *Journal of Gerontology*, 1969, 24, 470-474.

2   Bengtson (V.L.), Lovejoy (M.C.): Values, personality and social structure. *American Behavioral Scientist*, 1973, 16, 880-912.

3   Burgess (E.W.), Cavan (R.S.), Havighurst (R.J.): Your activities and attitudes. Science Research Associates, Chicago, 1949.

4   Bradburn (N.M.): The structure of psychological well-being. Chicago: Adline, 1969.

5   Cumming (E.), Dean (L.R.), Newell (D.S.): What is "morale"? A case history of a validity problem. *Human Organization*, 1958, 17, 3-8.

6   Gaitz (C.M.), Scott (J.): Age and the measurement of mental health. *Journal of Health and Social Behavior*, 1972, 13, 55-67.

7   Graney (M.J.): Happiness and social participation in old age (abstract). *Gerontologist*, 1973, 13, 3:2, 84.

8   Harman (H.H.): Modern factor analysis. Chicago: Univ. of Chicago Press, 1967.

9   Kutner (B.), Fanshel (D.), Togo (A.), Langer (T.S.): Five hundred over sixty. New York: Russell Sage Foundation, 1956.

10 Lawton (M.P.): The dimensions of morale. In: Kent (D.), Kastenbaum (R.), Sherwood (S.) Eds.: "Research, planning and action for the elderly: the power and potential of social science". New York: Behavioral Publications, 1972.

11 Lawton (M.P.): The Philadelphia Geriatric Center Morale Scale: a revision. *Journal of Gerontology*, 1975, vol. 30, n°. 1, 85-89.

12 Lawton (M.P.), Cohen (J.): The generality of housing impact on the elderly. *Journal of Gerontology*, 1974, 29, 194-204.

13 Maeda (D.), Asano (H.), Yaguchi (K.): Subjective well-being of old people: measurement by PGC Morale Scale. Unpublished manuscript.

14 Morris (J.N.), Sherwood (S.): A retesting and modification of the Philadelphia geriatric center morale scale. *Journal of Gerontology*, 1975, vol. 30, n°. 1, 77-84.

15 Neugarten (B.L.), Havighurst (R.J.), Tobin (S.S.): The measurement of life satisfaction. *Journal of Gerontology*, 1961, 16, 134-143.

16 Pierce (R.C.), Clark (M.M.): Measurement of morale in the elderly. *International Journal of Aging and Human Development*, 1973, 4, 83-101.

17 Rosow (I.), Breslau (N.): A Guttman health scale for the aged. *Journal of Gerontology*, 1966, 21, 556-559.

18 Schooler (K.): Residential physical environment and health of the aged. Final Report, USPHS Grant EC 00191. Waltham, MA: Brandeis Univ., 1970.

19 Srole (L.): Social integration and certain corollaries. *American Sociological Review*, 1956, 21, 709-716.

20 Thompson (W.E.), Streib (G.F.), Kosa (J.): The effect of retirement on personal adjustment: a panel analysis. *Journal of Gerontology*, 1960, 15, 165-169.

BRIEF ANXIETY RATING SCALE

SPECIFICITY

*   *

TYPE OF INSTRUMENT

| Ordinal rating scale |
| 12 items, 4 grades |

REFERENCE   **Wang (R.I.H.), Wiesen (R.L.), Treul (S.), Stockdale (S.)** · − A brief anxiety rating scale in evaluating anxiolytics. *Journal of Clinical Pharmacology,* 1976, 16, 2/3, 99-105.

Language: Original version published in English. Translation in French by L. Israël. **U.S.A.**

Location: Enclosed in volume two page 100
See ref. biblio n̲o̲ 5

For all information concerning the instrument write to the author at the following address:

Richard I.H. Wang,
Medical College of Wisconsin
Wood Veterans Administration Hospital
Milwaukee, Wisconsin 53193, U.S.A.

ORIGIN   The author was inspired by the works on the symptomatology of anxiety and its assessment by **Hamilton** (ref. 2), **Zung** (ref. 7) and **Wittenborn** (ref. 6). The symptoms corresponding to side effects of anxiolytics were systematically excluded, as their inclusion might have reduced the sensitivity of the instrument.

PURPOSE   To evaluate the degree of anxiety in patients under anxiolytic treatment by means of a short instrument, easy to administer and sensitive to therapeutic effects. To separate side effects due to medication.

POPULATION   In and out-patients of all ages affected by anxiety. The author particularly recommends additional use of his scale of side effects (13 items, see volume two) for older patients.

ADMINISTRATION   *Rater:* Physician. Possibly other qualified persons.

Time required: 10 minutes.

Training: Consists of learning to recognize anxiety from somatic symptoms due to treatment.

Scoring: Is based on a 4 point scale of growing severity ranging from 0 (no symptoms) to 3 (maximum intensity). The global score varies from 0 to 36.

VARIABLES

Subjective symptoms:
· Nervousness
· Restlessness
· Excitability
· Irritability
· Worrying
· Disturbed concentration
· Hostility

Somatic symptoms:
· Insomnia
· Palpitations
· Tremors
· Smoking
· Excessive perspiration

Side effects scale:
· Nausea, Burping-belching, Dry mouth,   · Ataxia, Anorexia, Dizziness, Daytime sleeping,
· Hypoactivity, Fatigue, Muscular weakness,   · Drowsiness, Depression

VALIDATION   Was done on male patients suffering from chronic anxiety, through a simple blind trial (ref. 5) covering:
External validity with a global clinical evaluation.
Concurrent validity with Hamilton's anxiety check-list of 13 items on side effects, at intervals throughout treatment.
Reliability: internal consistency of items.
Sensitivity to therapeutic effects.

APPLICATION   Diagnosis of anxiety state; following up the course of the illness over time; drug trials.

BIBLIOGRAPHY

1 Charalampous (K.D.), Tooley (W.), Yates (C.): A new benzodiazepine antianxiety agent. *J. Clin. Pharmacol.*, 1973, 13, 114.

2 Hamilton (M.): The assessment of anxiety states by rating. *Brit. J. Med. Psychol.*, 1959, 22, 50.

3 Holmberg (H.), Livsledt (B.): Clinical evaluation of a new benzodiazepine derivative, clorazepate. *Arznei-mittel - Forschung*, 1972, 22, 916.

4 Ricca (J.J.): Clorazepate dipotassium in anxiety: A clinical trial with diazepam and placebo controls. *J. Clin. Pharmacol.*, 1972, 12, 286.

5 Wang (R.I.H.), Wiesen (R.L.), Treul (S.), Stockdale (S.): A brief anxiety rating scale in evaluating anxiolytics. *J. Clin. Pharmacol.*, 1976, 16, 2/3, 99-105.

6 Wittenborn (J.R.): Reliability, validity and objectivity of symptom - rating scales. *J. Nerv. Ment. Dis.*, 1972, 145, 79.

7 Zung (W.W.K.): A rating instrument for anxiety disorders. *Psychosomatics,* 1971, 12, 371.

STANDARDIZED ASSESSMENT OF PATIENTS
WITH DEPRESSIVE DISORDERS (S.A.D.D.)

SPECIFICITY

> *

TYPE OF INSTRUMENT

> Nominal rating scale
> 60 items, 3-5 grades

REFERENCE	**World Health Organization** · – Schedule for a standardized assessment of patients with depressive disorders. Not published. Geneva: World Health Organization, March 1977.

Language: English, French, Bulgarian, Hindu, Japanese, Polish, German. **Switzerland**

Location: Enclosed in volume two page 101

For all information concerning the instrument or translation write to the author at the following address:

Norman Sartorius,
Director,
Division of Mental Health
W.H.O.
1211 Genèva 27, Switzerland

ORIGIN
Cooperative study by WHO evaluating depressive states in different countries.

PURPOSE
The instrument was designed as a protocol for the standard evaluation of patients with depressive disorders.

POPULATION
Adult persons of all ages from age 15 upwards hospitalized in psychiatric wards.

ADMINISTRATION
Rater: Psychologist, psychiatrist, trained general practitioner.
Time required: 30-40 minutes.
Training: Necessary.
Scoring: Is done on a 3 point and 5 point scale.

VARIABLES
Somatic and psychological symptoms of depressive states.
The instrument is composed of four parts:
   1. Identification data.
   2. Symptoms and signs of depressive state - psychiatric history
   3. Treatment in present episode.
   4. Diagnosis and classification.

VALIDATION
Using depressed patients, resulting in different publications particularly concerned with the evaluation of depressive states in different cultures (ref. 5).

OTHER WORKS
cited by author
A comparative study of depressive signs was carried out in five centres.
   Basel (Switzerland)
   Montreal (Canada)
   Nagasaki, Tokyo (Japan)
   Teheran (Iran)
There is a translation of depressive signs in the languages of these countries.

APPLICATION
Clinical: Therapeutic care planning
Research: Epidemiological studies. Drug trials

1 Bech. (P.), Gram (L.F.), Reisby (N.), Rafaelsen (O.J.):
   The W.H.O. depression scale: relationship to the
   Newcastle scales. *Acta Psychiat. Scand.*, 1980, 62, 140-
   153.

2 Gershon (E.S.), Mendlewicz (J.), Gastpar (M.), Bech
   (P.), Goldin (L.R.), Kielholz (P.), Rafaelsen (O.J.),
   Vartanian (F.), Bunney (W.E.Jr.): A collaborative study of genetic linkage of bipolar manic-depressive illness and red/green colour blindness. A project of the
   biological psychiatry collaborative programme of the
   World Health Organization. *Acta Psychiat. Scand.*,
   1980, 61, 319-338.

3 Jablensky (A.), Milenkov (K.), Temkov (I.): Depressive disorders and depressive symptoms among patients
   making a first contact with the mental health services.
   Paper prepared for presentation at the International
   Symposium of the Prevention and Treatment of Treatment for Depression, Washington, DC, 22-24 October
   1979.

4 Sartorius (N.): Description and classification of depressive disorders. *Pharmakopsychiat.*, 1974, 7, 76.

5 Sartorius (N.): Research on affective psychoses within
   the framework of the W.H.O. programme. In: "Origin,
   prevention and treatment of affective disorders". Proceedings of a seminar, Aaruhus University, Denmark,
   August 1978. 1979, 207-313.

6 Sartorius (N.): Collaboration between various medical
   and paramedical groups in the treatment of depression. In: Kielholz (P.) Ed.: "The general practitioner
   and his depressed patients". Bern, Stuttgart, Vienna:
   Hans Huber Publishers, 1980.

7 Sartorius (N.), Jablensky (A.), Gulbinat (W.), Ernberg
   (G.): Application of W.H.O. scales for the assessment
   of depressive states in different cultures. In: "Epidemiological research for the organization of extramural
   psychiatry". *Acta Psychiat. Scand.*, 1980, Suppl. 285,
   62.

8 Sartorius (N.), Jablensky (A.), Gulbinat (W.), Ernberg
   (G.): W.H.O. collaborative study: assessment of depressive disorders. Preliminary communication. *Psychological Medicine*, 1980, 10, 743-749.

9 World Health Organization: Mental disorders: glossary and guide to their classification in accordance
   with the ninth revision of the international classification of diseases. W.H.O. nonserial publication, 1978.

MANIA RATING SCALE

SPECIFICITY

| * |

TYPE OF INSTRUMENT

Ordinal rating scale
11 items, 5 grades

REFERENCE	**Bech (P.), Rafaelsen (O.J.), Kramp (P.), Bolwig (T.G.)** · – The Mania Rating Scale: Scale construction and inter-observer agreement. *Neuropharmacology,* 1978, 17, 6, 430-431.

Language: Original version in Danish. Translations in English, French, German. **Denmark**

Location: Enclosed in volume two page 102
See ref. biblio n° 4

For all information concerning the instrument or translations write to the author at the following address:

Per Bech,
Psychochemistry Institute
Rigshospitalet
9, Blegdamsvej
DK-2100 Copenhagen, Denmark

ORIGIN   Instrument constructed on the basis of the "Biegel mania state rating scale" (ref. 5) and the study of **Petterson** (ref. 10), with the addition of certain items.

PURPOSE   This instrument has been constructed with the purpose of quantifying the severity of manic states.

POPULATION   Patients of all ages presenting a mania state.

ADMINISTRATION *Rater:* Psychiatrist, psychologist or other skilled observer.

Time required: 15 to 30 minutes.

Training: Training in psychiatric interviewing.

Scoring: For each item 0-4 is scored with increasing intensity. The total score varies from 0, corresponding to total absence of the manic syndrome, to 44, representing the highest degree of severity of manic state.

VARIABLES   Eleven variables are described:
· Activity (motor)   · Self-esteem
· Activity (verbal)   · Contact
· Flight of ideas   · Sleep (average of last 3 nights)
· Voices/Noise level   · Sexual interest and activity
· Hostility/Destructiveness   · Activity (work and interests)
· Mood (feelings of well-being)

VALIDATION   They have included (ref. 4):
Correlation with the classification of patients by the diagnostic scale for affective disorders "Multi-Clad" (ref. 9).
Study on **inter-rater reliability**
Establishment of **norms** for clinical trials
· Inclusion criteria: total score above or equal to 15
· Partial response to treatment: total score from 6 to 14
· Full remission: total score less than 5
· No response to treatment: total score above or equal to 15.

OTHER WORKS   · Study on anti-manic effect of certain drugs (ref. 8).
cited by author · The Melancholia scale, simultaneous use of which is recommended by its authors in bipolar patients.

APPLICATION   **Research:** clinical trials.

Ia.12

1 Bech (P.), Allerup (P.), Rosenberg (R.): The Marke-Nyman temperament scale: evaluation of transferability by use of the Rasch item analysis. *Acta Psychiat. Scand.*, 1978, 57, 49-58.

2 Bech (P.), Bolwig (T.G.), Dein (E.), Jacobsen (O.), Gram (L.F.): Quantitative rating of manic states. *Acta Psychiat. Scand.*, 1975, 52, 1-6.

3 Bech (P.), Gram (L.F.), Dein (E.), Jacobsen (O.), Vitger (J.), Bolwig (T.G.): Quantitative rating of depressive states. *Acta Psychiat. Scand.*, 1975, 51, 161-170.

4 Bech (P.), Rafaelsen (O.J.), Kramp (P.), Bolwig (T.G.): The mania rating scale: scale construction and interobserver agreement. *Neuropharmacology*, 1978, 17, 430-431.

5 Biegel (A.), Murphy (D.L.), Bunney (W.): The mania-state rating scale. *Arch. Gen. Psychiat.*, 1971, 25, 256-262.

6 Hamilton (M.): A rating scale for depression. *J. Neurol. Neurosurg. Psychiat.*, 1960, 23, 56-62.

7 Hamilton (M.): Development of a rating scale for primary depressive illness. *Br. J. Soc. Clin. Psychol.*, 1967, 6, 278-296.

8 Jouvent (R.), Lecrubier (Y.), Puech (A.J.), Simon (P.), Widlöcher (D.): Antimanic effect of clonidine. *Am. J. Psychiatry*, October 1980, 137, 10, 1275,-1276.

9 Kramp (P.), Shapiro (R.W.), Rafaelsen (O.J.): Multiaxial classification system of affective disorders (MULTI-CLAD). In: Achté (K.), Aalberg (V.), Lönnqvist (J.) Eds: "Psychopathology of depression". Psychiatria Fennica Supplementum. 1980, 321-325.

10 Petterson (U.), Fyrö (B.), Sedvall (G.): A new scale for longitudinal rating of manic states. *Acta Psychiat. Scand.*, 1973, 49, 248-256.

IRRITABILITY - DEPRESSION - ANXIETY SCALE (I.D.A.)

SPECIFICITY

| * |

TYPE OF INSTRUMENT

Ordinal rating scale
18 items, 4 grades

REFERENCE   **Snaith (R.P.), Constantopoulos (A.A.), Jardine (M.Y.), Mc Guffin (P.)** · – A clinical scale for the self-assessment of irritability. *British Journal of Psychiatry,* 1978, 132, 164-171.

Language: Original version published in English. Translations in French, Flemish, Italian, Arabic, Swedish, Spanish.
Great Britain

Location: Enclosed in volume two page 103
See ref. biblio n° 9

For all information concerning the instrument or translation write to the author at the following address:

R.P. Snaith,
University of Leeds, Department of Psychiatry
15 Hyde Terrace
Leeds LS2 9LT, Great Britain

ORIGIN   The instrument comprises the items selected from the "Hostility and Direction of Hostility Questionnaire", by **Caine** et. al. (ref. 2) and from the "Buss-Durkee Inventory" (ref. 1) equating to the authors concept of irritability, and original items referring particularly to the states of depression and anxiety. The final selection derives from the study of correlations of that first version of the instrument with age, sex and 4 scales of depression, anxiety and irritability, inspired by **Hamilton** (ref. 5).

PURPOSE   To measure specifically irritability in a clinical context. Irritability is conceived as a momentary psychological state, characterized by impatience and poor control of inner tensions, directed towards others or towards oneself. The authors have held that it would be useful to combine its evaluation with that of depression and anxiety in order to throw light on the relations between these three states.

POPULATION   Patients of all ages in or out-patients, affected by depression and/or anxiety, possibly by other psychiatric afflictions and able to read and understand the items.

ADMINISTRATION   *Rater:* Self-administered.
Time required: 5 minutes.
Training: Not necessary.
Scoring: Relies on the actual state of the subject. If the item expresses a health or disease state, its scoring varies from 0-3 or from 3-0 respectively, as a frequency scale depicting growing or decreasing severity.

	Depression	Anxiety	Irritability Internal	External
Normal	0-3	0-5	0-4	0-3
Intermediate	4-6	6-8	5-7	4-6
Pathological state	7-15	9-15	8-12	7-12

VARIABLES   This scale evaluates 3 aspects:
· Depression (items 1, 3, 5, 9, 12)   · Irritability: directed outwards (items 4, 6, 13, 16)
· Anxiety (items 2, 7, 10, 14, 17)   · Irritability: directed inwards (items 8, 11, 15, 18)

VALIDATION   With in or out-patients showing signs of anxiety or depression, covering:
Construct validity by selection of items not depending on age or sex, but correlated to a considerable degree with corresponding scale inspired by Hamilton (depression, anxiety, irritability), and possessing a higher correlation with that scale than the three others taken separately.
Concurrent validity of the final version of the scale with the 4 sub-scales by Hamilton.
Sensitivity and discriminating as between healthy subjects and subjects with pathological charges whether improving moderately or severely affected, according to each of the 4 sub-scales.
Reliability: several studies of split-half. Study of the influence of previous psychiatric interview. These last studies were implemented with a population of depressives and a group of healthy subjects average age 35 years (ref. 9).

OTHER WORKS
cited by author   Comparison of different scales evaluating depression (ref. 6).
Construction of self administered scales of depression and anxiety (ref. 8).

APPLICATION   Monitoring of spontaneous course or changes induced by external agents. It is not a diagnostic instrument, although the scores of subscales give useful information of a diagnostic nature.

1 Buss (A.H.), Durkee (A.): An inventory for assessing different kinds of hostility. *Journal of Consulting Psychology*, 1957, 21, 343-349.

2 Caine (T.M.), Foulds (G.A.), Hope (K.): Manual of the hostility and direction of hostility questionnaire. University of London Press, 1967.

3 Gottschalk (L.A.), Gleser (G.C.), Springer (K.J.): Three hostility scales applicable to verbal samples. *Archives of General Psychiatry*, 1963, 9, 254-279.

4 Hamilton (M.): The assessment of anxiety states by rating. *British Journal of Medical Psychology*, 1959, 32, 50-55.

5 Hamilton (M.): Development of a rating scale for primary depressive illness. *British Journal of Social and Clinical Psychology*, 1967, 6, 278-296.

6 Kearns (N.P.), Cruickshank (C.A.), Mc Guigan (K.J.), Riley (S.A.), Shaw (S.P.), Snaith (R.P.): A comparison of depression rating scales. *British Journal of Psychiatry*, 1982, 141, 45-49.

7 Snaith (R.P.), Ahmed (S.N.), Mehta (S.), Hamilton (M.): The assessment of the severity of primary depressive illness. *Psychological Medicine*, 1971, 1, 143-149.

8 Snaith (R.P.), Bridge (G.W.K.), Hamilton (M.): The Leeds scales for the self-assessment of anxiety and depression. *British Journal of Psychiatry*, 1976, 128, 156-165.

9 Snaith (R.P.), Constantopoulos (A.A.), Jardine (M.Y.), Mc Guffin (P.): A clinical scale for the self-assessment of irritability. *British Journal of Psychiatry*, 1978, 132, 164-171.

10 Weissman (M.), Klerman (G.L.), Paykel (E.S.): Clinical evaluation of hostility in depression. *American Journal of Psychiatry*, 1971, 128, 3, 261-266.

MONTGOMERY AND ASBERG DEPRESSION RATING SCALE (M.A.D.R.S.)

SPECIFICITY

* *

TYPE OF INSTRUMENT

Ordinal rating scale
10 items,
7 scale steps

REFERENCE	**Montgomery (S.A.), Asberg (M.)** · – A new depression scale designed to be sensitive to change. *British Journal of Psychiatry,* 1979, 134, 382-389.
	Language: Original version published in English. Translated into French by D.P. Bobon (Clinique psychiatrique, Université de Liège, Belgium). Translated into other European languages and Chinese. **Great Britain**
	Location: Enclosed in volume two page 104 See ref. biblio nº 11
	For all information concerning the instrument or translation write to the author at the following address:
	Stuart Montgomery, Academic Department of Psychiatry St. Mary's Hospital Medical School London W9 3RL, Great Britain

ORIGIN
Developed from the 65 items Comprehensive Psychopathological Rating Scale (ref. 3, 12). The 17 most frequently occurring items were tested for sensitivity to change and the 10 most sensitive items were selected (ref. 11).

PURPOSE
The scale is designed to evaluate quickly and with precision the severity of depression and change in severity with treatment.

POPULATION
Depressed inpatients and out-patients.

ADMINISTRATION
Rater: Psychiatrist, psychologist, nurse, general practitioner.

Time required: 20 minutes to an hour, depending on patient's condition and ability of rater.

Training: One or two training sessions desirable.

Scoring: Each item is rated on a scale 0 to 6 of increasing severity. Alternate steps have severity definitions. Total score is from 0 to 60 and decrease in score represents improvement.

VARIABLES
The ten variables are specifically for the treatment of depression.
- Apparent sadness
- Reported sadness
- Inner tension
- Reduced sleep
- Reduced appetite
- Concentration difficulties
- Lassitude
- Inability to feel
- Pessimistic thoughts
- Suicidal thoughts

VALIDATION
Carried out in a population of patients suffering from endogenous or reactive depression, hospital inpatients and out-patients in England and Sweden.
Studies of intrinsic and **concurrent validity** with the "Hamilton Depression Scale" (ref. 9, 11).
Cross cultural studies (ref. 11, 13)
Inter-rater **reliability** studies (ref. 2, 11)
Further **validation studies** in progress.

OTHER WORKS
cited by author
Use in open and double blind studies of treatments for depression.

APPLICATION
Evaluation of results of treatment.
Therapeutic investigations.

1 Anderson (N.H.): Scales and statistics: parametric and non parametric. *Psychological Bulletin*, 1961, 58, 305-316.

2 Asberg (M.), Kragh-Sorensen (P.), Mindham (R.H.S.), Tuck (J.R.): International reliability and communicability of a rating scale for depression. *Psychological Medicine*, 1973, 3, 458-465.

3 Asberg (M.) Montgomery (S.), Perris (C.), Schalling (D.), Sedvall (G.): A comprehensive psychopathological rating scale. *Acta Psychiatrica Scandinavica*, 1978, Suppl. 271, 5-27.

4 Bobon (D.P.), Mendlewicz (J): Résultats préliminaires de l'adaptation francaise de l'échelle de schizophrénie de Montgomery. *Les Feuillets Psychiatriques de Liège*, 1981, 14, 4, 477-486.

5 Carroll (B.J.), Fielding (J.M.), Blashki (T.G.): Depression rating scales. A critical review. *Archives of General Psychiatry*, 1973, 28, 361-366.

6 Coppen (A.), Gupta (R.), Montgomery (S.), Ghose (K.), Bailey (J.), Burns (B.), De Ridder (J.J.): Mianserin hydrochloride: a novel antidepressant. *British Journal of Psychiatry*, 1976, 129, 342-345.

7 Feighner (J.P.), Robins (E.), Guze (S.B), Woodruff (R.A.), Winokur (G.), Munoz (R.): Diagnostic criteria for use in psychiatric research. *Archives of General Psychiatry*, 1972, 26, 57-63.

8 Gurney (C.), Roth (M.), Garside (R.F.), Kerr (T.A.), Schapira (K.): Studies in the classification of affective disorders: The relationship between anxiety states and depressive illnesses- Il. *British Journal of Psychiatry*, 1972, 121, 162-166.

9 Hamilton (M.): A rating scale for depression. *Journal of Neurology, Neurosurgery and Psychiatry*, 1960, 23, 56-62.

10 Hamilton (M.): Comparative value of rating scales. *British Journal of Clinical Pharmacology*, 1976, 3, 58-60.

11 Montgomery (S.A.), Asberg (M.): A new depression scale designed to be sensitive to change. *British Journal of Psychiatry*, 1979, 134, 382-389.

12 Montgomery, (S.), Asberg (M.), Jörnestedt (L.), Thoren (P.), Träskman (L.), Mc Auley (R.), Montgomery (D.), Shaw (P.): Reliability of the CPRS between the disciplines of psychiatry, general practice, nursing and psychology in depressed patients. *Acta Psychiat. Scand.*, 1978, Suppl. 271, 29-32.

13 Montgomery (S), Asberg (M.), Träskman (L.), Montgomery (D.): Cross-cultural studies on the use of CPRS in English and Swedish depressed patients. *Acta Psychiat. Scand.*, 1978, Suppl. 271, 33-37.

W.H.O. DEPRESSION SCALE

SPECIFICITY

*

TYPE OF INSTRUMENT

Rating scale
17 items

REFERENCE   **Bech (P.), Gram (L.F.), Reisby (N.), Rafaelsen (O.J.)** · – The W.H.O. depression scale. *Acta Psychiatrica Scandinavica,* 1980, 62, 2, 140-153.

Language: Original version published in English.
Denmark

Location: Enclosed in volume two page 106
See ref. biblio nº 4

For all information concerning the instrument write to the author at the following address:

Per Bech,
Psychochemistry Institute
Rigshospitalet
9, Blegdamsvej
DK-2100 Copenhagen, Denmark

ORIGIN   Instrument constructed from a combination of the WHO Depression Scale and the 2 Newcastle scales (ref. 4), each consisting of 10 items, with the purpose of making it possible to differentiate between the endogenous and the neurotic depressions, or between endogenous and the reactive depressions.

PURPOSE   To add to the WHO Depression Scale a dimension of diagnostic differentation between endogenous and reactive or neurotic depressions.

POPULATION   Depressed patients of all ages.

ADMINISTRATION   *Rater:* Psychiatrist, psychologist or another skilled observer.

Time required: 30 minutes.

Training: Training in psychiatric interviewing.

Scoring: The combination of the scales, in 3 degrees for the WHO scales or in 2 degrees for the Newcastle scale results in a half-point scoring system. The addition of the scores of the Newcastle I WHO and Newcastle II WHO gives a total score distinguishing the non-endogenous depressions from the endogenous depressions.

VARIABLES   Symptomatology of the present depressive syndrome.
Clinical history of the depression.

VALIDATION   Performed in a population of inpatients, mean age 52 years, included in a study on the clinical effects and the plasma levels of two anti-depressants, they have comprised:
· Studies on the correlation between the scores obtained and age, sex, plasma level.
· Studies on the scores as per the Hamilton Depression Scale and plasma levels as well as their correlation with the diagnostic classification by the Newcastle I WHO and the Newcastle II WHO scales.
· **Inter-rater reliability**.
· Study on patient distribution according to their score in relation to the diagnosis.

APPLICATION   **Clinical:**   Differential diagnosis of endogenous and reactive or neurotic depressions.
Research: Clinical trials.

1 Bech (P.): Depressive symptomatology and drug response. *Commun. Psychopharmacol.*, 1978, 2, 409-418.

2 Bech (P.), Allerup (P.), Gram (L.F.), Reisby (N.), Rosenberg (R.), Jacobsen (O.), Nagy (A.): The Hamilton depression scale: evaluation of objectivity using logistic models. *Acta Psychiat. Scand.*, 1981, 63, 290-299.

3 Bech (P.), Gram (L.F.), Dein (E.), Jacobsen (O.), Vitger (J.), Bolwig (T.G.): Quantitative rating of depressive states. *Acta Psychiat. Scand.*, 1975, 51, 161-170.

4 Bech (P.), Gram (L.F.) Reisby (N.), Rafaelsen (O.J.): The W.H.O. depression scale: relationship to the Newcastle scales. *Acta Psychiat. Scand.*, 1980, vol. 62, n°. 2, 140-153.

5 Bech (P.), Rafaelsen (O.J.): Personality and manic-melancholic illness. Paper read at the WPA Symposium "Psychopathology of depression", Helsinki, 1979.

6 Beck (A.T.), Ward (C.H.), Mendelson (M.), Mock (J.), Erbaugh (J.): An inventory for measuring depression. *Arch. Gen. Psychiat.*, 1961, 4, 561-571.

7 Carney (M.W.P.), Roth (M.), Garside (R.F.): The diagnosis of depressive syndromes and the prediction of ECT response, *Brit. J. Psychiat.*, 1965, 111, 659-674.

8 Carney (M.W.P.), Sheffield (B.F.): Depression and the Newcastle scales: their relationship to Hamilton's scale. *Brit. J. Psychiat.*, 1972, 121, 35-40.

9 Carroll (B.J.): Neuroendocrine procedures for the diagnosis of depression. In: Garattini (S.) Ed.: "Depressive disorders". Stuttgart: F.K. Schattauer, 1978, 231-236.

10 Checkley (S.A.): Hormones and classification of depressive illness. *Lancet*, 1979, 1, 1081.

11 Ferguson (G.A.): Statistical analysis in psychology and education. New York: Mc Graw-Hill, 1976.

12 Garside (R.F.), Roth (M.): Multivariate statistical methods and problems of classification in psychiatry. *Brit. J. Psychiat.*, 1978, 133, 53-57.

13 Gram (L.F.), Bech (P.), Reisby (N.), Jorgensen (O.S.): Methodology in studies on plasma level/effect relationship of tricyclic antidepressants. In: Usdin (E.) Ed.: "Clinical pharmacology in psychiatry." North-Holland, New York: Elsevier, 1980.

14 Gurney (C.): Diagnostic scales for affective disorders. Proceedings of the fifth World Conference of Psychiatry, Mexico City, 1971.

15 Gurney (C.), Roth (M.), Garside (R.F.), Kerr (T.A.), Schapira (K.): Studies in the classification of affective disorders. The relationship between anxiety state and depressive illness. *Brit. J. Psychiat.*, 1972, 121, 162-166.

16 Hamilton (M.): Development of a rating scale for primary depressive illness. *Brit. J. Soc. Clin. Psychol.*, 1967, 6, 278-296.

17 Hamilton (M.): Prediction of response to ECT in depressive illness. In: Angst (J.) Ed.: "Classification and prediction of outcome of depression." Stuttgart: F.K. Schattauer Verlag, 1974, 273-279.

18 Kendell (R.E.): The classification of depressive illness. Maudsley Monograph n°. 18. London: Oxford University Press, 1968.

19 Kendell (R.E.): The classification of depressions. A review of contemporary confusion. *Brit. J. Psychiat.*, 1976, 129, 15-28.

20 Kendell (R.E.), Post (F.): Depressive illnesses in late life. *Brit. J. Psychiat.*, 1973, 122, 615-617.

21 Kerr (T.A.), Roth (M.), Schapira (K.), Gurney (C.): The assessment and prediction of outcome in affective disorders. *Brit. J. Psychiat.*, 1972, 121, 167-174.

22 Kielholz (P.), Terzani (S.), Gastpar (M.): Treatment for therapy resistant depressions. *Int. Pharmacopsychiat.*, 1979, 14, 94-100.

23 Kragh-Sorensen (P.), Hansen (C.E.), Asberg (M.): Plasma levels of nortriptyline in the treatment of endogenous depression. *Acta Psychiat. Scand.*, 1973, 49, 444-456.

24 Kramp (P.), Shapiro (R.W.), Rafaelsen (O.J.): Multi-Axial Classification System of Affective Disorders (MULTI-CLAD). Paper read at the WPA Symposium "Psychopathology of depression", Helsinki, 1979.

25 Nelson (J.C.), Charney (D.C.), Vingiano (A.W.): False-positive diagnosis with primary-affective-disorder criteria. *Lancet*, 1978, 11, 1252-1253.

26 Perris (C.): The course of depressive psychoses. *Acta Psychiat. Scand.*, 1968, 44, 238-248.

27 Post (F.): The management and nature of depressive illnesses in late life: a follow-through study. *Brit. J. Psychiat.*, 1972, 121, 393-404.

28 Rao (V.A.R.), Coppen (A.): Classification of depression and response to amitriptyline therapy. *Psychol. Med.*, 1979, 9, 321-325.

29 Reisby (N.), Gram (L.F.), Bech (P.), Nagy (A.), Petersen (G.O.), Ortmann (J.), Ibsen (I.), Dencker (S.J.), Jacobsen (O.), Krautwald (O.), Sondergaard (I.), Christiansen (J.): Imipramine: clinical effects and pharmacokinetic variability. *Psychopharmacology*, 1977, 54, 263-272.

30 Reisby (N.), Gram (L.F.), Bech (P.), Sihm (F.), Krautwald (O.), Elly (J.), Ortman (J.), : Clomipramine: Plasma levels and clinical effects. *Commun. Psychopharmacol.*, 1979, 3, 341-351.

31 Roth (M.), Gurney (C.), Garside (R.F.), Kerr (T.A.): Studies in the classification of affective disorders. *Brit. J. Psychiat.*, 1972, 121, 147-161.

32 Sartorius (N.): Depressive disorders: a major public health problem. In: Ayd (F.J.), Taylor (I.J.) Eds: "Mood disorders". Ayd Medical Communication, Baltimore, 1978, 1-8.

33 Siegel (S.): Non-parametric statistics. New York: Mc Graw-Hill, 1956.

34 Walter (C.J.S.): Drug plasma levels and clinical effect. *Proc. Roy. Soc. Med.*, 1971, 64, 282-285.

SELF RATING ANXIETY SCALE (S.A.S.)

SPECIFICITY

*

TYPE OF INSTRUMENT

Ordinal rating scale
20 items, 4 grades

REFERENCE	**Zung (W.W.K.)** · – How normal is anxiety? (Current concepts). Upjohn Company, 1980.
	Language: Original version published in English. Translations in Chinese, Dutch, French, German, Italian and Siamese. **U.S.A.**
	Location: Enclosed in volume two page 107 See ref. biblio n° 14
	For all information concerning the instrument or translations write to the author at the following address:
	William Zung, Dpt of Psychiatry, Duke University Medical Center, Veterans Administration Hospital Durham, North Carolina 27705, U.S.A.

ORIGIN	The instrument derives from a revision made by the author of diagnostic criteria of anxiety, analysis of interview records of anxious patients with the aim of formulating appropriate items, and also works by **Feighner** (ref. 1), by **Hamilton** (ref. 3) and **F.D.A.** (ref. 2).
PURPOSE	To measure anxiety conceived as a clinical entity, by self-administration, the advantage of which has been shown by a number of works to be: · information directly and entirely from the patient, objective and standardized; · rapid administration not requiring qualified staff; · easy scoring which may be repeated in any medical context.
POPULATION	Patients of all ages suffering from anxiety.
ADMINISTRATION	*Rater:* Self administration. *Time required:* 3 minutes. *Training:* It is necessary to give the patient instructions. *Scoring:* Done for each item according to a scale of growing severity of 4 grades. The total score, divided by the total maximum score of 80 and converted to a percentage, is an index of anxiety.
VARIABLES	Affective symptoms: 5 items. Somatic symptoms: 15 items.
VALIDATION	Done in different populations in or out-patients of different ages (ref. 14): **Face validity:** including physical and psychological symptoms. **Validity of content:** all physical and psychic symptoms of the syndrome brought together. **Concurrent validity** in relation to the Taylor Manifest Anxiety Scale (T.M.A.S.) in anxious patients as well as subjects affected by coronary insufficiency; in relation to Hamilton's anxiety scale during anxiolytic drug trials. **Discriminative sensibility** for normal and anxious subjects, for each item and for the global score. **Reliability:** Split-half and internal consistency. **Norms** differentiating populations, with regard to age and source, in cardiac and psychiatric patients.
OTHER WORKS cited by author	Study of age groups (younger than 19, aged 19-64, over 65) Study of large population of out-patients and those at the time of admission to hospital which can be used prospectively as a screening tool, studies in cardiology, drug trials, transcultural studies: USA, Nigeria, Taiwan, Korea. Construction of a similar inventory for completion by an observer (Anxiety Status Inventory).
APPLICATION	Diagnostic and clinical studies of anxiety. Screening of pathological anxiety Drug trials.

1 Feighner (J.P.), Robins (E.), Guze (S.B.), Woodruff (R.A. Jr.), Winokur (G.), Munoz (R.): Diagnostic criteria for use in psychiatric research. *Arch. Gen. Psychiatry*, 1972, 26, 57-63.

2 Guidelines for the conduct of clinical trials. FDA Guidelines for psychotropic drugs. *Psychopharmacol. Bull.*, 1974, 10, 70-91.

3 Hamilton (M.): The assessment of anxiety states by rating. *Br. J. Med. Psychol.*, 1959, 32, 50.

4 Jegede (R.O.): Psychometric attributes of the self-rating anxiety scale. *Psychol. Rep.*, 1977, 40, 303-306.

5 Ko (Y.H.): Mental health of college students. *Bulletin of Mental Health Society of the Republic of China*, 1972, 17, 11-17.

6 Lader (M.), Marks (I.): Clinical anxiety. New York: Grune and Stratton, 1971.

7 Miao (E.): An exploratory study on college freshmen mental health status. *Acta Psychologica Taiwanica*, 1976, 18, 129-148.

8 Rosenman (R.H.), Friedman (M.), Straus (R.) et al.: Coronary heart disease in the western collaborative group study: a follow-up experience of a 4 ½ years. *J. Chron. Dis.*, 1970, 23, 173-190.

9 Taylor (J.): A personality scale of manifest anxiety. *J. Abnorm. and Soc. Psychol.*, 1953, 48, 285-290.

10 Wang (S.G.): A study of anxiety with the self-rating anxiety scale on psychiatric out-patients. *Neuropsychiatry*, 1978, 17, 179-191.

11 Zung (W.W.K.): A rating instrument for anxiety disorders. *Psychosomatics,* 1971, 12, 371-379.

12 Zung (W.W.K.): The differentiation of anxiety and depressive disorders: a psychopharmacological approach. *Psychosomatics*, 1973, 24, 362-366.

13 Zung (W.W.K.): Assessment of anxiety disorders; qualitative and quantitative approaches. In: Fann (W.E.), Karacan (I.), Pokorny (A.), Pokorny (A.), Williams (R.) Eds: "Phenomenology and treatment of anxiety". New York: Spectrum Publications, 1979.

14 Zung (W.W.K.): How normal is anxiety? (Current concepts). Upjohn Company, 1980.

CARROLL RATING SCALE (C.R.S.)

SPECIFICITY

* *

TYPE OF INSTRUMENT

Check-list 52 items

REFERENCE	**Carroll (B.J.), Feinberg (M.), Smouse (P.E.), Rawson (S.G.), Greden (J.F.)** · − The Carroll rating scale for depression. 1 - Development, reliability and validation. 2 - Factor analyses of the feature profiles. 3 - Comparison with other rating instruments. *British Journal of Psychiatry,* 1981, 138, 194-200 (1), 201-204 (2), 205-209 (3).

Language: Original version published in English.
U.S.A.

Location: Enclosed in volume two page 78
See ref. biblio n° 6, 9, 18

For all information concerning the instrument write to the author at the following address:

Bernard J. Carroll,
Department of Psychiatry
University of Michigan
Ann Arbor, Michigan 48109, U.S.A.

ORIGIN   The instrument was inspired by **Hamilton**'s Scale of Depression of 17 items (ref. 12, 13) and by studies of the author concerned with depression scales (ref. 7).

PURPOSE   To measure the intensity of depression by a self-administered test complementary to that of Hamilton.

POPULATION   Depressed adults, other psychiatric patients and aged persons not presenting with cognitive disorders.

ADMINISTRATION   *Rater:* Self-administration.

Time required: 10 minutes.

Training: Not necessary.

Scoring: Each item requires an answer of the yes-no type to each of the 2 proposed situations.

VARIABLES   The various symptoms of depression.

VALIDATION   Carried out in a population composed of university employees aged 18-64, from different socio-economic background - and of subjects suffering from depression, covering (ref. 6):
Concurrent validity (ref. 9) with other scales of depression, e.g. Scale by Hamilton (ref. 13)
Depression Inventory by Beck (ref. 4).
External validity in relation to clinical rating of the severity of depression.
Reliability: Test-retest, Split-half, Internal consistency of items with the total score.
Sensitivity discriminating depressed and non depressed subjects.

APPLICATION   **Clinical:**   Prognosis and screening of depressive state.
Research: Drug trials
            Longitudinal follow-up
            Outcome

1   Aitken (R.C.B.): Measurement of feelings using visual analogue scales. *Proceedings of the Royal Society of Medicine*, 1969, 62, 989-993.

2   Bailey (J.), Coppen (A.): A comparison between the Hamilton rating scale and the Beck inventory in the measurement of depression. *British Journal of Psychiatry*, 1976, 128,486-489.

3   Beck (A.T.): Depression: clinical, experimental and theoretical aspects. London: Harper and Row, 1967.

4   Beck (A.T.), Ward (C.H.), Mendelson (M.), Mock (J.), Erbaugh (J.): An inventory for measuring depression. *Archives of General Psychiatry*, 1961, 28, 361-366.

5   Carroll (B.J.), Feinberg (M.), Greden (J.F.), Haskett (R.F.), James (N.), Steiner (M.), Tarika (J.): Diagnosis of endogenous depression: comparison of clinical, research and neuroendocrine criteria. *Journal of Affective Disorders*, 1980, 2, 177-194.

6   Carroll (B.J.), Feinberg (M.), Smouse (P.E.), Rawson (S.G.), Greden (J.F.): The Carroll rating scale for depression. I: Development, reliability and validation. *British Journal of Psychiatry*, 1981, 138, 194-200.

7   Carroll (B.J.), Fielding (J.M.), Blashki (T.G.): Depression rating scales: a critical review. *Archives of General Psychiatry*, 1973, 28, 361-366.

8   Feinberg (M.): Presentation at panel, affective disorders clinics: new concept in outpatient care. Annual meeting. Atlanta: American Psychiatric Association, 1978.

9   Feinberg (M.), Carroll (B.J.), Smouse (P.E.), Rawson (S.G.): The Carroll rating scale for depression. III: Comparison with other rating instruments. *British Journal of Psychiatry*, 1981, 138, 205-209.

10   Feinberg (M.), Carroll (B.J.), Smouse (P.), Rawson (S.), Haskett (R.), Steiner (M.), Albala (A.), Zelnick (T.): Comparison of physician and self-ratings of depression. Society of Biological Psychiatry, 34th annual meeting, abstract 80, 1979.

11   Folstein (M.F.), Luria (R.E.): Reliability, validity, and clinical application of the visual analogue mood scale. *Psychological Medicine*, 1973, 3, 479-486.

12   Hamilton (M.): A rating scale for depression. *Journal of Neurology, Neuro-surgery and Psychiatry*, 1960, 23, 56-62.

13   Hamilton (M.): Development of a rating scale for primary depressive illness. *British Journal of Social and Clinical Psychology*, 1967, 6, 278-296.

14   Hedlund (J.L.), Vieweg (B.W.): The Hamilton rating scale for depression: a comprehensive review. *Journal of Operational Psychiatry*, 1979, 10, 149-165.

15   Luria (R.E.): The validity and reliability of the visual analogue mood scale. *Journal of Psychiatric Research*, 1975, 12, 51-57.

16   Mowbray (R.M.): Rating scales for depression. In: Davies (B.M.), Carroll (B.J.), Mowbray (R.M.) Eds: "Depressive illness. Some research studies". Springfield: Thomas, 1972.

17   Prusoff (B.A.), Klerman (G.L.), Paykel (E.S.): Concordance between clinical assessments and patients' self-report in depression. *Archives of General Psychiatry*, 1972, 26, 546-552.

18   Smouse (P.E.), Feinberg (M.), Carroll (B.J.), Park (M.H.), Rawson (S.G.): The Carroll rating scale for depression. II: Factor analyses of the feature profiles. *British Journal of Psychiatry*, 1981, 138, 201-204.

19   Spitzer (R.L.), Endicott (J.), Robins (E.): Research diagnostic criteria (RDC) for a selected group of functional disorders. 3rd ed. New York State Psychiatric Institute, 1977.

20   Van Der Geer (J.P.): Introduction to multivariate analysis for the social sciences. San Francisco: Freeman, 1971.

21   Weissman (M.M.), Myers (J.K.): Rates and risks of depressive symptoms in a United States urban community. *Acta Psychiatrica Scandinavica*, 1978, 57, 219-231.

22   Zung (W.W.K.): A self-rating depression scale. *Archives of General Psychiatry*, 1965, 12, 63-70.

MELANCHOLIA RATING SCALE

SPECIFICITY

*

TYPE OF INSTRUMENT

Ordinal rating scale
11 items, 5 grades

REFERENCE   **Bech (P.), Rafaelsen (O.J.)** · – The Melancholia scale: Development, consistency, validity and utility. In: Sartorius (N.), Ban (T.): "Depression rating scales", 1982.

         Language: Original version in Danish. Translations in English, French, German, Spanish, Italian, Japanese.
                               Denmark

         Location: Enclosed in volume two page 108
                               See ref. biblio nº 1

         For all information concerning the instrument or translations write to the author at the following address:

         Per Bech,
         Psychochemistry Institute
         Rigshospitalet
         9, Blegdamsvej
         DK-2100 Copenhagen, Denmark

ORIGIN   Instrument constructed on the basis of the "Cronholm-Otteson Depression Scale" (ref. 3) and the six quantitative items of the Hamilton Depression Scale (ref. 5, 6).

PURPOSE   This instrument has been constructed with the purpose of quantifying the severity of depressive states, i.e. to identify the depressive patient and to measure the response to treatment with an antidepressant.

POPULATION   Patients of all ages presenting a depressive state.

ADMINISTRATION   *Rater:* Psychiatrist, psychologist or another skilled observer.

     Time required: 15-30 minutes.

     Training: Training in psychiatric interviewing.

     Scoring: Each item is scored from 0-4 on a scale of increasing intensity. The total score varies from 0, corresponding to total absence of the depressive syndrome, to 44, representing the most severe degree of this syndrome.

VARIABLES   Eleven variables are assessed:

- Activity (motor)
- Activity (verbal)
- Retardation (intellectual)
- Anxiety (psychic)
- Suicidal impulses
- Lowered mood
- Self-depreciation and guilt feeling
- Emotional retardation
- Sleep disturbances
- Tiredness and pain
- Work and interests

VALIDATION   They have included (ref. 2):
Concurrent validity with Hamilton Depression Scale, with the Hamilton Anxiety Scale, and the Newcastle Scales.
Inter-observer reliability, studies on internal consistency.
Correlation studies with plasma levels of antidepressant, age, and sex.
Establishment of **norms** for clinical trials:
- Inclusion criteria: total score above or equal to 15
- Partial response to treatment: total score from 6 to 14
- Complete remission: total score from 0 to 5
- No response to treatment: total score above or equal to 15.

OTHER WORKS
cited by author   Simplified version of the scale with a scoring system of 2 grades: present-absent.
Mania scale the simultaneous use of which is recommended by the authors in bipolar patients.
Papers on the Newcastle scales.

APPLICATION   These tests are screening tests to indicate abnormalities (including visual and hearing defects).
Research: Clinical trials.

1 Bech (P.), Rafaelsen (O.J.): The melancholia scale: development, consistency, validity and utility. In: Sartorius (N.), Ban (T.): "Depression rating scales". 1982.

2 Carney (M.W.P.), Roth (M.), Garside (R.F.): The diagnosis of depressive syndromes and prediction of ECT response. *Brit. J. Psychiat.*, 1965, 111, 659-674.

3 Cronholm (B.), Ottosson (J.O.): Experimental studies of the therapeutic action of electroconvulsive therapy in endogenous depression. The role of the electrical stimulation and of the seizure studied by variation of stimulus and modification by lidocaine of seizure discharge. *Acta Psychiat. Neurol. Scand.*, 1960., Suppl. 145, 69-97.

4 Gurney (C.): Diagnostic scales for affective disorders. Proceedings of the Fifth World Conference of Psychiatry, Mexico City, 1971, 330.

5 Hamilton (M.): A rating scale for depression. *J. Neurol. Neurosurg. Psychiat.*, 1960, 23, 56-62.

6 Hamilton (M.): Development of a rating scale for primary depressive illness. *Brit. J. Soc. Clin. Psychol.*, 1967, 6, 278-296.

GERIATRIC DEPRESSION SCALE (G.D.S.)

SPECIFICITY

* * *

TYPE OF INSTRUMENT

Check-list 30 items

REFERENCE

Brink (T.L.), Yesavage (J.A.), Lum (O.), Heersema (P.H.), Adey (M.), Rose (T.L.) · – Screening tests for geriatric depression. *Clinical Gerontologist,* 1982, 1, 1, 37-43.

Yesavage (J.A.), Brink (T.L.), Rose (T.L.), Lum (O.), Huang (V.), Adey (M.), Leirer (O.) · – Development and validation of a geriatric depression screening scale: A Preliminary report. *Journal of Psychiatric Research,* 1983, 17, 1, 37-49.

Language: Original version published in English. Translations in French, Spanish and German.
U.S.A.

Location: Enclosed in volume two page 80
See ref. biblio n° 2

For all information concerning the instrument or translations, write to the author at the following addresses:

Jerome Yesavage,
Dpt of Psychiatry and Behavioral Sciences,
Stanford University Medical Center
Stanford, California, 94305 U.S.A.

T.L. Brink,
1044 Sylvan,
San Carlos, California 94070
U.S.A.

ORIGIN
One hundred questions were first selected by a team of clinicians and investigators working in the field of psychogeriatrics to characterise aged depressed people. Then a study took place with two populations composed of elderly people affected by depression or healthy, 30 questions out of the initial 100, correlating highest with the total score, were retained.

PURPOSE
The instrument is designed to detect depression in aged subjects being sensitive to their specific complaints.

POPULATION
Aged depressed population.

ADMINISTRATION
Rater: Self-administration
Time required: 5 minutes.
Training: Brief.
Scoring: Each question requires an answer of the yes-no type, assessed 1 or 0. The total score varies from 0-30.

VARIABLES
Depression only.

VALIDATION
Carried out with 3 groups of geriatric patients: normal and those undergoing anti-depressant treatment, classified according to "Research Diagnostic Criteria" (R.D.C.) as depressed, affected by a moderate or severe syndrome, covering:
Concurrent validity with the self-evaluation scale by Zung and the depression scale by Hamilton (ref. 8, 9, 20).
Discriminative sensitivity among normal, moderately and severely depressed persons, assessed according to the "Research Diagnostic Criteria" (ref. 18) among depressed dements, or non-dements according to assessment by clinician; among patients with or without organic depression among alcoholics depressed or not, between before and after treatment.
Reliability: internal consistency between items and between each item and the global score. Split-half and test-retest at one week intervals.

OTHER WORKS
cited by author
Scaling in 3 groups: normal subjects, moderately depressed, very depressed.

APPLICATION
Screening, Contribution to diagnosis, Drug trials.

1 Brink (T.L.): Geriatric psychotherapy. New York: Human Sciences Press, 1979.

2 Brink (T.L.), Yesavage (J.A.), Lum (O.), Heersema (P.H.), Adey (M.), Rose (T.L.): Screening tests for geriatric depression. *Clinical Gerontologist*, 1982, 1, 1, 37-43.

3 Carroll (B.J.), Fielding (J.M.), Blashki (T.G.): Depression rating scales: a critical review. *Archives of General Psychiatry*, 1973, 28, 361-366.

4. Comfort (A.): The practice of geriatric psychiatry. New York: Elsevier, 1980.

5 Cutler (N.R.), Heiser (J.F.): The tricyclic antidepressants. *Journal of the American Medical Association*, 1978, 240, 2264-2266.

6 Fillenbaum (G.G.), Pfeiffer (E.): The mini-mult: a cautionary note. *Journal of Consulting and Clinical Psychology*, 1976, 44, 698-703.

7 Gurland (B.J.): The comparative frequency of depression in various adult age groups. *Journal of Gerontology*, 1976, 31, 283-292.

8 Hamilton (M.): A rating scale for depression. *Journal of Neurology, Neurosurgery and Psychiatry*, 1960, 23, 56-62.

9 Hamilton (M.): Development of a rating scale for primary depressive illness. *British Journal of Social and Clinical Psychology*, 1967, 6, 278-296.

10 Kline (N.S.): Treatment of depression. *Journal of the American Medical Association*, 1978, 240, 2287-2288.

11 Lesse (S.): Masked depression. New York: Aronson, 1974.

12 Liston (E.H.): Occult presenile dementia. *Journal of Nervous and Mental Disease*, 1977, 164, 263-267.

13 Miller (N.): Psychopathology in the aged. In: Cole (J.O.), Barrett (J.E.) Eds.: "Psychopathology in the aged". New York: Wiley, 1978, 120-121.

14 Myers (J.K.), Weissman (M.M.): Use of a self-report symptom scale to detect depression in a community sample. *American Journal of Psychiatry*, 1980, 137, 1081-1084.

15 Pfeiffer (E.): Drugs and the elderly. Los Angeles: University of Southern California, 1974.

16 Raft (D.), Spencer (R.F.), Toomey (T.), Brogan (D.): Depression in medical outpatients: the use of the Zung scale. *Diseases of the Nervous System*, 1977, 38, 999-1004.

17 Scott (J.), Gaitz (C.M.): Ethnic and age differences in mental measurements. *Diseases of the Nervous System*, 1975, 36, 389-393.

18 Spitzer (R.L.), Endicott (J.), Robins (E.): Research diagnostic criteria: rationale and reliability. *Archives of General Psychiatry*, 1978, 35, 773-782.

19 Von Praag (H.M.): Psychotropic drugs in the aged. *Comprehensive Psychiatry*, 1977, 18, 429-443.

20 Zung (W.W.K.): A self-rating depression scale. *Archives of General Psychiatry*, 1965, 12, 63-70.

21 Zung (W.W.K.): The measurement of depression. Columbus OH: Merrill, 1975.

COGNITIVE FUNCTIONS

Ib.1	Histoire du Lion	BARBIZET	1965
Ib.2	Visual Retention Test	BENTON	1965
Ib.3	Shaw Blocks Test	LESTER	1967
Ib.4	Memory Battery	BARBIZET	1968
Ib.5	Three-dimensional Constructive Praxis Test	BENTON	1968
Ib.6	Information-Memory-Concentration Test	BLESSED-ROTH	1968
Ib.7	Dementia Scale	BLESSED-ROTH	1968
Ib.8	Scale for the Measurement of Memory	WILLIAMS	1968
Ib.9	Praxies Grapho-Motrices	ANDREY	1969
Ib.10	Simple Non-Language Test of New Learning	FOWLER	1969
Ib.11	Short-Term Memory Test	DANA	1970
Ib.12	Screening Test for Organic Brain Disease	NAHOR	1970
Ib.13	Wechsler Adult Intelligence Scale	WECHSLER	1970
Ib.14	Geriatric Interpersonal Evaluation Scale	PLUTCHIK	1971
Ib.15	Embedded Figures Test	WITKIN	1971
Ib.16	Mental Test Score	HODKINSON	1972
Ib.17	Set Test	ISAACS	1972
Ib.18	Simple Methods of Testing Ability	SILVER	1972
Ib.19	Dementia Screening Scale	HASEGAWA	1974
Ib.20	Echelle de Développement de la Pensée Logique	LONGEOT	1974
Ib.21	Abbreviated Mental Test	QURESHI	1974
Ib.22	Mini Mental State	FOLSTEIN	1975
Ib.23	Ischemia Score	HACHINSKI	1975
Ib.24	Short Portable Mental Status Questionnaire	PFEIFFER	1975
Ib.25	Batterie de Vigilance en Institution	ISRAEL	1976
Ib.26	Philadelphia Geriatric Center Mental Status Questionnaire	FISHBACK	1977
Ib.27	Cognitive Capacity Screening Examination	JACOBS	1977
Ib.28	Confusion Assessment Schedule	SLATER	1977
Ib.29	Modified Tooting Bec Questionnaire	DENHAM	1978
Ib.30	Echelle d'Efficience Intellectuelle	JANIN	1978
Ib.31	Stimulus Recognition Test	BRINK	1979
Ib.32	Misplaced Objects Task	CROOK	1979
Ib.33	Extended Scale for Dementia	HERSCH	1979
Ib.34	Kendrick Battery for the Detection of Dementia in the Elderly	KENDRICK	1979
Ib.35	Galveston Orientation and Amnesia Test	LEVIN	1979
Ib.36	Check-list Differentiating Pseudo-dementia from Dementia	WELLS	1979
Ib.37	Orientation Scale for Geriatric Patients	BERG	1980
Ib.38	Hierarchic Dementia Scale	COLE	1980
Ib.39	Batterie de Vigilance en Ambulatoire	ISRAEL	1980
Ib.40	Echelle Clinique d'Aptitudes Intellectuelles	ISRAEL	1980
Ib.41.	Batterie de Fluidité à l'usage des Généralistes	ISRAEL	1980
Ib.42	Batterie de Mémoire en Ambulatoire	ISRAEL	1980
Ib.43	Examen Psychologique pour Personnes Agées Hospitalisées	ISRAEL	1980
Ib.44	Guild Memory Test	GILBERT	1981
Ib.45	Shopping List Task	MAC CARTHY	1981
Ib.46	Memory Activity Scale	SIGNORET	1982
Ib.47	Bilan d'Evaluation du Syndrome Démentiel	ISRAEL	1982

HISTOIRE DU LION
LION'S STORY

SPECIFICITY

* *

TYPE OF INSTRUMENT

Psychometric test
22 items

REFERENCE	**Barbizet (J.), Truscelli (D.)** · – L'histoire du Lion: considérations sur la fabulation. *La Semaine des Hôpitaux,* 1965, n° 28, 1688-1694.

Language: Original version in French.
France

Location: Enclosed in volume two page 5
See ref. biblio n° 4

ORIGIN — Modification of test by **Lesage.**

PURPOSE — Memory test designed to detect confabulation as well as memory impairment.

POPULATION — All adults.

ADMINISTRATION — *Rater:* Psychologist or physician.

Time required: Three minutes.

Training: Clinical training desirable.

DESCRIPTION — The test is a story told to the person tested, consisting of 22 items of information which are to be recalled immediately, after one hour, after a day and one week later. Interviewer scores omissions by aid of a grid and notes errors and confabulation distorting the sense of the story.

Scoring: One point per item recalled correctly.

VARIABLES — The following activities are assessed:
· Immediate memory
· Ability to synthesize
· Recall
· Delayed memory
· Attention
· Language

VALIDATION — This test has provided the basis for work to be carried out allowing differentiation of clinical categories (chronic ethyl alcohol intoxication, cortical trauma, dementia, cerebral tumours, vascular deficiencies). Qualitative scoring of replies to this test allows confabulation mechanisms to be discriminated in addition to the main memory contents.

OTHER WORKS cited by author — Standardization was done on elderly out-patients using an abbreviated form of the story (20 items) (ref. 4).

APPLICATION — **Clinical:** Diagnosis, prognosis.
Research: Drug trials, if the test is administered in a battery of memory tests.
Neuro-psychological research on memory.

1 Barbizet (J.): Etudes sur la mémoire: première série. Paris: L'Expansion Scientifique Française, 1964.

2 Barbizet (J.): Etudes sur la mémoire: deuxième série. Paris: L'Expansion Scientifique Française, 1966.

3 Barbizet (J.), Grison (B.).: Etude des fonctions supérieures. *Concours Médical*, 17 janvier 1970, n°. 3.

4 Barbizet (J.), Truscelli (D.): L'histoire du Lion (considérations sur la fabulation). *La Semaine des Hôpitaux*, 1965, n°. 28, 1688-1694.

5 Delay (J.): Les maladies de la mémoire. Paris: Presses Universitaires de France, 1949.

6 Dupré (E.): Traité de l'imagination et de l'émotivité. Paris: Payot, 1925.

7 Hunter (M.L.): Memory. Harmondsworth, Middlesex: Penguin Books, 1964, 144-153.

VISUAL RETENTION TEST

SPECIFICITY

* *

TYPE OF INSTRUMENT

Non verbal
psychometric test
10 items

REFERENCE	**Benton (A.L.)** · – Manuel pour l'application du test de rétention visuelle. Applications cliniques et expérimentales. 2ème édition francaise. – Paris: Centre de Psychologie Appliquée, 1965.

Language: Original version published in English. Translated into French and other languages.
U.S.A.

Location: Enclosed in volume two page 6
See ref. biblio n° 3

For all information concerning the instrument write to the publisher at the following address:

Editions du Centre de Psychologie Appliquée
48, avenue Victor Hugo
75783 Paris Cedex 16, France

ORIGIN
This instrument is a revised version of the original **Benton** test (ref. 1 and 2) revealing critical reflections of the author on the work of **Jacobs** (ref. 4) and **Thurstone** (ref. 8) pertaining to memory.

PURPOSE
The Revised Visual Retention Test was developed to help distinguish between patients with and without organic cerebral injuries.

POPULATION
All persons capable of understanding instructions.

ADMINISTRATION
Rater: Psychologist.
Time required: 5 minutes.
Training: Knowledge of the test necessary.

DESCRIPTION
The test consists of three parallel forms. Each one comprises ten drawings of one or more shapes. There are four methods of administration A, B, C and D:
A. The drawing is exhibited for ten seconds to the patient who reproduces it immediately from memory.
B. The drawing is shown for five seconds to the patient who then reproduces it immediately.
C. The patient copies the drawings.
D. The drawing is exhibited to the patient for ten seconds and he reproduces it from memory after a delay of fifteen seconds.
There is another oral procedure by multiple choice, designed for patients with physical handicaps, but this procedure does not allow qualitative analysis of the results.
Scoring: **quantitative** a score given for successful test, from 0 to 10.
     qualitative detailed analysis of the type of error is carried out, with 6 categories scored: omission and addition - distortion - perseveration - rotation - displacement - size error.

VARIABLES
The test involves two types of mental activities:
 · Visuo-spatial ability
 · Immediate or delayed visual memory.

VALIDATION
Validity and accuracy of the instrument have been studied (ref. 3).
Standardization was carried out with children and adults (age 15 to 64) for administration "A" (ref. 3).
Norms for persons above the age of 65 have been compiled by Poitrenaud in 1972, (ref. 6).

OTHER WORKS
cited by author
Reference is made to the "Science Citation Index" for studies using the Visual Retention Test.

APPLICATION
Clinical: This instrument used in diagnostic work enables detection of patients suffering from organic cerebral injuries.
Research: Studies of normal deterioration due to aging or in connection with pathological disturbance.

1 Benton (A.L.): a visual retention test for clinical use. *Archives of Neurology and Psychiatry,* 1945, 54, 212-216.

2 Benton (A.L.): Manuel pour l'application du test de rétention visuelle. 1ᵉ édition française. Paris: Centre de Psychologie Appliquée, 1960.

3 Benton (A.L.): Manuel pour l'application du test de rétention visuelle. Applications cliniques et expérimentales. 2ᵉ édition française. Paris: Centre de Psychologie Appliquée, 1965.

4 Jacobs (J.): Experiments on "prehension". *Mind,* 1887, 12, 75-79.

5 Poitrenaud (J.): La "mesure" des déficits intellectuels pathologiques chez le sujet âgé. *Gazette Médicale de France,* 1968, 75, 3371-3396.

6 Poitrenaud (J.), Barrère (H.): Etude sur la signification diagnostique de certaines erreurs de reproduction au V.R.T. de Benton. *Revue de Psychologie Appliquée,* 1ᵉ trim. 1972, vol. 22, n°. 1, 43-56.

7 Poitrenaud (J.), Clément (F.): La détérioration physiologique dans le test de rétention visuelle de Benton: résultats obtenus par 500 sujets normaux. *Psychol. Franç.,* 1965, 10, 359-368.

8 Thurstone (L.L.): Primary mental abilities. Psychometric monograph, n° 1. Chicago: University of Chicago Press, 1938.

SHAW BLOCKS TEST

SPECIFICITY

*

TYPE OF INSTRUMENT

Non verbal psychometric test

REFERENCE	**Lester (D.)** · – The Shaw Blocks Test: A description. *Journal of Clinical Psychology,* 1967, Vol. XXIII, nº 1, 88-89.
	Language: Original version published in English. **U.S.A.**
	Location: Enclosed in volume two page 8 See ref. biblio nº 8

For all information concerning the instrument write to the author at the following address:

David Lester,
Dpt of Psychology
New Jersey
Stockton State College
Pomona, New Jersey 08240, U.S.A.

ORIGIN

The instrument was inspired by several previous studies, notably those of **Bromley** (ref. 1, 2), **Heim** (ref. 3, 4), **Howson** (ref. 5).

PURPOSE

A non verbal test conceived with the goal of evaluating intelligence in a manner which does not penalize original or creative responses.

POPULATION

Children, adults of all ages.

ADMINISTRATION

Rater: A person with experience of psychological testing.

Time required: 10 to 30 minutes depending upon the subject.

Training: The use of the test requires several hours of practice.

DESCRIPTION

The subject is seated and given four cylindrical blocks with different weights, heights and lengths. Each block has a circular hole and a rectangular notch cut out which differ in size. Each block has the name of an animal printed on it (with the print differing in size) and a letter of the alphabet. The subject has to arrange the blocks in logical sequences based upon any attribute of the blocks. The subject is asked to devise as many sequences as possible in 12 minutes, and to give the logical basis for each sequence.

The evaluation of the performance takes account of the degree of originality of the logical basis for the sequence and the objectivity of the basis. The scoring system is indicated by the author in the articles cited.

VARIABLES

Intelligence, creativity, originality, rigidity.

VALIDATION

The test has been given to children, young adults (students) and the elderly.

Concurrent validity has been explored using the Miller Analogies Test (ref. 11), the California Test of Mental Maturity, the WAIS (ref. 10) and the Graduate Record Exam (ref. 7).

Reliability: split-half (ref. 7).

Norms established only for children aged 8 to 14 years of age.

APPLICATION

This test is on the whole an experimental instrument for the evaluation of intelligence, for clinical research and to supplement conventional tests of intelligence.

1 Bromley (D.B.): Notes on the Shaw Test. *Brit. J. Psychol.*, 1955, 46, 310-311.

2 Bromley (D.B.): Some experimental tests of the effect of age on creative intellectual output. *J. Geront.*, 1956, 11, 74-82.

3 Heim (A.W.), Lester (D.): Performance of children on the Shaw Blocks Test. *Perceptual and Motor Skills*, 1964, 19, 740.

4 Heim (A.W.), Watts (K.P.): Further study of children's Shaw Blocks Test performance. *Perceptual and Motor Skills*, 1965, 21, 80.

5 Howson (J.D.): Intellectual impairment associated with brain – injured patients as revealed in the Shaw Test of abstract thought. *Canad. J. Psychol.*, 1948, 2, 123-133.

6 Lester (D.): The Lester point-score for the Shaw Blocks Test. Manuscript, 1965.

7 Lester (D.): Consistency, and validity of the Shaw Blocks Test: a preliminary study. *Perceptual and Motor Skills*, 1966, 22, 134.

8 Lester (D.): The Shaw Blocks Test: a description. *Journal of Clinical Psychology*, January 1967, vol. XXIII, n°. 1, 88-89.

9 Lester (D.): The Shaw Test: simultaneous measures of intelligence, originality, and rigidity. *Perceptual and Motor Skills*, 1967, 24, 1106.

10 Lester (D.), Bird (K.), Brown (K.), Massa (J.): Validity of Shaw Blocks Test. *Perceptual and Motor Skills*, 1973, 37, 442.

11 Miller Analogies Test. Revised Manual. New York: Psychological Corporation., 1960.

MEMORY BATTERY

SPECIFICITY

* *

TYPE OF INSTRUMENT

Psychometric test
6 sub-tests

REFERENCE	**Barbizet (J.), Cany (E.)** · – Clinical and psychometrical study of a patient with memory disturbances. *International Journal of Neurology,* 1968, 7, 44-54.
	Language: Original version published in English. **France**
	Location: Enclosed in volume two page 9 See ref. biblio nº 3

ORIGIN

This original test was developed by the author in association with tests adapted from the literature (ref. 5, 6, 7).

PURPOSE

This instrument is designed as a memory test, to be used as a part of assessments of intellectual function. More precisely, it differentiates problems in new learning and retention capability from memory difficulties due to a loss of previous learning.

POPULATION

Adults of all ages suffering from cerebral injuries.

ADMINISTRATION

Rater: Psychologist or speech therapist.

Time required: 25 minutes.

Training: Training in psychology necessary.

DESCRIPTION

This battery consists of five verbal tests and one performance test:
· Auditory-verbal: Digit Span (Weschler)
                            Lion Story (Barbizet)
                            Words (Rey)
                            Recognition (Rey)
· Visual-verbal: Objects of Kim
· Visuo-motor: Peg board

Scoring: Score is established from raw scores varying from one test to another. Norms are given in reference No 1.

VARIABLES

Four aspects of memory are measured:
· Immediate memory
· Recall
· Learning
· Retention

VALIDATION

Norms have been established for different populations (ref. 3).

APPLICATION

Clinical: This instrument may be used for establishing organicity and more particularly to separate objective from subjective troubles in head injuries. It allows distinction between memory disorders of cortical or hippocampal-mammillary origin from global amnesia.

1 Barbizet (J.): Etudes sur la mémoire: première série. Paris: L'Expansion Scientifique Française, 1964.

2 Barbizet (J.): Etudes sur la mémoire: deuxième série. Paris: L'Expansion Scientifique Française, 1966

3 Barbizet (J.), Cany (E.): Clinical and psychometrical study of a patient with memory disturbances. *International Journal of Neurology*, 1968, 7, 44-54.

4 Barbizet (J.), Truscelli (D.): L'histoire du Lion (consi-dérations sur la fabulation). *La Semaine des Hôpitaux*, 1965, n°. 28, 1688-1694.

5 Rey (A.): L'examen clinique en psychologie. Paris: P.U.F., 1958.

6 Rey (A.): Les troubles de la mémoire et leur examen psychométrique. Bruxelles: Dessart, 1966.

7 Wechsler (D.): A standardized memory scale for clinical use. *The Journal of Psychology*, 1945, 19, 87-95.

THREE-DIMENSIONAL CONSTRUCTIONAL PRAXIS TEST

SPECIFICITY

* *

TYPE OF INSTRUMENT

Non verbal test
3 sub-tests

REFERENCE	**Benton (A.L.)** · – Test de praxie constructive tridimensionnelle. Manuel. Paris: Centre de Psychologie Appliquée, 1968.

Language: Original version published in English. Translated into French.
U.S.A.

Location: See ref. biblio n° 5

For all information concerning the instrument write to the publisher at the following address:

Editions du Centre de Psychologie Appliquée
48, avenue Victor Hugo
75783 Paris Cedex 16, France

ORIGIN
The instrument is a revised version of the **Benton** and **Fogel** (ref. 7) clinical test of three-dimensional constructional praxis which itself was a revised and standardized form of the original **Critchley** (ref. 8) test.

PURPOSE
This test was designed to evaluate three-dimensional constructional capability in patients, especially in neurological clinics.

POPULATION
Adult, young and aged in and out-patients.

ADMINISTRATION
Rater: Psychologist.
Time required: 5 minutes per sub-test.
Training: Knowledge of the test.
Scoring: There are 3 systems of scoring. In the standard scoring system, number and type of errors observed in the 3 sub-tests (omissions, additions, substitutions, displacement) are taken into account together with the time taken.
The second scoring system differs in the level of emphasis on errors of displacement.
In the third system a total of points is given to the patient, corresponding to the number of correctly placed blocks in all three sub-tests.

DESCRIPTION
Test material consists of three wooden model structures which are presented to the patient one by one. The patient is asked to construct an exact replica by selecting appropriate blocks from among the set of blocks presented on a plate. The three models are the following:
Sub-test   I : a pyramid with 6 cubes size 2.5 cm
Sub-test II : a structure of 8 blocks in 4 levels
Sub-test III : a structure of 15 blocks in 4 levels
A parallel form proposed by Benton (ref. 6) exists in which the proposed stimuli are actual size photographs of model-structures, described above.

VARIABLES
Three-dimensional constructional ability, visuo-spatial ability.

VALIDATION
Was carried out on three groups of patients (patients without cerebral pathology, patients suffering from injuries of the left or right hemisphere) and involved the following (ref. 5):
Inter-rater reliability and concordance of parallel forms.
Norms for distribution of scores have been given for adults aged from 16 to 60, normal or suffering from cerebral injuries.

OTHER WORKS
cited by author
Science Citation Index.

APPLICATION
Instrument for clinical use and research allowing detection of deterioration in three-dimensional constructional ability which may be considered as an indication of organic cerebral pathology.

Ib.5

1 Ajuriaguerra (J. de), Zazzo (R.), Granjon (N.): Le phénomène d'accolement (closing-in) dans un syndrome d'apraxie oxycarbonée. *Encéphale*, 1949, 38, 1-20.

2 Arrigoni (G.), De Renzi (E.): Constructional apraxia and hemispheric locus of lesion. *Cortex*, 1964, 1, 170-197.

3 Benton (A.L.): Test de rétention visuelle. Paris: Centre de Psychologie Appliquée, 1965.

4 Benton (A.L.): Differential behavioral effects in frontal lobe disease. *Neuropsychologia*, 1968, 6.

5 Benton (A.L.): Test de praxie constructive tri-dimensionnelle: manuel. Paris: Centre de Psychologie Appliquée, 1968.

6 Benton (A.L.): Test de praxie constructive tridimensionnelle: forme pour alternative la clinique et la recherche. *Revue de Psychologie Appliquée*, ler trim. 1973, vol. 23, n°. 1, 1-5.

7 Benton (A.L.), Fogel (M.L.); Three-dimensional constructional praxis: a clinical test. *Arch. Neurol.*, 1962, 7, 347-354.

8 Critchley (M.): The Parietal lobes. London: Arnold, 1953.

9 Domrath (R.P.): Constructional praxis and visual perception in young school children. Ph. D. Thesis, Univ. Iowa, 1965.

10 Fogel (M.L.): The Intelligence quotient as an index of brain damage. *Amer. J. Orthopsychiat.*, 1964, 34, 555-562.

11 Hecaen (H.), Ajuriaguerra (J. de), Massonet (J.): Les troubles visuo-constructifs par lésion pariéto-occipitale droite. *Encéphale*, 1951, 40, 122-179.

12 Hecaen (H.), Penfield (W.), Bertrand (C.), Malmo (R.): The syndrome of apractognosia due to lesions of the minor cerebral hemisphere. *Arch. Neurol. Psychiat.*, 1956, 75, 400-434.

13 Mc Fie (J.), Piercy (M.F.), Zangwill (O.L.): Visual spatial agnosia associated with lesions of the right hemisphere. *Brain*, 1950, 73, 167-190.

14 Paterson (A.), Zangwill (O.L.): Disorders of visual space perception associated with lesions of the right hemisphere. *Brain*, 1944, 67, 331-358.

15 Rey (A.): L'examen psychologique dans les cas d'encéphalopathie traumatique. *Arch. Psychol.*, 1941, 28, 215-285.

INFORMATION-MEMORY-CONCENTRATION TEST (I.M.C.T.)

SPECIFICITY

* * *

TYPE OF INSTRUMENT

Psychometric test

REFERENCE	**Blessed (G.), Tomlinson (B.E.), Roth (M.)** · – The association between quantitative measures of dementia and of senile change in the cerebral grey matter of elderly subjects. *British Journal of Psychiatry,* 1968, 114, 797-811.

Language: Original version in English.
Great Britain

Location: Enclosed in volume two page 11
See ref. biblio nº 2

For all information concerning the instrument write to the author at the following address:

Martin Roth,
Department of Psychiatry
University of Cambridge Clinical School
Addenbrooke's Hospital, Hills Road
Cambridge CB2 2QQ, Great Britain

ORIGIN
This instrument was inspired by other works of the same author (ref. 3, 8).

PURPOSE
This test was devised as a dual purpose instrument for clinical experimental use with populations suffering from severe dementia and with normals.

POPULATION
All aged persons, regardless of mental state.

ADMINISTRATION
Rater: Physician, psychologist, nurse or a social worker.
Time required: 25 to 30 minutes.
Training: Necessary for nurses and social workers.

DESCRIPTION
The test consists of 27 questions or verbal trials.
Scoring: The total score varies from 0 to 37.

VARIABLES
Orientation, secondary memory, concentration, performance.

VALIDATION
Studies carried out on patients in psychogeriatric wards have included testing **concurrent validity** with the Roth and Hopkins (ref. 8) dementia scale.

OTHER WORKS
cited by author
Different unpublished works dealing with research into correlation between neurobiological findings and mental disorders.

APPLICATION
Clinical: Differential diagnosis between functional and organic forms of mental disorders in the aged.
Research: Correlation between mental functioning and post-mortem neuropathological and neuro-chemical findings.

1 Arab (A.): Plaques séniles et artériosclérose céré-brale; absence de rapports de dépendance entre les deux processus; étude statistique. *Rev. Neurol.*, 1954, 91, 22.

2 Blessed (G.), Tomlinson (B.E.), Roth (M.): The Association between quantitative measures of dementia and of senile change in the cerebral grey matter of elderly subjects. *Brit. J. of Psychiatry*, 1968, 114, 797-811.

3 Hopkins (B.), Roth (M.): Psychological test performance in patients over sixty. II: Paraphrenia, arteriosclerotic psychosis and acute confusion. *J. Ment. Sci.*, 1953, 99, 451.

4 Kay (D.W.K.), Beamish (P.), Roth (M.): Old age mental disorder in Newcastle – upon – Tyne. I: A study of prevalence. *Brit. J. Psychiat.*, 1964, 110, 146.

5 Kay (D.W.K.), Roth (M.): Physical accompaniments of mental disorder in old age. *Lancet*, 1955, ii, 740.

6 Newton (R.D.): Identity of Alzheimer's disease and senile dementia and their relation to senility. *J. Ment. Sci.*, 1948, 94, 225.

7. Roth (M.): The natural history of mental disorders in old age. *J. Ment. Sci.*, 1955, 101, 281.

8 Roth (M.), Hopkins (B.): Psychological test performance in patients over sixty. I: Senile psychosis and the affective disorders of old age. *J. Ment. Sci.*, 1953, 99, 439.

9 Roth (M.), Morrissey (J.D.): Problems in the diagnosis and classification of mental disorder in old age. *J. Ment. Sci.*, 1952, 98, 66.

10 Shapiro (M.B.), Post (F.), Löfving (B.), Inglis (J.): "Memory function" in psychiatric patients over sixty; some methodological and diagnostic implications. *J. Ment. Sci.*, 1956, 102, 233.

11 Sjgören (H.), Sourander (P.), Svennerholm (L.): Clinical, histological and chemical studies on presenile and senile neuropsychiatric diseases. Proceedings of fifth Internat.Congress Neuropathology, Zurich, September 1965. Excerpta Medica Internat. Congr. Series, n°. 100, 555.

12 Wolf (A.): Clinical neuropathology in relation to the process of aging. In: Birren (J.E.) Ed.: "The process of aging in the nervous system". Springfield, Illinois, 1959.

DEMENTIA SCALE

SPECIFICITY

* * *

TYPE OF INSTRUMENT

Scale of 22 items
with 4 grades

REFERENCE	**Blessed (G.), Tomlinson (B.E.), Roth (M.)** · – The association between quantitative measures of dementia and of senile change in the cerebral grey matter of elderly subjects. *British Journal of Psychiatry,* 1968, 114, 797-811.

Language: Original version published in English.
Great Britain

Location: Enclosed in volume two page 110
(Reference is made to bibliography from the preceeding Ib.6.)

For all information concerning the instrument write to the author at the following address:

Martin Roth,
Department of Psychiatry
University of Cambridge Clinical School
Addenbrooke's Hospital, Hills Road
Cambridge CB2 2QQ, Great Britain

ORIGIN

This instrument was derived from other work by the same author (ref. 8).

PURPOSE

This scale was devised both for clinical and experimental purposes in order to make up for the deficiencies in available measures and be suitable for assessment of unimpaired individuals in addition to persons suffering from severe dementia.

POPULATION

Populations of all ages regardless of the state of their mental health, preferably hospitalized.

ADMINISTRATION

Rater: Physician, psychologist or nurse.

Time required: 35 to 40 minutes.

Training: Necessary.

Scoring: Maximum score is 28 points.

VARIABLES

Competence for activities of everyday life.

VALIDATION

Validity studies were carried out on a population of patients hospitalized in psychogeriatric wards and in general hospitals (ref. 2).
Validity: Studies of correlation with radiological measures of cerebral atrophy detected by scanner.
Test-retest and inter-rater reliability.

OTHER WORKS
cited by author

Different unpublished works looking at the correlation between neurobiological findings and mental disorders.

APPLICATION

Clinical: Differential diagnosis between functional and organic forms of mental disorders in the aged.
Research: Correlation between mental functioning and quantitative measures of post-mortem neuropathological and neurochemical findings.

SCALE FOR THE MEASUREMENT OF MEMORY

SPECIFICITY

```
* *
```

TYPE OF INSTRUMENT

Psychometric test
5 sub-tests

REFERENCE Williams (M.) · – The measurement of memory in clinical practice. *British Journal of Social and Clinical Psychology,* 1968, 7, 19-34.

Language: Published in English.
Great Britain

Location: Enclosed in volume two page 12
See ref. biblio nº 15

For all information concerning forms B and C of the instrument write to the author at the following address:

Moyra Williams,
Fulbown and Addenbrooke's Hospital
Cambridge CB2 2QQ, Great Britain

ORIGIN This battery of test was inspired by critical analyses of numerous authors on the measurement of memory and its relation to organic pathology (ref. 2, 4, 7, 9, 10, 11, 12, 16, 19). This battery comprises original tests as well as tests adapted from **Wechsler** (ref. 10), **Rey-Davis** (ref. 17) and **Walton** (ref. 8).

PURPOSE The test was developed to measure memory capacities of subjects in four dimensions and to study differential sensitivity of these dimensions to numerous variables such as age and organic cerebral pathology, in order to allow staff to reach a more precise diagnosis of the nature and origin of memory disorders in adults.

POPULATION Young and aged adults, in or out-patients.

ADMINISTRATION *Rater:* Psychologist, physician.

Time required: About 10 minutes.

Training: Knowledge of the test.

Scoring: One point per item. A score is calculated for each test. Comparison of test results allows diagnosis to be made, differentiating between organic and functional forms of memory disorders.

DESCRIPTION The test consists of five sub-tests:
1. Memory for numbers (digit span forward and backward)
2. Rey-Davis non-verbal learning
3. Meanings (8 words)
4. Delayed recall and recognition of 9 figures.
   Recognition test is carried out in case of partial or total failure with the test of delayed recall.
5. Memory for past events in personal life.
The test contains three parallel forms A, B and C.

VARIABLES The battery measures the following aspects of memory:
1. Immediate memory   4. Delayed recall
2. Non verbal learning   5. Long term memory
3. Verbal learning

VALIDATION Equivalence of A, B and C forms as well as differential sensitivity of sub-tests have been verified. Norms are supplied (ref. 15).

APPLICATION This test is intended for clinical use, permitting the assessment of four memory functions and enabling differential diagnosis between memory disorders of functional and organic origin.

Ib.8

1 Bartlett (F.C.): Remembering. London: Cambridge University Press, 1932.

2 Eysenck (H.J.), Halstead (H.): The memory function: a factorial analysis. *Am. J. Psychiat.*, 1945, 102, 2.

3 Ingham (J.G.): Memory and intelligence. *Br. J. Psychol.*, 1952, 43, 20.

4 Milner (B.): The memory defect in bilateral hippocampal lesions. *Psychiat. Res. Rep.*, 1959, II.

5 Rey (A.): L'examen psychologique dans les cas d'encéphalopathie traumatique. *Arch. Psychol.*, 1941, 28, 215-285.

6 Ribot (T.): Diseases of memory. London: Kegan Paul, 1885.

7 Talland (G.A.): Deranged memory: psychonomic study of the amnesia syndrome. New York: Academic Press, 1965.

8 Walton (D.) et al.: The modified word-learning test. *Brit. J. Med. Psychol.*, 1959, 32, 213.

9 Wechsler (D.): The measurement of adult intelligence. Baltimore: Williams and Wilkins, 1939.

10 Wechsler (D.): A standardized memory scale for clinical use. *J. Psychol.*, 1945, 19, 87.

11 Wells (F.L.), Martin (H.A.A.): A method of memory examination. *Am. J. Psychiat.*, 1923, 3, 243.

12 Westropp (C.), Williams (M.): Health and happiness in old age. London: Methuen and Co, 1960.

13 Williams (M.): Memory defects associated with cerebral lesions. D. Phil. thesis. Oxford, 1954.

14 Williams (M.): The measurement of mental performance in older people. (Published by Nuffield Foundation and obtainable from the author).

15 Williams (M.): The measurement of memory in clinical practice. *Brit. J. Soc. Clin. Psychol.*, 1968, 7, 19-34.

16 Zangwill (O.L.): Clinical tests of memory impairment. *Proc. R. Soc. Med.*, 1943, 36, 576.

17 Zangwill (O.L.): Some clinical applications of the Rey-Davis performance test. *J. Ment. Sci.*, 1946, 92, 19.

18 Zangwill (O.L.): Amnesia and the generic image. *Q. J. Exp. Psychol.*, 1950, 2, 7.

19 Zwerling (I.), Titchener (J.), Gottschalk (L.), Levine (M.), Culbertson (W.), Cohen (S.F.), Silver (H.): Emotions and surgical illness. *Am. J. Psychiat.*, 1955, 112, 270.

PRAXIES GRAPHO-MOTRICES
GRAPHO-MOTOR PRAXIS

SPECIFICITY

* *

TYPE OF INSTRUMENT

Non verbal
psychometric test
17 items

REFERENCE	Andrey (B.) · – Les praxies grapho-motrices. *Bulletin de Psychologie Scolaire,* 1969, 111-131.

Language: Original version published in French
France

Location: Enclosed in volume two page 14
See ref. biblio n° 1

For all information concerning the instrument write to the author or the publisher at the following addresses:

Bernard Andrey   Imprimerie du Néron,
2, rue Très Cloîtres   Avenue Grugliasco
38000 Grenoble, France   38130 Echirolles, France

ORIGIN

The instrument was inspired by works of **Bender** (ref. 2) from a developmental perspective and from the "Gestalt" theory.

PURPOSE

This instrument is designed for clinical use and is intended to study stages and modalities in graphic presentation of space in normal and mentally retarded children.

POPULATION

Children older than three, and all adults.

ADMINISTRATION

Rater: Psychologist.

Time required: Time available - 15 to 30 minutes.

Training: Not needed.

Scoring: From statistical tables and sample drawings. Qualitative scoring determines the stage of disintegration through analysis of different phenomena: inclusions, additions, orthogonal structure, superimpositions, circular shapes.

DESCRIPTION

It consists copying geometric drawings of different forms representing two or three dimensional space. The subject is asked to reproduce these drawings from the model in front of him.

VARIABLES

Processes of visuo - motor integration. Two mental activities are involved:
· Perceptual mode or structural stage
· Operational mode

VALIDATION

Standardization was carried out on persons of 60 to 82 years of age.
Comparative tables of different stages and processes. Works have also been carried out with children aged 3, 3.5, 4, 5, 6, 7, 9 and 11. The standardization norms are available in the Department of Psychology, University of Grenoble.

OTHER WORKS
cited by author

Other studies have been carried out at the Geriatric and Gerontological Hospital Services in Grenoble (Service Hospitalier de Gériatrie et Gérontologie) for clinical use.

Numerous memory research studies have also been performed by postgraduate students in Psychopathology (ref. 3, 5, 6) at Grenoble University.

APPLICATION

Clinical: To detect possible deterioration in different types of cerebral disorders.
Research: Comparative studies of disorganisation in spatial representation in patients suffering from neurological injuries and healthy aged subjects.

1 Andrey (B.): Les praxies grapho-motrices. *Bull. Psychol. Scol.*, décembre 1969, n°. 6, 111, 131.

2 Bender (L.): A visual motor gestalt test and its clinical use. New York: American Orthopsychiatric Association, 1938.

3 Delassus (C.): Troubles spatiaux et atteinte fonctionnelle des hémisphères cérébraux. Mémoire non publié. Grenoble: Université des Sciences Sociales, 1966.

4 Le Men (G.): Les troubles spatiaux dans les lésions hémisphériques. Mémoire non publié. Grenoble: Université des Sciences Sociales, 1973.

5 Luirard (C.): Les praxies grapho-motrices chez les malades mentaux. Mémoire non publié. Grenoble: Université des Sciences Sociales, 1968.

6 Pelletier (C.): Etude comparative entre débiles endogènes et débiles exogènes au travers de praxies graphomotrices de B. Andrey. Mémoire non publié. Grenoble: Université des Sciences Sociales, 1973.

7 Piaget (J.), Inhelder (B.): La représentation de l'espace chez l'enfant. Paris: Presses Universitaires de France, 1948.

8 Vereecken (P.): Spatial development: constructive praxia from birth to the age of 7. Groningen: J.B. Wolters, 1961.

SIMPLE NON-LANGUAGE TEST OF NEW LEARNING

SPECIFICITY

* *

TYPE OF INSTRUMENT

Psychometric test
10 **non-verbal** items

REFERENCE	**Fowler (R.S.)** · − A simple non-language test of new learning. *Perceptual and Motor Skills,* 1969, 29, 895-901.

Language: Published in English.
             U.S.A.

Location: Enclosed in volume two page 15
             See ref. biblio n̲o̲ 7

For all information concerning the instrument write to the author at the following address:

Roy Fowler,
Department of Physical Medicine and Rehabilitation
University of Washington School of Medicine
Seattle, Washington, U.S.A.

ORIGIN   Non-verbal test inspired by paired associate learning from **Wechsler** (ref. 20).

PURPOSE   The test was developed to evaluate learning ability.

POPULATION   All in and out-patients.

ADMINISTRATION   *Rater:* Physician, psychologist.
                 Time required: 20 minutes.
                 Training: Knowledge of the test.

DESCRIPTION   At first presentation, subject is presented with ten pairs of images: six pairs are of objects frequently associated, such as pipe and matches or fork and knife, and four pairs of objects not logically associated, such as pliers and a sugar cube or cigar and red rubber ball.
                 At second presentation, one image of the pair is hidden. The subject is invited to find it on the basis of its associated image.
                 The test is repeated twice. Order of presentation and recall may vary but are standardized.
                 Scoring: The score corresponds to the number of correctly produced pairs.

VARIABLES   Short-term recognition and learning.

VALIDATION   Carried out on healthy volunteer subjects divided into age groups it has included:
                 Concurrent validity with paired associates of Wechsler (ref. 7).
                 Standardization was carried out and may be found in the reference quoted.

APPLICATION   Non-verbal and experimental test for clinical use allows evaluation of recognition and learning capacities of subjects, especially among those suffering from cortical injuries or disturbances in verbal expression.

1 Caldwell (B.M.), Watson (R.I.): An evaluation of psychologic effects of sex hormone administration in aged women. 1: Results of therapy after six months. *J. Gerontol.*, 1952, 7, 228-244.

2 Caldwell (B.M.), Watson (R.I.): An evaluation of sex hormone replacement in aged women. *J. Genet. Psychol.*, 1954, 85, 181-200.

3 Cohen (J.): Wechsler memory scale performance of psychoneurotic, organic, and shizophrenic groups. *J. Consult. Psychol.*, 1950, 14, 371-375.

4 Fordyce (W.): Psychological assessment and management. In: Krusen (F.), Kottke (F.), Ellwood (P.) Eds.: "Handbook of physical medicine and rehabilitation". Philadelphia: Saunders, 1965, 137-164.

5 Fordyce (W.): Psychology and rehabilitation. In: Licht (S.) Ed.: "Rehabilitation and medicine". New Haven: Elizabeth Licht, 1968, 129-151.

6 Fordyce (W.), Jones (R.): The efficacy of oral and pantomime instructions for hemiplegic patients. *Arch. Phys. Med. and Rehab.*, 1966, 47, 676-680.

7 Fowler (R.S.): A simple non-language test of new learning. *Perceptual and Motor Skills*, 1969, 29, 895-901.

8 Howard (A.): Diagnostic value of the Wechsler memory scale with selected groups of institutionalized patients. *J. Consult. Psychol.*, 1950, 14, 376-380.

9 Klebanoff (S.G.): Psychological changes in organic brain lesions and ablations. *Psychol. Bull.*, 1945, 42, 585-623.

10 Meyer (V.): Psychological effects of brain damage. In: Eysenck (H) Ed.: "Handbook of abnormal psychology". New York: Basic Books, 1961, 529-565.

11 Rapaport (D.), Gill (M.M.), Schafer (R.): Diagnostic psychological testing. Chicago: Year Book Publ., 1945, vol. 1.

12 Reitan (R.): Certain differential effects of left and right cerebral lesions in human adults. *J. Comp. Physiol. Psychol.*, 1955, 48, 474-477.

13 Riklan (M.), Levita (E.): Laterality of subcortical involvement and psychological functions. *Psychol. Bull.*, 1965, 64, 217-224.

14 Shipley (W.C.): A self-administering scale for measuring intellectual impairment and deterioration. *J. Psychol.*, 1940, 9, 371-377.

15 Sines (L.K.): Intelligence test correlates of Shipley-Hartford performance. *J. Clin. Psychol.*, 1958, 14, 399-404.

16 Sines (L.K.), Simmons (H.): The Shipley-Hartford scale and the Doppelt short form as estimators of WAIS IQ in a state hospital population. *J. Clin. Psychol.*, 1959, 15, 452-453.

17 Stone (C.), Girdner (J.), Albrecht (R.): An alternate form of the Wechsler memory scale. *J. Psychol.*, 1946, 22, 199-206.

18 Teuber (H.L.): Effects of brain wounds implicating right or left hemisphere in man. In: Mountcastle (V.) Ed.: "Interhemispheric relations and cerebral dominance". Baltimore: John Hopkins Press, 1962, 131-157.

19 Wechsler (D.): Retention defect in Korsakoff's psychosis. *Psychiat. Bull.*, 1917, 2, 403-451.

20 Wechsler (D.): A standardized memory scale for clinical use. *J. Psychol.*, 1945, 19, 87-95.

21 Williams (M.): Mental testing in clinical practice. Oxford: Pergamon, 1965.

SHORT TERM MEMORY TEST

SPECIFICITY

* * *

TYPE OF INSTRUMENT

Psychometric test
5 items

REFERENCE	**Dana (L.A.), White (L.), Merlis (S.)** · – A new approach to measuring short-term memory in geriatric subjects: a pilot study. *Psychological Reports,* 1970, 27, 8-10.
	Language: Published in English. **U.S.A.**
	Location: See ref. biblio n⁰ 2

ORIGIN

This original test follows upon a critical review of the existing instruments in this field, more particularly **Cameron** (ref. 1), **Gilbert** (ref. 3), **Kamin** (ref. 4), **Kriauciunas** (ref. 5), **Maxwell** (ref. 6), **Pelz** et al. (ref. 7), **Wechsler** (ref. 8).

PURPOSE

This instrument was developed to measure short-term memory in disabled aged persons.

POPULATION

Elderly inpatients suffering from psychiatric disorders or senile dementia.

ADMINISTRATION

Rater: Physician, psychologist, nursing staff.

Time required: 10 to 20 minutes.

Training: Knowledge of the test.

DESCRIPTION

The material consists of a three-dimensional doll's house divided into five parts, such as the bedroom the kitchen, etc., and with five dolls representing a traditional family.
The subject and the rater, alternately, place one doll into a room.
When one or more dolls have been placed, the house is hidden by a curtain. The subject then, after a delay of 10 seconds, recalls the persons placed (father, mother, son, etc.) and where the rooms were.

VARIABLES

Short-term recall.
Topographical memory.

VALIDATION

Test-retest reliability (ref. 2), was done on patients hospitalized in geriatric wards, suffering from psychiatric disorders.

APPLICATION

Clinical primarily.
This instrument enables measuring capacities for short-term recall in aged deteriorated patients.

1 Cameron (D.E.): Loss of memory. *Postgraduate Medicine*, 1966, 40, 202-209.

2 Dana (L.A.), White (L.), Merlis (S.): A new approach to measuring short-term memory in geriatric subjects: a pilot study. *Psychological Reports*, 1970, 27, 8-10.

3 Gilbert (J.G.), Levee (R.F.), Catalano (F.L.): A preliminary report on a new memory scale. *Perceptual and Motor Skills*, 1968, 27, 277-278.

4 Kamin (L.J.): Differential changes in mental abilities in old age. *Journal of Gerontology*, 1957, 12, 66-70.

5 Kriauciunas (R.): Short-term memory and age. *Journal of the American Geriatrics Society*, 1968, 16, 83-93.

6 Maxwell (A.E.): Trends in cognitive ability in the older age ranges. *Journal of Abnormal Psychology*, 1961, 63, 449-452.

7 Pelz (K.), Pike (F.), Ames (L.B.): A proposed battery of childhood tests for discriminating between different levels of intactness of function in elderly subjects. *Journal of Genetic Psychology*, 1962, 100, 23-40.

8 Wechsler (D.): A standardized memory scale for clinical use. *Journal of Psychology*, 1945, 19, 87-95.

SCREENING TEST FOR ORGANIC BRAIN DISEASE

SPECIFICITY

* *

TYPE OF INSTRUMENT

Non verbal
psychometric test
8 items

REFERENCE	**Nahor (A.), Benson (D.F.)** · – A screening test for organic brain disease in emergency psychiatric evaluation. *Behavioral Neuropsychiatry,* 1970, 2, 23-36.
	Language: Published in English. **U.S.A.**
	Location: Enclosed in volume two page 16 See ref. biblio n° 9

ORIGIN

This test is inspired by numerous works on association between grapho-motor activities and organic cerebral pathology (ref. 1, 2, 3, 4, 5, 6, 7, 8, 10, 11).

PURPOSE

This instrument was designed to detect organic cerebral disorders through psychiatric examination.

POPULATION

All ages, in or out-patients.

ADMINISTRATION

Rater: Physician, psychologist.

Time required: 10 minutes.

Training: Not necessary.

DESCRIPTION

The test consists of 8 items:
· With the first five, the subject is asked to reproduce a drawing: a flower, two simple and two complexe geometric forms.
· With the last three items, the subject is asked to draw a freehand circle, a cube and a clock indicating 5.20.

Scoring: Scoring is essentially qualitative. The rater himself estimates the quality of the drawings. Unimpaired individuals succeed in all the tests.

VARIABLES

Graphic ability as an indicator of organic brain disease.

VALIDATION

Was carried out on 4 groups of adult subjects: neurotics, psychotics, subjects with proven organic cerebral disorders and consultants in a psychiatric hospital service for behavioural disturbances. **Validity** and **discriminative sensitivity** (ref. 9) were tested.

APPLICATION

Clinical: The instrument is designed to detect organic cerebral disorders in hospitalized patients. Incorporated into a battery of tests, this instrument may contribute towards medical diagnosis distinguishing organic from functional disorders.

1 Arrigoni (G.), DeRenzi (E.): Constructional apraxia and hemispheric locus of lesion. *Cortex*, 1964, 1, 178-197.

2 Benton (A.L.): A visual retention test for clinical use. *Arch. Neurol. and Psych.*, 1945, 45, 212-216.

3 Critchley (M.): The parietal lobes. London: Arnold, 1953.

4 Goodenough (F.L.): The measurement of intelligence by drawing. New York: World Book Company, 1926.

5 Heimburger (R.F.), Reitan (R.M.): Easily administered written test for localizing brain lesions. *J. Neurosurg.*, 1961, 18, 301-312.

6 Kleist (K.): Der gung und der gegenwartige Stand der Apraxiaforschung. *Ergebn. Neurol. Psychiat.*, 1912, 1, 342-452.

7 Kleist (K.): Gehirnpathologie. Leipzig: Barth, 1934.

8 McFie (J.), Zangwill (O.L.): Visual constructive disabilities associated with lesions of the left cerebral hemisphere. *Brain*, 1960, 83, 243-260.

9 Nahor (A.), Benson (F.): A screening test for organic brain disease in emergency psychiatric evaluation. *Behavioral Neuropsychiatry*, 1970, vol. 2, n°. 1-2, 23-26.

10 Piercy (M.), Hecaen (H.), Ajuriaguerra (J.): Constructional apraxia associated with unilateral cerebral lesions - left and right cases compared. *Brain*, 1960, 83, 225-242.

11 Reitan (R.): The effects of brain lesions on adaptive abilities in human beings. Indiana University Medical Center, 1959.

WECHSLER ADULT INTELLIGENCE SCALE (W.A.I.S.)

SPECIFICITY

** * **

TYPE OF INSTRUMENT

Psychometric test
11 sub-tests

REFERENCE	**Wechsler (D.)** · − Echelle d'Intelligence de Wechsler pour Adultes: WAIS. 2e édition. Paris: Centre de Psychologie Appliquée, 1970.

Language: Original version in English. Translated into French, and several other languages.
U.S.A.

Location: Enclosed in volume two page 17
See ref. biblio nº 5

For all information concerning the instrument write to the editor at the following address:

Psychological Corporation
New-York 17
New-York, U.S.A.

ORIGIN
This test is a revision of the Wechsler-Bellevue Intelligence Scale (1939), (ref. 3).

PURPOSE
This test was developed to evaluate intellectual functioning in various fields and to assess mental deterioration.

POPULATION
Young and older adults capable of understanding the instructions.

ADMINISTRATION
Rater: Psychologist.
Time required: 1 hour to 1 hour 30 minutes.
Training: Knowledge of psychometric techniques adapted for aged persons.

DESCRIPTION
This scale comprises eleven sub-tests: six form a verbal scale, five others constitute a performance scale. All eleven sub-tests are included in the full scale.

Verbal sub-tests:
· Information, Comprehension
· Arithmetic
· Similarities
· Digit Span
· Vocabulary

Performance sub-tests:
· Digit Symbol
· Picture Completion
· Block Design
· Picture Arrangement
· Object Assembly

Two abridged forms of the WAIS have been developed, one by Britton in 1966, (ref. 1) designed to differentiate clinical categories and the other by Hafner in 1978 (ref. 2) designed for aged persons.

Scoring: Raw scores obtained on the Verbal Scale, Performance Scale and the Full scale may be transformed into standard scores. Conversion tables allow determination of the Intelligence Quotient for each particular scale. It is also possible to calculate deterioration index.

VARIABLES
Four factors saturate the test:
· Verbal comprehension
· Visuo-spatial ability
· Attention - concentration
· Logical thinking

VALIDATION
Reliability: split-half. **Standardization** (ref. 4, 5).

OTHER WORKS
cited by author
Official list figures in the "Science Citation Index".

APPLICATION
This instrument is intended for clinical and experimental use and may be used in diagnosis, prognosis, epidemiological studies as well as applied or fundamental research work.

1 Britton (P.G.), Savage (R.D.): A short form of the WAIS for use with the aged. *Brit. J. Psychiat.*, 1966, 112, 417-418.

2 Hafner (J.L.), Gorotto (L.V.), Curnutt (R.H.): The development of a WAIS short form for clinical populations. *J. Clin. Psychol.*, 1978, vol. 34, n°. 4, 935-937.

3 Wechsler (D.): The measurement and appraisal of adult intelligence. Baltimore: Williams and Wilkins, 1939.

4 Wechsler (D.): Manual for the Wechsler adult intelligence scale. New York: Psychological Corporation, 1955.

5 Wechsler (D.): Echelle d'intelligence de Wechsler pour adultes: WAIS. 2e édition. Paris: Centre de Psychologie Appliquée, 1970.

GERIATRIC INTERPERSONAL EVALUATION SCALE (G.I.E.S.)

SPECIFICITY

* * *

TYPE OF INSTRUMENT

Psychometric test 16 items

REFERENCE	**Plutchik (R.), Conte (H.), Lieberman (M.)** · − Development of a scale (GIES) for assessment of cognitive and perceptual functioning in geriatric patients. *Journal of the American Geriatrics Society,* 1971, Vol. 19, nₒ 7, 614-623.

Language: Original version published in English.
U.S.A.

Location: Enclosed in volume two page 20
See ref. biblio nₒ 3

For all information concerning the instrument write to the author at the following address:

Robert Plutchik
Department of Psychiatry
Albert Einstein College of Medicine
of Yeshiva University
1300 Morris Park Avenue
Bronx, New York 10461, U.S.A.

ORIGIN

This verbal battery was inspired by the "Mental Status Questionnaire" by **Kahn** (ref. 2), the "Rapid Approximate Intelligence Test" by **Wilson** (ref. 7) and the "Minimal Social Behavior Scale" by **Dinoff** (ref. 1).

PURPOSE

This instrument was developed to guide care planning and to evaluate its effects. This evaluation is made through assessment of the cognitive abilities of the subject.

POPULATION

Hospitalized deteriorated aged patients.

ADMINISTRATION

Rater: Psychologist or therapist.

Time required: 20 to 30 minutes.

Training: Training in interviewing techniques.

DESCRIPTION

Test battery consists of 16 essentially verbal items (temporal orientation, analogies, repetition of numbers, comprehension, mental arithmetic and card games). The subject is tested in the context of a semi-structured interview.

Scoring: One point per correct item.

VARIABLES

Cognitive, intellectual and perceptuomotor functions.

VALIDATION

Was done on aged persons hospitalized in geriatric wards, suffering from mental disease (ref. 4).
Study of **reliability:** Split-half
Study of discriminative **sensitivity** between physically well and socially integrated patients and others who were not.

APPLICATION

Evaluation of drug and non-drug therapies.

1 Dinoff (M.), Raymaker (H.), Morris (J.R.): The reliability and validity of the minimal social behavior scale and its use as a selection device. *J. Clin. Psychol.*, 1962, 18, 441-444.

2 Kahn (R.L.), Goldfarb (A.I.), Pollock (M.), Gerber (I.E.): The relationship of mental and physical status in institutionalized aged persons. *Amer. J. Psychiat.*, 1960, 117, 120-124.

3 Plutchik (R.), Conte (H.), Lieberman (M.): Development of a scale (GIES) for assessment of cognitive and perceptual functioning in geriatric patients. *Journal of the American Geriatrics Society*, 1971, vol. 19, n°. 7, 614-623.

4 Plutchik (R.), Conte (H.), Lieberman (M.), Bakur (M.), Grossman (J.), Lehrman (N.): Reliability and validity of a scale for assessing the functioning of geriatric patients. *Journal of the American Geriatrics Society*, 1970, 18, 491-500.

5 Richman (L.): Sensory training for geriatric patients. *Am. J. Occupat. Therapy*, 1969, 23, 254-257.

6 Tate (M.W.): Statistics in education and psychology. New York: The Macmillan Company, 1965.

7 Wilson (I.C.): Rapid approximate intelligence test. *Am. J. Psychiat.* 1967, 123, 1289-1290.

8 Zwerling (I.), Plutchik (R.), Hotz (M.), Kling (R.), Rubin (L.), Grossman (J.), Siegel (B.): Effects of a procaine preparation (Gerovital H 3) in hospitalized geriatric patients: a double-blind study. *Journal of the American Geriatrics Society*, 1975, vol. XXIII, n°. 8, 355-359.

EMBEDDED FIGURES TEST

SPECIFICITY

| * * |

TYPE OF INSTRUMENT

| **Non verbal**
psychometric test
12 items |

REFERENCE	**Witkin (H.A.), Oltman (P.K.), Raskin (E.), Karp (S.A.)** · – Manual for embedded figures test, children embedded figures test, and group embedded figures test. Palo Alto, CA: Consulting Psychologists Press, 1971.

Language: Original version published in English.
                U.S.A.

Location: See ref. biblio n° 76

For all information concerning the instrument write to the publisher at the following address:

Consulting Psychologists Press
577 College Avenue
Palo Alto, CA 94306, U.S.A.

ORIGIN
The test figures were inspired by the work of **Gottschaldt** (ref. 19). Colour has been added to the figures.

PURPOSE
A test of the cognitive style field dependence-independence.

POPULATION
Young and older adults without visual or psychomotor impairment.

ADMINISTRATION
Rater: Psychologist.
Time required: Approximately 20 minutes.
Training: Knowledge of the test is necessary.
Scoring: The mean time needed to find the simple figures in each item.

DESCRIPTION
The test consists of two types of figures: simple and complex geometric figures. The complex figure includes the simple figure, but in such a way that the structure of the complex figure does not permit the immediate perception of the simple one. There are 12 items, where the simple and complex figures vary from item to item. For each item, the rater shows the subject the simple figure for 10 seconds; after the subject identifies it, the complex figure is shown. The subject then tries to locate the simple figure within the complex figure as quickly as possible. Maximum time allowed per item is three minutes. Two forms exist (ref. 75).

VARIABLES
Field dependence-independence cognitive style (F.D.I.C.S.).

VALIDATION
Included in the users' manual (Ref. 76).

OTHER WORKS
cited by author
See "Science Citation Index".

APPLICATION
Clinical and experimental use to assess the field dependence-independence cognitive style.

1 Axelrod (S.), Cohen (L.D.): Senescence and embedded - figures performance in vision and touch. *Perceptual and Motor Skills*, 1961, 12, 283-288.

2 Bennett (D.H.): Perception of the upright in relation to body image. *The Journal of Mental Science*, 1956, 102, 487-506.

3 Berry (J.W.): Independence and conformity in subsistence-level societies. *Journal of Personality and Social Psychology*, 1967, 7, 415-418.

4 Bertini (M.): Traits somatiques, aptitudes perceptives et traits supérieurs de personnalité. Paper read at International Congress of Psychology, Bonn, Germany, 1960.

5 Bruininks (R.H.): Auditory and visual perceptual skills related to the reading performance of disadvantaged boys. *Perceptual and Motor Skills*, 1969, 29, 179-186.

6 Davis (J.M.), Mc Court (W.F.), Solomon (P.): Sensory deprivation: 1: effects of social contact. – 2: effects of random and visual stimulation Paper read at American Psychiatric Association meeting. Philadelphia, 1958.

7 Dawson (J.L.M.): Cultural and physiological influences upon spatial-perceptual processes in West Africa. Part I. *International Journal of Psychology*, 1967, 2, 115-128.

8 Dawson (J.L.M.): Cultural and physiological influences upon spatial-perceptual processes in West Africa. Part II. *International Journal of Psychology*, 1967, 2, 171-185.

9 Dawson (J.L.M.): Theoretical and research bases of bio-social psychology. An inaugural lecture from the Chair of Psychology, University of Hong-Kong. *Supplement to the Gazette*, 1969, vol. 16, n°. 3, 1-10.

10 Dyk (R.B.), Witkin (H.A.): Family experiences related to the development of differentiation in children. *Child Development*, 1965, 30, 21-55.

11 Eagle (M.), Goldberger (I.), Breitman (M.): Field dependence and memory for social vs. neutral and relevant vs. irrelevant incidental stimuli. *Perceptual and Motor Skills*, 1969, 29, 903-910.

12 Fenchel (G.H.): Cognitive rigidity as a behavioral variable manifested in intellectual and perceptual tasks by an outpatient population. Unpublished doctoral dissertation. New York University, 1958.

13 Fiebert (M.): Cognitive styles in the deaf. *Perceptual and Motor Skills*, 1967, 24, 319-329.

14 Fitzgibbons (D.), Goldberger (L.), Eagle (M.): Field dependence and memory for incidental material. *Perceptual and Motor Skills*, 1965, 21, 743-749.

15 Gardner (R.W.), Jackson (D.N.), Messick (S.J.): Personality organization in cognitive controls and intellectual abilities. *Psychological Issues*, 1960, 2, 4, Monograph 8.

16 Goldstein (A.G.), Change (J.E.): Effects of practice on sex-related differences in performance on embedded – figures. *Psychonomic Science*, 1965, 3, 361-362.

17 Goodenough (D.R.), Eagle (C.A.): A modification of the embedded – figures test for use with young children. *Journal of Genetic Psychology*, 1963, 103, 67-74.

18 Goodenough (D.R.), Karp (S.A.): Field dependence and intellectual functioning. *Journal of Abnormal and Social Psychology*, 1961, 63, 241-246.

19 Gottschaldt (K.): Uber den Einfluss der Erfahrung auf die Wahrnehmung von Figuren 1, uber den Einfluss gehaufter Eingragung von Figuren auf ihre Sichtbarkeit in umfassenden Konfigurationen. *Psychol. Forsch.*, 1926, 8, 261-317.

20 Hustmyer (F.E.Jr), Karnes (E.): Background autonomic activity and "analytic perception". *Journal of Abnormal and Social Psychology*, 1964, 68, 467-468.

21 Jackson (D.N.): A short form of Witkin's embedded-figures test. *Journal of Abnormal and Social Psychology*, 1956, 53, 254-255.

22 Jackson (D.N.): Independence and resistance to perceptual field forces. *Journal of Abnormal and Social Psychology*, 1958, 56, 279-281.

23 Jahoda (G.): Supernatural beliefs and changing cognitive structures among Ghanaian university students. *Journal of Cross-Cultural Psychology*, 1970, 1, 115-130.

24 Karp (S.A.): Field dependence and overcoming embeddedness. *Journal of Consulting Psychology*, 1963, 27, 294-302.

25 Karp (S.A.), Kissin (B.), Hustmyer (F.E.): Field dependence as a predictor of alcoholic therapy dropouts. *Journal of Nervous and Mental Disease*, 1970, 150, 77-83.

26 Karp (S.A.), Konstadt (N.L.): Alcoholism and psychological differentiation: long-range effect of heavy drinking on field dependence. *Journal of Nervous and Mental Disease*, 1965, 140, 412-416.

27 Karp (S.A.), Pardes (H.): Psychological differentiation (field dependence) in obese women. *Psychosomatic Medicine*, 1965, 27, 238-244.

28 Karp (S.A.), Poster (D.), Goodman (A.): Differentiation in alcoholic women. *Journal of Personality*, 1963, 31, 386-393.

29 Karp (S.A.), Silberman (L.), Winters (S.): Psychological differentiation and socioeconomic status. *Perceptual and Motor Skills*, 1969, 28, 55-60.

30 Karp (S.A.), Winters (S.), Pollack (I.W.):Field dependence among diabetics. *Archives of General Psychiatry*, 1969, 21, 72-76.

31 Karp (S.A.), Witkin (H.A.), Goodenough (D.R.): Alcoholism and psychological differentiation: Effect on achievement of sobriety on field dependence. *Quarterly Journal of Studies on Alcohol*, 1965, 26, 580-585.

32 Karp (S.A.), Witkin (H.A.), Goodenough (D.R.): Alcoholism and psychological differentiation: the effect of alcohol on field dependence. *Journal of Abnormal Psychology*, 1965, 70, 262-265.

33 Kato (N.): The validity and reliability of new rod-and-frame test. *Japanese Psychological Research*, 1965, 7, 120-125.

34 Konstadt (N.), Forman (E.): Field dependence and external directedness. *Journal of Personality and Social Psychology*, 1965, 1, 490-493.

35 Kraidman (E.): Developmental analysis of conceptual and perceptual functioning under stress and non-stress conditions. Unpublished doctoral dissertation. Clark University, 1959.

36 Lapidus (L.B.): The relation between cognitive control and reactions to stress: a study of mastery in the anticipatory phase of childbirth. Unpublished doctoral dissertation. New-York University, 1968.

37 Linton (H.B.): Relations between mode of perception and tendency to conform. Unpublished doctoral dissertation. Yale University, 1952.

38 Loeff (R.G.): Embedding and distracting field contexts as related to the field dependence dimension. Unpublished master's thesis. Brooklyn College, 1961.

39 Luborsky (L.): Individual differences in cognitive style as a determinant of vasoconstrictive orienting responses. In: "Mechanisms of orienting reaction in man": transactions of an International Colloquium held under the auspices of the Slovak Academy of Sciences, Bratislava and Smolensk, September 1965, 73-90.

40 Mac Arthur (R.S.): Some differential abilities of northern Canadian native youth. *International Journal of Psychology*, 1968, 3, 43-51.

41 Messick (S.), Damarin (F.): Cognitive styles and memory for faces. *Journal of Abnormal and Social Psychology*, 1964, 69, 313-318.

42 Minard (J.G.), Mooney (W.): Psychological differentiation and perceptual defense: studies of the separation of perception from emotion. *Journal of Abnormal and Social Psychology*, 1969, 74, 131-139.

43 Nebelkopf (E.B.), Dreyer (A.S.): Perceptual structuring: cognitive style differences in the perception of ambiguous stimuli. *Perceptual and Motor Skills*, 1970, 30, 635-639.

44 Oltman (P.K.): Field dependence and arousal. *Perceptual and Motor Skills*, 1964, 19, 441.

45 Pascual-Leone (J.): Cognitive development and cognitive style: a general psychological integration. Unpublished Ph. D. dissertation. University of Geneva, Switzerland and York University, Canada, 1969.

46 Pollack (M.), Kahn (R.L.), Karp (E.), Fink (M.): Individual differences in the perception of the upright in hospitalized psychiatric patients. Paper read at Eastern Psychological Association, New York, 1960.

47 Rosenberg (S.): Cognitive styles and overt symptomatology in schizophrenia. Unpublished Ph. D. dissertation, Columbia University, 1966.

48 Scallon (R.J.), Herron (W.G.): Field articulation of enuretic boys and their mothers. *Perceptual and Motor Skills*, 1969, 28, 407-413.

49 Schaffer (M.C.): Parent-child similarity in psychological differentiation. Unpublished doctoral dissertation. Purdue University, 1969.

50 Schimek (J.G.): Cognitive style and defenses: a longitudinal study of intellectualization and field independence. *Journal of Abnormal Psychology*, 1968, 73, 575-580.

51 Schonbar (R.A.): Differential dream recall frequency as a component of "life style". *Journal of Consulting Psychology*, 1965, 29, 468-474.

52 Schwartz (D.W.), Karp (S.A.): Field dependence in a geriatric population. *Perceptual and Motor Skills*, 1967, 24, 495-504.

53 Scott (T.H.), Bexton (W.H.), Heron (W.), Doane (B.K.): Cognitive effects of perceptual isolation. *Canadian Journal of Psychology*, 1959, 13, 200-209.

54 Silverman (A.J.), Cohen (S.I.), Shmavonian (B.M.), Greenberg (G.): Psychophysical investigations in sensory deprivation: the body-field dimension. *Psychosomatic Medicine*, 1961, 23, 48-61.

55 Silverstone (S.), Kissin (B.): Field dependence in essential hypertension and peptic ulcer. *Journal of Psychosomatic Research*, 1968, 12, 157-161.

56 Stelle (W.W.): Field dependence and reactive-process schizophrenia. Master's thesis. College of William and Mary, 1968.

57 Thurstone (L.L.): A factorial study of perception. Chicago: University of Chicago Press, 1944.

58 Tobias (J.): The relationship of cognitive patterns to the adaptive behavior of mentally retarded adults. Research studies series from associated Educational Services Corp., Selected Academic Readings, 1968, 1-125.

59 Tryon (R.C.): Reliability and behavior domain validity: reformulation and historical critique. *Psychological Bulletin*, 1957, 54, 229-249.

60 Weiner (M.): Effects of training in space orientation on perception of the upright. *Journal of Experimental Psychology*, 1955, 49, 367-373.

61 Werner (H.): The concept of development from a comparative and organismic point of view. In: Harris (D.B.). Ed.: "The concept of development: an issue in the study of human behavior". Minnesota: University of Minnesota Press, 1957, 125-148.

62 Winestine (M.C.): Twinship and psychological differentiation. *Journal of the American Academy of Child Psychiatry*, 1969, 8, 436-455.

63 Witkin (H.A.): The effect of training and of structural aids on performance in three tests of space orientation. Report n°. 80. Washington, DC: Division of Research, Civil Aeronautics Administration, 1948.

64 Witkin (H.A.): Perception of body position and of the position of the visual field. *Psychological Monographs*, 1949, 63, n°. 302, 1-46.

65 Witkin (H.A.): Individual differences in ease of perception of embedded figures. *Journal of Personality*, 1950, 19, 1-15.

66 Witkin (H.A.): Further studies of perception of the upright when the direction of the force acting on the body is changed. *Journal of Experimental Psychology*, 1952, 43, 9-20.

67 Witkin (H.A.): Psychological differentiation and forms of pathology. *Journal of Abnormal Psychology*, 1965, 70, 317-336.

68 Witkin (H.A.): Asch (S.E.): Studies in space orientation. IV: Further experiments on perception of the upright with displaced visual fields. *Journal of Experimental Psychology*, 1948, 38, 762-782.

69 Witkin (H.A.), Birnbaum (J.), Lomonaco (S.), Lehr (S.), Herman (J.L.): Cognitive patterning in congenitally totally blind children. *Child Development*, 1968, 39, 768-786.

70 Witkin (H.A.), Dyk (R.), Faterson (H.F.), Goodenough (D.R.), Karp (S.A.): Psychological differentiation. New York: John Wiley and Sons, 1962.

71 Witkin (H.A.), Goodenough (D.R.), Karp (S.A.): Stability of cognitive style from childhood to young adulthood. *Journal of Personality and Social Psychology*, 1967, 7, 291-300.

72 Witkin (H.A.), Karp (S.A.), Goodenough (D.R.): Dependence in alcoholics. *Quarterly Journal of Studies on Alcohol*, 1959, 20, 493-504.

73 Witkin (H.A.), Lewis (H.B.), Hertzman (M.), Machover (K.), Meissner (P.), Wapner (S.): Personality through perception. New York: Harper, 1954.

74 Witkin (H.A.), Lewis (H.B.), Weil (E.): Affective reactions and patient-therapist interactions among more differentiated and less differentiated patients early in therapy. *The Journal of Nervous and Mental Disease*, 1968, 146, 193-208.

75 Witkin (H.A.), Oltman (P.K.): Cognitive style. *International Journal of Neurology*, 1967, 6, 119-137.

76 Witkin (H.A.), Oltman (P.K.), Raskin (E.), Karp (S.A.): Manual for embedded figures test, children's embedded figures test, and group embedded figures test. Palo Alto, California: Consulting Psychologists Press, 1971.

77 Wolf (A.): Body rotation and the stability of field dependence. *Journal of Psychology*, 1965, 59, 211-217.

78 Zuckerman (M.): Field dependency as a predictor of responses to sensory and social isolation. *Perceptual and Motor Skills*, 1968, 27, 757-758.

MENTAL TEST SCORE

SPECIFICITY

| * * * |

TYPE OF INSTRUMENT

| Questionnaire |
| 10 questions |

REFERENCE   **Hodkinson (H.M.)** · – Evaluation of a mental test score for assessment of mental impairment in the elderly. *Age and Ageing,* 1972, 1, 233-238. ·

Language: Original version published in English.
                      Great Britain

Location: Enclosed in volume two page 45
                 See ref. biblio nº 3

For all information concerning the instrument write to the author at the following address:

        H.M. Hodkinson,
        Northwick Park Hospital
        Harrow Middlesex, Great Britain

ORIGIN   This instrument was derived from the psychometric test by **Blessed** and **Roth** (ref. 1) containing 26 questions.

PURPOSE   To reduce the test to 10 questions. Preserves the same discriminative power as the original questionnaire.

POPULATION   Elderly inpatients.

ADMINISTRATION   *Rater:* Physician, psychologist, nurse or non-qualified nursing staff.

Time required: 3 minutes.

Training: Not necessary.

Scoring: One point for each correct answer. The total score of 0 to 10 enables separation of confused or demented patients from normals.

VARIABLES   Three variables assessed:
       · Memory
       · Orientation
       · General information

VALIDATION   Was carried out on a population of elderly persons age over 65 years and involved the following (ref. 3):
Concurrent validity with the original instrument of 26 questions.
Reliability: study of internal consistency.
Discriminative power of each question.

APPLICATION   **Clinical:** Differentiation between normal and pathological subjects. The instrument does not differentiate between confusion and dementia.

1 Blessed (G.), Tomlinson (B.E.), Roth (M.): The association between quantitative measures of dementia and of senile change in the cerebral grey matter of elderly subjects. *Br. J. Psychiat.*, 1968, 114, 797.

2 Denham (M.J.), Jefferys (P.M.): Routine mental assessment in elderly patients. *Modern Geriatrics*, 1972, 2, 275.

3 Hodkinson (H.M.): Evaluation of a mental test score for assessment of mental impairment in the elderly. *Age and Ageing*, 1972, 1, 233-238.

4 Lloyd (C.M.): Royal College of Physician's study of mental impairment in the elderly. Report of findings of pilot study. London: Royal College of Physicians, 1970.

SET TEST

SPECIFICITY

* * *

TYPE OF INSTRUMENT

Psychometric test,
4 sub-test

REFERENCE	**Isaacs (B.), Akhtar (A.J.)** · – The Set Test: a rapid test of mental function in old people. *Age and Ageing,* 1972, vol. 1, 222-226.
	Language: Original version published in English. **Great Britain**
	Location: See ref. biblio n⁰ 2

For all information concerning the instrument write to the author at the following address:

Bernard Isaacs,
Department of Geriatric Medicine
The Hayward Building, Selly Oak Hospital
Raddlebarn Road
Birmingham B29 6JD, Great Britain

ORIGIN | Not specified by the authors.

PURPOSE | The instrument was devised for non-specialist staff with the aim of obtaining a rapid quantifiable measure of the ability of elderly persons to recall and express.

POPULATION | Elderly persons in institutions or in the community who are not deaf or aphasic.

ADMINISTRATION | *Rater:* Physician, psychologist, nurse, non-specialist care staff.

Time required: 4 to 5 minutes.

Training: Minimal.

Scoring: The subject is requested to recall all the colours of which he can think. The score is one point for every correct recall with a maximum of 10 points. The test is repeated for animals, fruits and towns. The maximum score is 40 points. Demented subjects score less than 15 points. Normal subjects score more than 25 points.

VARIABLES | Mental flexibility, recall ability, alertness.

VALIDATION | In a group of healthy subjects aged 65 and over living at home (ref 2) the test results were found to be in conformity with the Mill Hill Vocabulary Test and Raven's Progressive Coloured Matrices and with the Crichton Rating Scale (ref. 5).
Means and standard deviations were obtained by sex for two age groups, 65-74 and over 75 (ref. 4).

APPLICATION | **Clinical:** Rapid evaluation of the capacity of recall in elderly subjects. Included in a battery of tests it can assist the diagnosis and screening of dementia.
Research: Included in a test battery it is useful in epidemiological studies.

1 Akhtar (A.J.), Andrews (G.), Caird (F.I.), Fallon (R.J.): Urinary tract infections in the elderly. A population study. *Age and Ageing*, 1972, 1, 48.

2 Isaacs (B.), Akhtar (A.J.): The set test: a rapid test of mental function in old people. *Age and Ageing*, 1972, 1, 222-226.

3 Isaacs (B.), Kennie (A.T.): The set test as an aid to the detection of dementia in old people. *Brit. J. Psychiat.*, 1973, 123, 467-470.

4 Raven (J.C.): Guide to using the coloured progressive matrices. Ed. revised. London: H.K.Lewis, 1956.

5 Robinson (R.A.): The organisation of a diagnostic and treatment unit for the aged in a mental hospital. In "Psychiatric disorders in the aged". Manchester: Geigy (U.K.), 1965.

SIMPLE METHODS OF TESTING ABILITY

SPECIFICITY

| * * * |

TYPE OF INSTRUMENT

Psychometric test
16 items

REFERENCE   **Silver (C.P.)** · – Simple methods of testing ability in geriatric patients. *Gerontologia Clinica,* 1972, 14,110-122.

Language: Original version published in English.
Great Britain

Location: Enclosed in volume two page 21
See ref. biblio nº 5

For all information concerning the instrument write to the author at the following address:

C.P. Silver,
The London Hospital (Mile End)
Bancroft Road
London E1 4DG, Great Britain

ORIGIN   The author was inspired by various neurological studies (ref. 1, 3, 4, 7, 9).

PURPOSE   The test has been introduced with the object of detecting motor and sensory deficits.

POPULATION   Elderly people at home or in institutions.

ADMINISTRATION   *Rater:* Doctor, nurse, qualified or auxiliary, therapist and even untrained observer.
Time required: 15 minutes.
Training: No training necessary. A sheet of instructions accompanies the test.

DESCRIPTION   The test comprises two parts, verbal and practical.
The 12 verbal items account for a maximum of 26 points and concern memory, speech and orientation which are evaluated by questions which have a bearing on every day life.

The practical part of the test accounts for 14 points and comprises two sub-tests. In the second sub-test the subject is asked to first insert six differently shaped objects through appropriately shaped openings in a box and then to construct a pyramid from different sized rings.

A sensory examination (hearing-vision) is also carried out. Three minutes per test must not be exceeded.

VARIABLES
· Memory
· Orientation
· Speech
· Perceptual abnormalities and apraxia.
· Vision
· Hearing

VALIDATION   Carried out on a population composed of hospitalized geriatric patients and a group of subjects of the same age in good health attending a club (ref. 5).
Inter-observer reliability. Serious discrepancies did not arise when tests on the same subjects were conducted by two judges (an English occupational therapist and a doctor from overseas) and by panels of 5 observers (ref. 5).

APPLICATION   This test has the clinical aim of evaluating the cognitive and sensory capacities of elderly persons and indicating their degree of independence. It is used in hospital patients to assess the likelihood of discharge home.
Experience has shown that, if the total score was below 3+ points (maximum score 40) return home was rarely possible.

1 Inglis (J.): A paired associate learning test for use with elderly psychiatric patients. *J. Ment. Sci.*, 1959, 105, 440-443.

2 Irving (G.), Robinson (R.A.), Mc Adam (W.): The validity of some cognitive tests in the diagnosis of dementia. *Brit. J. Psychiat.*, 1970, 117, 149-156.

3 Isaacs (B.): The diagnostic value of tests with toys in old people. *Gerontologia Clinica*, 1963, 5, 8-22.

4 Isaacs (B.), Walkey (F.A.): The measurement of mental impairment in geriatric practice. *Gerontologia Clinica*, 1964, 6, 114-123.

5 Silver (C.P.): Simple methods of testing ability in geriatric patients. *Geront. Clin.*, 1972, 14, 110-122.

6 Silver (C.P.): The assessment of dependency. *Modern Geriatrics*, 1975, 5, 9, 24-29.

7 Slater (E.), Roth (M.): Clinical psychiatry. London: Bailliere, Tindall and Cassel, 1969.

8 Walton (D.): The diagnostic and predictive accuracy of the modified word learning test in psychiatric patients over 65. *J. Ment. Sci.*, 1958, 104, 1119-1122.

9 Walton (D.), Black (D.A.): The validity of a psychological test of brain damage. *Brit. J. Med. Psychol.*, 1957, 30, 270-279.

DEMENTIA SCREENING SCALE

SPECIFICITY

* * *

REFERENCE	Instrument not published. **Hasegawa (K.)** · − Validity and reliability of rating scales for psycho-geriatric assessment. The study on Hasegawa's dementia scale. Kawasaki: Dpt of Psychiatry, St Marianna University, 1974.

Language: Original version in Japanese. Translated into English and French.
Japan

Location: English translation enclosed in volume two page 46
See ref. biblio n⁰ 5

For all information concerning the instrument write to the author at the following address:

Kazuo Hasegawa,
Dpt of Psychiatry
St. Marianna University
School of Medicine
2095 Sugao Takatsu-Ku, Kawasaki, Japan 213

ORIGIN — Original instrument inspired by the memory scale of **Kaneko** (ref. 8), I.M.C. of **Blessed** (ref. 2), **Guttman** and **Markson's** scale (ref. 12) and the Mental Ageing Scale of **Schinfuku** (ref. 17).

PURPOSE — The aim was to design a short and rapid instrument which would differentiate between those who are demented and those who are not.

POPULATION — Elderly in and out-patients.

ADMINISTRATION — *Rater:* Physician, psychologist.

Time required: 10 to 20 minutes.

Training: Not necessary.

Scoring: Varies for each item: a good reply is scored 2-2.5, 3 or 3.5 points depending on difficulty of the question. The total score varies from 0 to 32.5.

VARIABLES — The following aspects are assessed:
- · Orientation (2 items)
- · Memory recall (4 items)
- · Memory retention (2 items)
- · Mental Control (2 items)
- · Arithmetic (1 item).

VALIDATION — Was carried out on a population of demented and non-demented elderly persons and included:
Construct validity from determination of scores for each item in 2 sessions: observation of the curve of cumulative frequency by a simple scoring method, followed by weighting of score for each question according to difficulty.
Concurrent validity with different performance tests: Kohs blocks, Bender-Gestalt and WAIS. Discriminative **sensitivity** between demented and non-demented subjects. **Sensitivity** to degrees of severity of dementia clinically established by Kaneko's classification. (ref. 8).
Establishment of **norms** defining 4 groups by global score: normal (31-32.5), borderline cases (22-30.5), pre-dementia (10.5-21.5), dementia (0-10) (ref. 5).

OTHER WORKS
cited by author — Epidemiological survey carried out on 5.000 elderly persons aged over 65, living in the district of Tokyo.
Studies of cognitive functions of centenarian subjects in comparison with the demented.

APPLICATION — **Clinical:** Mainly contribution to diagnosis.
Research on dementia

1 Bender (L.): A visual motor gestalt test and its clinical use. New York: American Orthopsychiatric Association, 1938.

2 Blessed (G.), Tomlinson (B.E.), Roth (M.): The association between quantitative measures of dementia and of senile change in the cerebral grey matter of elderly subjects. *Brit. J. Psychiat.*, 1968, 114, 797-811.

3 Bremer (J.): A social psychiatric investigation of a small community in northern Norway. *Acta Psychiat. Scand.*, 1952, Suppl. 62.

4 Essen-Moller (E.): Individual traits and morbidity in a Swedish rural population. *Acta Psychiat. Scand.*, 1956, Suppl. 100.

5 Hasegawa (K.): Validity and reliability of rating scales for psychogeriatric assessment: the study on Hasegawa's dementia scale. Kawasaki: Dpt of Psychiatry, St Marianna University, 1974. Unpublished.

6 Kahn (R.L.), Goldfarb (A.I.), Pollack (M.), Peck (A.): Brief objective measures for the determination of mental status in the aged. *Amer. J. Psychiat.*, 1960, 117, 326-328.

7 Kameyama (M.) et al.: Neurotransmitters in the aged. Paper read at WPA regional symposium, Kyoto, Japan, 1982.

8 Kaneko (J.), Ito (M.), Sugiura (S.): Psychiatric disorders among the elderly residing in the community. *Jap. Geriat. Med.*, 1956, 3, 131.

9 Kay (D.W.K.), Beamish (P.), Roth (M.): Old age mental disorders in Newcastle-upon-Tyne. *Brit. J. Psychiat.*, 1964, 110, 146.

10 Maeda (D.): Community-oriented care for elderly. In: Hasegawa (K.), Nasu (S.) Eds.: "Handbook of gerontology". Tokyo: Iwasaki Publishing Co., 1975, 478.

11 Makyiya (H.): Epidemiological investigation of psychiatric disorders of old age in Sashiki-village, Okinawa. *Keio J. Med.*, 1978, 55, 503.

12 Markson (E.W.), Levitz (G.): A Guttman scale to assess memory loss among the elderly. *Gerontologist*, Autumn 1973, Part. I. 337-340.

13 Miyoshi (K.) et al.: Neuropathological aspects of the disorders of aging: studies of the tri-dimensional structures. Paper read at WPA regional symposium, Kyoto, Japan, 1982.

14 Nielsen (J.): Geronto-psychiatric period-prevalence investigation in a geographically delimited population. *Acta Psychiat. Scand.*, 1962, 38, 308.

15 Palmore (E.): The honorable elders. Durham, NC: Duke University Press, 1975, 133.

16 Primrose (E.J.R.): Psychological illness: a community study. London: Tavistock, 1962.

17 Shinfuku (N.): Psychiatric study of the subnormal aged in "Longevity Village". *Seishin Igaku Kenkyusho Gyosekishu*, 1959, 1, 303.

18 Wechsler (D.): Manual for the Wechsler adult intelligence scale. New York: Psychological Corporation, 1955.

ECHELLE DE DEVELOPPEMENT DE LA PENSEE LOGIQUE (E.P.L.)
LOGICAL THINKING DEVELOPMENT SCALE

SPECIFICITY

** * ***

TYPE OF INSTRUMENT

Non verbal
psychometric test
5 sub-tests

REFERENCE	**Longeot (F.)** · – L'échelle de développement de la pensée logique. Issy-les-Moulineaux: Editions Scientifiques et Psychotechniques, 1974.

Language: Original version published in French.
France

Location: Enclosed in volume two page 22
See ref. biblio n° 5

For all information concerning the instrument write to the publisher at the following address:

Etablissements d'Applications Psychotechniques
6 bis, rue André Chenier
92130 Issy-les-Moulineaux, France

ORIGIN
: The author adapted and standardized the tests of **Piaget** and **Inhelder** (ref. 1, 9, 10, 11).

PURPOSE
: This battery of tests was devised to evaluate the structural operational level of subjects within the framework of clinical examinations or in applied or fundamental research.

POPULATION
: All persons capable of understanding instructions.

ADMINISTRATION
: *Rater:* Psychologist.
Time required: 1 hour to 1 hour 30 minutes.
Training: Knowledge of techniques of Piaget and Inhelder's operational tests.

DESCRIPTION
: This battery of tests is composed of five logical tests containing items of different levels of complexity:
Conservation of volume and weight-volume dissociation.
Permutation: the subject anticipates then carries out permutations of three and four different colour chips and should give exact prediction of the number of possible permutations with five and six colours.
Quantification of probabilities: the subject has in front of him two sets of chips. Each set is composed of chips marked or not marked with a cross. At each item, the subject is asked to point out the set where the chances are the highest of finding on the first trial a chip marked with a cross.
Mechanical curves: the test demands coordination of the two systems of reference in spatial representation:
A horizontal cylinder covered with a piece of paper which may move freely around its axis by means of a handle, and a pencil touching the paper which may be moved along a shaft placed horizontally above the cylinder.
The subject is required to trace, on a piece of paper wrapped around the cylinder, the results of movement of the cylinder and the pencil, combined or not, according to a pattern.
Pendulum: the subject has to specify the variable (length of the rope, weight, momentum, height of launching) which determines the frequency of pendulum movement.
Scoring: Six scores per subject. The structural level of performance (stage) in each test and the modal stage for the total of tests, is qualitatively assessed.

VARIABLES
: Logical thinking, one general factor, structural operational level (21% of the variance) and two group factors:
Combined group operations of the I.N.R.C. group (Identical, Negation, Reversibility, Correlative).
Factor distinguishing pre-or infra-logical level from the logico-mathematical one.

VALIDATION
: Construct validity was calculated (ref. 2). Standardization for children 9 to 16 years of age (ref. 3).

OTHER WORKS
cited by author
: Works by Ohlmann (ref. 8) and Marendaz (ref. 7).

APPLICATION
: This instrument is intended for clinical and experimental use allowing determination of the structural level of functioning of subjects and assessment of variability of such functioning. The test evaluates in elderly subjects disintegration of the operational structure, its processes and severity of this disintegration.

1 Inhelder (B.), Piaget (J.): De la logique de l'enfant à la logique de l'adolescent. Paris: P.U.F., 1974.

2 Lautrey (J.): La variabilité intra-individuelle du niveau de développement opératoire et ses implications théoriques. *Bulletin de Psychologie*, 1980, 345, 685-696.

3 Longeot (F.): Aspects différentiels de la psychologie génétique. BINOP, 1967.

4 Longeot (F.): Psychologie différentielle et théorie opératoire de l'intelligence. Paris: Dunod, 1969.

5 Longeot (F.): L'échelle de développement de la pensée logique. Issy-les-Moulineaux: Editions Scientifiques et Psychotechniques, 1974.

6 Longeot (F.): Les stades opératoires de Piaget et les facteurs de l'intelligence. Grenoble: P.U.G., 1978.

7 Marendaz (C.): Dépendance-indépendance à l'égard du champ, pensée opératoire et sénescence. Thèse doc. 3e cycle: U.E.R. de Psycho: Grenoble, 1981.

8 Ohlmann (Th.), Mendelsohn (P.): Variabilité intra-individuelle des activités opératoires et dépendance – indépendance à l'égard du champ. *L'Année Psychologique*, 1982, 82.

9 Piaget (J.), Inhelder (B.): Le développement des quantités physiques chez l'enfant. Neufchâtel: Delachaux et Niestlé, 1941.

10 Piaget (J.), Inhelder (B.): La genèse de l'idée de hasard chez l'enfant. Paris: P.U.F., 1951.

11 Piaget (J.), Inhelder (B.), Szeminska (A.): La géométrie spontanée de l'enfant. Paris: P.U.F., 1948.

ABBREVIATED MENTAL TEST (A.M.T.)

SPECIFICITY

* * *

TYPE OF INSTRUMENT

Questionnaire
10 items

REFERENCE	**Qureshi (K.N.), Hodkinson (H.M.)** · − Evaluation of a ten-question mental test in the institutionalized elderly. *Age and Ageing,* 1974, 3, 152-157.

Language: Original version published in English.
                  Great Britain

Location: Enclosed in volume two page 47
              See ref. biblio n⁰ 7

For all information concerning the instrument write to the author at the following address:

    K.N. Qureshi,
    Northwick Park Hospital
    Harrow, Middlesex, Great Britain

ORIGIN

This instrument was derived from the dementia scale of **Roth** and **Hopkins** (ref. 8).

PURPOSE

To elaborate an abbreviated assessment questionnaire adapted to institutionalized populations where mental tests are often difficult and burdensome to administer.

POPULATION

Elderly institutionalized patients only.

ADMINISTRATION

Rater: Physician, psychologist, nurse, paramedical nursing staff.

Time required: 3 minutes.

Training: Not necessary.

Scoring: 1 point for each correct answer.

VARIABLES

This questionnaire explores mainly three aspects commonly connected with the dementia syndrome
    · Recognition of time
    · Recognition of place
    · Recognition of persons.

VALIDATION

Was carried out on a population of persons over 60 years of age (the average age was 78 years) and institutionalized for at least two weeks (ref. 7):
Concurrent **validity** with the Roth and Hopkins scale (ref. 8) and with Denham's questionnaire (ref. 2).
Reliability: test-retest.

APPLICATION

Purely clinical: contribution to diagnosis and determination of the degree of severity of dementia.

1 Blessed (G.), Tomlinson (B.E.), Roth (M.): The association between quantitative measures of dementia and of senile change in the cerebral grey matter of elderly subjects. *Brit. J. Psychiatry*, 1968, 114, 797-811.

2 Denham (M.J.), Jefferys (P.M.): Routine mental assessment in elderly patients. *Mod. Geriatr.*, 1972, 2, 275-279.

3 Hodkinson (H.M.): Evaluation of a mental test score for assessment of mental impairment in the elderly. *Age and Ageing*, 1972, 1, 233-238.

4 Hodkinson (H.M.): Mental impairment in the elderly. *J. R. Coll. Physicians Lond.*, 1973, 7, 305-317.

5 Isaacs (B.), Walkey (F.A.): Measurement of mental impairment in geriatric practice. *Gerontol. Clin.*, 1964, 6, 114-123.

6 Isaacs (B.), Walkey (F.A.): A survey of incontinence in elderly hospital patients. *Gerontol. Clin.*, 1964, 6, 367-376.

7 Qureshi (K.N.), Hodkinson (H.M.): Evaluation of a ten-question mental test in the institutionalized elderly. *Age and Ageing*, 1974, 3, 152-157.

8 Roth (M.), Hopkins (B.): Psychological test performance in patients over 60. I: Senile psychosis and affective disorders of old age. *J. Ment. Sci.*, 1953, 99, 439-450.

9 Wilson (L.A.), Brass (W.): Brief assessment of the mental state in geriatric domiciliary practice. *Age and Ageing*, 1973, 2, 91-101.

MINI-MENTAL STATE

SPECIFICITY

| ✳ ✳ ✳ |

TYPE OF INSTRUMENT

| Psychometric test |
| 11 sub-tests |

REFERENCE	**Folstein (M.F.), Folstein (S.E.), Mc Hugh (P.R.)** · – "Mini-Mental State": A practical method for grading the cognitive state of patients for the clinician. *Journal of Psychiatric Research,* 1975, 12, 189-198.
	Language: Original version published in English. Translated into Spanish and Portuguese. **U.S.A.**
	Location: Enclosed in volume two page 23 See ref. biblio n° 3
	For all information concerning the instrument or translations write to the author at the following address:
	Marshal Folstein, Osler 320 Johns Hopkins Hospital Dpt of Psychiatry and Behavior Sciences 600 N. Wolfe Street Baltimore, Maryland 21205, U.S.A.

ORIGIN	The authors were inspired by a publication of **Kirby** and **Meyer** in 1917.
PURPOSE	This instrument was devised to enable quantification of cognitive potential and screening of possible functional disorders.
POPULATION	All elderly inpatients or out-patients, regardless of the type of pathology.
ADMINISTRATION	*Rater:* Physician, psychologist, nurse, social worker, non-specialized interviewer. *Time required:* 10 minutes. *Training:* One session of training in administration of the test is necessary.
DESCRIPTION	The test consists of two parts: verbal and performance. Four verbal sub-tests have a maximum score of 21 points and evaluate orientation in time, memory and attention. Two performance sub-tests have a maximum score of 9 points and involve naming of objects, execution of written or spoken orders, writing, and copying a complex polygon. The total score has a maximum of 30 points. A score below 24 points indicates cognitive disorders.
VARIABLES	· Orientation, registration and recall. · Attention, concentration, calculation. · Language, motor skill items including: naming, repetition, understanding, reading, writing, and copying a design.
VALIDATION	Carried out on a population of psychiatric elderly patients suffering from dementia, mood disorders and other mental disturbance and on a group of subjects in good health (ref. 3). **Concurrent validity** with the WAIS **Reliability:** test-retest at 24 hr intervals carried out with two raters and test-retest at 28 day interval carried out with one rater. **Inter-group sensitivity:** with four groups of elderly subjects: normal, demented, persons with cognitive disorders and depressed persons without such disorders.
OTHER WORKS cited by author	Surveys in institutions.
APPLICATION	**Clinical:** This clinical instrument allows discrimination between disturbed subjects and the general population. It may be used for diagnostic and prognostic purposes. **Research:** Surveys, longitudinal studies and drug trials. As an educational device to teach the cognitive aspect of the Mental Status Examination.

Ib.22

1 Anthony (J.C.), Le Resche (L.A.), Niaz (U.), Korff (M.R.von), Folstein (M.F.): Limits of the "mini-mental state" as a screening test for dementia and delirium among hospital patients. *Psychological Medicine*, 1982, 12, 2, 397-408.

2 De Paulo (J.), Folstein (M.F.), Gordon (B.): Psychiatric screening on a neurological ward. *Psychological Medicine*, 1980, 10, 125-132.

3 Folstein (M.F.), Folstein (S.E.), Mc Hugh (P.R.): "Mini-Mental State". A practical method for grading the cognitive state of patients for the clinician. *J. Psychiat. Res.*, 1975, vol. 12, 189-198.

4 Halstead (H.): A psychometric study of senility. *J. Ment. Sci.*, 1943, 89, 363.

5 Kiloh (L.G.): Pseudo-dementia. *Acta Psychiat. Scand.*, 1961, 37, 336.

6 Post (F.): The clinical psychiatry of late life. Oxford: Pergamon Press, 1965.

7 Roth (M.): The clinical interview and psychiatric diagnosis. Have they a future in psychiatric practice? *Comp. Psychiat.*, 1967, 8, 427.

8 Shapiro (M.B.), Post (F.), Löfving (B.), Inglis (J.): "Memory functions» in psychiatric patients over sixty, some methodological and diagnostic implications. *J. Ment. Sci.*, 1956, 102, 233.

9 Withers (E.), Hinton (J.): Three forms of the clinical tests of the sensorium and their reliability *Brit. J. Psychiat.*, 1971, 119, 1.

ISCHEMIA SCORE

SPECIFICITY

*   *

TYPE OF INSTRUMENT

Check list
9 to 13 items

REFERENCE

Hachinski (V.C.), Iliff (L.D.), Zilhka (E.), Du Boulay (G.H.), Mc Allister (V.L.), Marshall (J.), Russell (R.W.R.), Symon (L.) · − Cerebral blood flow in dementia. *Archives of Neurology,* 1975, 32, 632-637.

Language: Original version published in English.
Canada

Location: Enclosed in volume two page 81
See ref. biblio nọ 6

For all information concerning the instrument write to the author at the following address:

V.C. Hachinski,
Sunnybrooks Hospital,
University of Toronto Clinic
2075, Bayview Avenue
Toronto, Ontario M4N 3M5, Canada

ORIGIN

Scale devised by **Hachinski** et al (ref. 6) in the course of a study of cerebral blood flow in dementia, within the term of reference of the works of **Mayer-Gross** et al (ref. 14). The ischemia score was revised by **Rosen** et al (ref. 17).

PURPOSE

This instrument was developed to differentiate between arteriopathic and degenerative dementia.

POPULATION

Patients suffering from dementia.

ADMINISTRATION

Rater: Physician.

Time required: 5 minutes.

Training: Medical training necessary.

Scoring: Every item is scored either 0, 1 or 2 depending on the field it evaluates. The higher the total score, the greater the possibility of a vascular aetiology.

VARIABLES

The instrument contains the following variables:
· Medical history and evolution of present illness.   · Psychiatric state
· Medical antecedents   · Neurological state

VALIDATION

Carried out on subjects suffering from senile dementia, arteriopathics or both, (ref. 6):
Concurrent validity with anatomic and pathological diagnosis
External validity and discriminative sensitivity between arteriopathic, degenerative and mixed dementias.
Study on the cerebral blood flow in different aetiological types of dementia. Ischemia score was used in combination with the Blessed and Roth (ref. 1) scale.

APPLICATION

Clinical: Diagnosis of dementia. Criteria for inclusion in drug trials for purpose of having homogeneous groups.

1 Blessed (G.), Tomlinson (B.E.), Roth (M.): The association between quantitative measures of dementia and of senile change in the cerebral grey matter of elderly subjects. *Br. J. Psychiatry.*, 1968, 114, 797-811.

2 Corsellis (J.A.N.): Mental illness and the ageing brain. London: Oxford University Press, 1962.

3 Fazekas (J.F.), Bessman (A.N.), Cotsonas (N.J.) et al.: Cerebral hemodynamics in cerebral arteriosclerosis. *J. Gerontol.*, 1953, 8, 137-143.

4 Freyham (F.A.), Woodford (R.B.), Kety (S.S.): Cerebral blood flow and metabolism in psychosis of senility. *J. Nerv. Ment. Dis.*, 1951, 113, 445-456.

5 Gustafson (L.), Hagberg (B.), Ingvar (D.H.): Psychiatric symptoms and psychological test results related to regional cerebral blood flow in dementia with early onset. In: Meyer (J.S.) et al. Eds: "Research on cerebral circulation". Springfield, Ill.: Charles C. Thomas Publisher, 1972, 291-300.

6 Hachinski (V.C.), Iliff (L.D.), Zilhka (E.), Du Boulay (G.H.), Mc Allister (V.L.), Marshall (J.), Russell (R.W.R.), Symon (L.): Cerebral blood flow in dementia. *Arch. Neurol.*, Sept. 1975, vol. 32, 632-637.

7 Iliff (L.D.), Zilhka (E.), Bull (J.W.D.), et al.: Effect of changes in cerebral blood flow on proportion of high and low flow tissue in the brain. *J. Neurol. Neurosurg. Psychiatry*, 1974, 37, 631-635.

8 Ingvar (D.H.), Gustafson (L.): Regional cerebral blood flow in organic dementia with early onset. *Acta Neurol. Scand.*, 1970, 43, Suppl. 46, 42-73.

9 Ingvar (D.H.), Obist (W.), Chirian (E.), et al.: General and regional abnormalities of cerebral blood flow in senile and "presenile" dementia. *Scand. J. Clin. Lab. Invest.*, 1968, Suppl. 102, XIIB.

10 Kay (D.W.K.), Beamish (P.), Roth (M.): Old age disorders in Newcastle – upon – Tyne. *Br. J. Psychiatry*, 1964, 110, 146-158.

11 Kety (S.S.): Human cerebral blood flow and oxygen consumption as related to ageing. *Assoc. Res. Nerve Dis. Proc.*, 1956, 35, 31-45.

12 Lassen (N.A.), Feinberg (I.), Lane (M.H.): Bilateral studies of cerebral oxygen uptake in young and aged normal subjects and in patients with organic dementia. *J. Clin. Invest.*, 1960, 39, 491-500.

13 Lassen (N.A.), Munck (O.), Tottery (E.R.): Mental function and cerebral oxygen consumption in organic dementia. *Arch. Neurol. Psychiatry*, 1957, 77, 126-133.

14 Mayer-Gross (W.), Slater (E.), Roth (M.): Clinical psychiatry. 3rd ed. London: Bailliere, Tindall and Cassell, 1969.

15 Newton (R.D.): The identity of Alzheimer's disease and senile dementia and their relationship to senility. *J. Ment. Sci.*, 1948, 94, 225-249.

16 O'Brien (M.D.), Mallet (B.L.): Cerebral cortex perfusion rates in dementia. *J. Neurol. Neurosurg. Psychiatry*, 1970, 33, 497-500.

17 Rosen (W.G.), Terry (R.D.), Fuld (P.A.), Katzman (R.), Peck (A.): Pathological verification of ischemic score in differentiation of dementias. *Ann. Neurol.*, 1980, 7, 486-488.

18 Rothschild (D.): Neuropathologic changes with arteriosclerotic psychosis and their psychiatric significance. *Arch. Neurol. Psychiatry*, 1942, 48, 417-436.

19 Simard (D.), Olesen (J.), Paulson (O.), et al.: Regional cerebral blood flow and its regulation in dementia. *Brain*, 1971, 273-288.

20 Sokoloff (L.): Cerebral hemodynamics in cerebral arteriosclerosis. *J. Gerontol.*, 1953, 8, 137-143.

21 Tomlinson (B.E.), Blessed (G.), Roth (M.): Observations on the brains of non-demented old people. *J. Neurol. Sci.*, 1968, 7, 331-356.

22 Tomlinson (B.E.), Blessed (G.), Roth (M.): Observations on the brains of demented old people. *J. Neurol. Sci.*, 1970, 11, 205-242.

23 Wilkinson (I.M.S.), Browne (D.R.G.): The influence of anesthesia and of arterial hypocapnia on regional blood flow in the normal human cerebral hemisphere. *Br. J. Anaesth.*, 1970, 42, 472-482.

24 Wilkinson (I.M.S.), Bull (J.W.D.), Du Boulay (G.H.), et al.: Regional blood flow in the normal cerebral hemisphere. *J. Neurol. Neurosurg. Psychiatry*, 1969, 32, 367-378.

SHORT PORTABLE MENTAL STATUS QUESTIONNAIRE (S.P.M.S.Q.)

SPECIFICITY

* * *

TYPE OF INSTRUMENT

Questionnaire
10 questions

REFERENCE	**Pfeiffer (E.)** · – A short portable mental status questionnaire for the assessment of organic brain deficit in elderly patients. *Journal of the American Geriatrics Society,* oct. 1975, vol. 23, n̊ 10, 433-441.

Language: Original version published in English.
U.S.A.

Location: Enclosed in volume two page 48
See ref. biblio n̊ 13

For all information concerning the instrument write to the author at the following address:

Eric Pfeiffer,
Medical Center
Suncoast Gerontology Center, Box 50
12901 North 30th Street
Tampa, Florida 33612, U.S.A.

ORIGIN

The instrument was inspired by the clinical memory scale of **Wechsler** (ref. 14) and works of **Kahn** et al (ref. 5, 6).

PURPOSE

Assessment of the presence and intensity of intellectual disorders of organic origin in elderly persons, by means of a concise, easy to handle, simple to score instrument.

POPULATION

All elderly persons.

ADMINISTRATION

Rater: physician, psychologist, nurse, social worker.

Time required: 2 minutes.

Training: Not necessary.

Scoring: 1 point per question.
The presence of cognitive disorders and their grading as severe, medium or light is assessed from the number of errors (ref. 13).

VARIABLES

This questionnaire explores the following activities:
· Short-term memory   · Orientation
· Long-term memory   · Ability to conduct serial operations

VALIDATION

Was carried out on a population of elderly persons, local residents, institutionalized patients or outpatients, and involved the following (ref. 13):
External validity in respect to psychiatric clinical diagnosis
Concurrent validity with OARS (ref. 2).
Test-retest reliability

OTHER WORKS
cited by author

Numerous drug trials, clinical studies and surveys

APPLICATION

Clinical: **Research:**
Functional diagnosis   Drug trials
Prognosis   Interviews - surveys.

1 Abdo (E.), Dills (J.), Shectman (H.) et al.: Elderly wo-men in institutions versus those in public housing: comparison of personal and social adjustments. *Journal of the American Geriatrics Society*, 1973, 21, 81.

2 Center for the Study of Aging and Human Develop-ment. Duke University: Multidimensional functional assessment: the OARS methodology. 2nd edition. Duke University: Center for the Study of Aging and Human Development, 1978.

3 Goldfarb (A.): Predicting mortality in the institutiona-lized aged. *Arch. Gen. Psychiat.*, 1971, 21, 172.

4 Gregory (R.J.): A survey of residents in five nursing and rest homes in Cumberland County, North Caro-lina. *Journal of the American Geriatrics Society*, 1970, 18, 501.

5 Kahn (R.L.), Goldfarb (A.I.), Pollack (M.), et al.: The relationship of older persons: In: "Old age in the mo-dern world". Report persons. *Am. J. Psychiat.*, 1960, 117, 120.

6 Kahn (R.L.), Goldfarb (A.I.), Pollack (M.), et al.: Brief objective measures for the determination of mental status in the aged. *Am. J. Psychiat.*, 1960, 117, 326.

7 Kay (D.W.), Beamish (P.), Roth (M.): Old age mental disorders in Newcastle – upon – Tyne. I. A study of prevalence. *Brit. J. Psychiat.*, 1964, 110, 146.

8 Lowenthal (M.F.), Berkman (P.L.) et al.: Aging and mental disorders in San Francisco. San Francisco: Jos-sey-Bass, 1967.

9 Nielsen (J.): Geronto-psychiatric period-prevalence investigation in a geographically delimited popula-tion. *Acta Psychiat. Neurol. Scandinav.*, 1962, 38, 307.

10 Pasamanick (B.): A survey of mental disease in an ur-ban population. VI: An approach to total prevalence by age. *Mental Hyg.*, 1962, 46, 567.

11 Peak (D.T.): Older Americans Resources and Services Program (OARS): clinical operations. Paper presented at the Annual Meeting of the Gerontological Society, Miami Beach, November 5-9 1973.

12 Pfeiffer (E.): Multidimensional quantitative asses-sment of three populations of elderly. Paper presented at the Annual Meeting of the Gerontological Society, Miami Beach, November 5-9 1973.

13 Pfeiffer (E.): A short portable mental status question-naire for the assessment of organic brain deficit in el-derly patients. *Journal of the American Geriatrics So-ciety*, 1975, vol. 23, n° 10, 433-441.

14 Wechsler (D.): A standardized memory scale for clini-cal use. *J. Psychol.*, 1945, 19, 87.

15 Wechsler (D.): Measurement and evaluation of intel-ligence of older persons. In: "Old age in the modern world". Report of the 3rd Congress Internat. Assoc. of Gerontology. Edinburgh: Livingston, 1954, 257-278.

16 Whanger (A.D.): A study of the institutionalized el-derly of Durham County. Paper presented at the An-nual Meeting of the Gerontological Society, Miami Beach, November 5-9, 1973.

BATTERIE DE VIGILANCE EN INSTITUTION
VIGILANCE BATTERY FOR ELDERLY INPATIENTS

SPECIFICITY

| * * * |

TYPE OF INSTRUMENT

| Psychometric test
7 sub-tests |

| REFERENCE | **Israël (L.), Ohlmann (Th.)** · – Mise au point et étalonnage d'une batterie d'épreuves psycho-métriques pour l'examen des personnes âgées. *Gerontology,* 1976, vol. XXII, n° 3, 141-156. |

Language: Published in French.
              France

Location: Enclosed in volume two page 24
              See ref. biblio n° 3
              Apply to the author

For all information concerning the instrument write to the author at the following address:

     Liliane Israël
     Pavillon Chissé, C.H.R.U.
     38700 La Tronche,
     Grenoble, France

| ORIGIN | Sub-tests have been inspired by several well known authors **Zazzo** (ref. 12), **Wechsler** (ref. 11), **Rey** (ref. 9), **Thurstone** (ref. 10), the tests have been modified and adapted to the elderly population. |

| PURPOSE | Elderly over 65 years-institutionalized (homes for elderly). |

| POPULATION | Elderly inpatients living in institutions. |

| ADMINISTRATION | *Rater:* Psychologist.
Time required: 20-25 minutes according to subject.
Training: Psychological training is necessary. |

| DESCRIPTION | Seven short and non tiring tests |

· **4 verbal tests**
   ordering object
   repetition of digits
   memory recall
   fluency

· **3 graphic tests**
   coding
   crossing
   punching holes

Rating is established from a raw score which is adjusted either to a standard score or a factor score.

| VARIABLES | The variable are one general factor, vigilance (51% of explained variance) and three group factors:
   · Memory (21% of explained variance)
   · Fluency (15% of explained variance)
   · Psychomotor activity (13% of explained variance) |

| VALIDATION | On elderly persons living in institutions (ref. 3).
Construct validity: factor analysis of principal components of Hotteling (explained variance: 75.2%).
Standardization: not published yet. |

| OTHER WORKS
cited by author | Many drug trials (ref. 1, 2, 3, 4, 5, 6, 7, 8). Total 1600 observations. |

| APPLICATION | This instrument allows the measurement of change in individuals over time and particularly during drug trials. |

1 Israel (L.): Application des techniques psychométriques à l'étude des thérapeutiques à visée cérébrale en milieu gériatrique. Thèse doc. 3ᵉ cycle: UER de psycho.: Grenoble, 1977, 157 p.

2 Israel (L.): Application of psychometric techniques to the study of treatment affecting brain functioning. In: "Drugs studies in CVD and PVD": proceedings of the international symposium, Geneva, May 25-26 1981. Paris: Pergamon Press, 1982, 89-95.

3 Israel (L.), Ohlmann (Th.): Mise au point et étalonnage d'une batterie d'épreuves psychométriques pour l'examen des personnes âgées. *Gerontology*, 1976, vol. XXII, n°. 3, 141-156.

4 Israel (L.), Ohlmann (Th.): The application of psychometric technique in the study of treatments affecting brain functioning. According to a new methodology. Communication présentée au XIᵉ Congrès International de Gérontologie, Tokyo, 1978.

5 Israel (L.), Ohlmann (Th.), Delomier (Y.), Hugonot (R.): Etude contrôlée multicentre d'un nouveau traitement de l'insuffisance circulatoire cérébrale effectuée à l'aide d'une méthode originale. *Revue de Gériatrie*, septembre 1977, tome 2, n°. 5, 323.

6 Israel (L.), Ohlmann (Th.), Delomier (Y.), Hugonot (R.): Etude psychométrique de l'activité d'un extrait végétal au cours des états d'involution sénile. *Lyon Méditerranée Médical*, octobre 1977, tome XIII, n°. 16, 1197.

7 Israel (L.), Ohlmann (Th.), Hugonot (R.): Etude de l'action de médications à visée cérébrale. Une nouvelle méthodologie: le banc d'essais comparatifs. *Revue de Gériatrie*, 1976, tome 1, n°. 1, 46-57.

8 Israel (L.), Ohlmann (Th.), Hugonot (R.): Activité d'un alcaloïde de la petite pervenche jugée à partir d'épreuves psychométriques chez des personnes âgées. *Revue de Gériatrie*, mai 1978, tome 3, n°. 3, 169.

9 Rey (A.): Les troubles de la mémoire et leur examen psychométrique. Bruxelles: Dessart, 1966.

10 Thurstone (L.L.): Primary mental abilities. Paris: Centre de Psychologie Appliquée, 1953.

11 Wechsler (D.): La mesure de l'intelligence de l'adulte. 4ᵉ éd. Paris: P.U.F., 1973, 291 p.

12 Zazzo (R.): Le test des deux barrages. *Actualités pédagogiques et psychologiques*, 1964, vol. 7, 254.

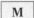 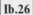

PHILADELPHIA GERIATRIC CENTER MENTAL STATUS QUESTIONNAIRE (P.G.M.S.Q.)

SPECIFICITY

*	*	*

TYPE OF INSTRUMENT

Questionnaire
35 items

REFERENCE	**Fishback (D.B.)** · – Mental status questionnaire for organic brain syndrome with a new visual counting test. *Journal of the American Geriatrics Society,* 1977, vol. 25, nº 4, 167-170.

Language: Original version published in English.
U.S.A.

Location: Enclosed in volume two page 49
See ref. biblio nº 6

For all information concerning the instrument write to the author at the following address:

David Fishback,
Philadelphia Geriatric Center
5391 Old York Road
Philadelphia, Pennsylvania 19141, U.S.A.

ORIGIN
Instrument derived from questionnaires of **Kahn** et al (ref. 13) and of **Pfeiffer** (ref. 15) to which have been added original questions suggested by experience at the Philadelphia Geriatric Center (P.G.C.).

PURPOSE
To establish a functional classification of intellectual problems related to organic brain syndrome, by means of a questionnaire and a visual counting test.

POPULATION
People with organic brain syndrome, ambulatory or bedridden.

ADMINISTRATION
Rater: Patient questioned by medical doctor, nurse or aide.

Time required: 10 minutes.

Training: Not necessary.

Scoring: Each good response gets one point. The total score determines 5 levels of gravity: complete dementia (0) severe (1-10), moderate (11-20), mild or benign (21-33), absence of deficiency or not impaired (34-35).

VARIABLES
The instrument makes note of the following variables.
· Orientation for time of day or night
· Orientation for place, awareness of objects in room, eyeglasses, dental plates
· Recognition of others, including family
· Continence (bladder, bowel)
· General Information
· Perception

· Being able to feed oneself
· Being able to dress oneself
· Memory of recent events
· Memory of old events
· Rapidity of answers and span of attention
· Intelligence

VALIDATION
Tests on nursing home and hospital patients as to their behavior (ref. 6).
Empirical confirmation by clinical findings of degree of severity of dementia.

OTHER WORKS
cited by author
· Many papers on arterial hypertension, treatment of arterial hypertension in old age nursing home (ref. 4, 5).
· Biological psychiatry (ref. 14).
· An interesting discovery was that some accurate visual counting was present in senile dementia cases except those of the most severe type.

APPLICATION
Contribution to the diagnostic differences and grades of dementia. It was noted that patients with mild senile dementia are better when kept with a similar group than with patients with moderate or severe dementia. This helped to lessen mental regression.

1 Fishback (D.B.): A new objective circulation time test (fluorescein method). *J. Lab. and Clin. Med.*, 1941, 26, 1966.

2 Fishback (D.B.): Scientific exhibit. American Medical Association, Atlantic City Session, June 8-12 1942.

3 Fishback (D.B.): A new test for vasopressor substances in hypertension. *Am. J. M. Sci.*, 1950, 219, 517.

4 Fishback (D.B.): Fluorescein circulation time and the treatment of hypertension in the aged. *Journal of the American Geriatrics Society*, 1973, vol. 21, n°. 11, 495-503.

5 Fishback (D.B.): An approach to the treatment of hypertension in the aged. *Angiology*, april 1976, vol. 27, n°. 4, 212-218.

6 Fishback (D.B.): Mental status questionnaire for organic brain syndrome, with a new visual counting test. *Journal of the American Geriatrics Society*, 1977, vol. 25, n°. 4, 167-170.

7 Fishback (D.B.), Castor (L.H.): The use of chlorothiazide or hydrochlorothiazide with reserpine in the office treatment of hypertension. *Diseases of the Chest*, august 1961, vol. 40, n°. 2, 203-209.

8 Fishback (D.B.), Castor (L.H.): Effective hypertension therapy with least side effects: observations on mebutamate and hydrochlorothiazide.. *J. Am. Geriatrics Soc.*, 1963, 11, 432.

9 Fishback (D.B.), Castor (L.H.): Polythiazide and reserpine combined in the office treatment of hypertension. *Angiology*, 1964, 15, 196.

10 Fishback (D.B.), Castor (L.M.): Fluorescein circulation time and treatment in hypertension. *Angiology*, january 1965, vol. 16, n°. 1, 21-28.

11 Fishback (D.B.), Guttman (S.A.), Abramson (E.B.): An objective method of determining blood velocity (fluorescein method). *Am. J. M. Sci.*, 1942, 203, 535.

12 Gesell (A.), Amatruda (C.S.): Developmental diagnosis. 2nd ed. New York: Harper and Row, 1947.

13 Kahn (R.L.), Goldfarb (A.I.), Pollack (M.), Peck (A.): Brief objective measures for the determination of mental status in the aged. *Am. J. Psychiatry*, 1960, 117, 326-328.

14 Krouse (T.B.), Fishback (D.B.): Vasoconstrictor activity of the sera of psychotic patients. *The Clinical Proceedings of the Jewish Hospital*, june 1951, vol. 4, n°. 2, 56-58.

15 Pfeiffer (E.): A short portable mental status questionnaire for the assessment of organic brain deficit in elderly patients. *Journal of the American Geriatrics Society*, 1975, 23, 433.

16 Shakespeare (W.): As you like it, Act II, Scene 7, line 139.

17 Shakespeare (W.): Othello, Act II, Scene 3, line 241.

COGNITIVE CAPACITY SCREENING EXAMINATION

SPECIFICITY

| * * |

TYPE OF INSTRUMENT

| Questionnaire |
| 30 items |

| **REFERENCE** | **Jacobs (J.W.), Bernhard (M.R.), Delgado (A.), Strain (J.J.)** · − Screening for organic mental syndromes in the medically ill. *Annals of Internal Medicine,* 1977, 86, 40-46. |

Language: Published in English.
            U.S.A.

Location: Enclosed in volume two page 50
            See ref. biblio n° 6

For all information concerning the instrument write to the author at the following address:

John Jacobs,
Montefiore Hospital and Medical Center
111 East 210th Street
Bronx, New York 10467, U.S.A.

ORIGIN

The text coincides with the works and reflections of numerous authors on the links between cognitive activity and organic brain pathology (ref. 1, 5, 8, 10, 12, 13, 14, 17).

PURPOSE

Brief Cognitive Screening Examination designed to make a quick diagnosis of diffuse organic mental syndromes, particularly delirium and diffuse dementia (e.g. Alzeheimer's Disease).

POPULATION

Young and old adults, out-patients or institutionalized patients, without deafness or affection of speech.

ADMINISTRATION

Rater: Physician, psychologist, mental health professional.

Time required: 5 minutes.

Training: Familiarization with the test.

Scoring: 1 point per successful item. The maximum score is 30 points. In subjects who are not mentally retarded, an organic brain syndrome must be considered if the grade is lower than 20 points.

VARIABLES

The test studies different facets of intellectual activity:
· Orientation   · Short term and middle term memory
· Flow of thought   · Attention-concentration
· Calculation   · Logical reasoning

VALIDATION

The **inter-rater reliability** and the concurrent **validity** have been checked (ref. 6).

OTHER WORKS cited by author

Kaufman (ref. 8) has stressed the importance of this questionnaire for screening examination.

APPLICATION

This clinical tool makes possible a rapid clinical screening of many subjects for a diagnosis of diffuse organic brain syndrome and differentiation in longitudinal studies between acute and chronic affections.

1   Cobb (S.), Ruesch (J.): A series of tests for the measurement of disturbed "consciousness". *Trans. Am. Neurol. Assoc.*, 1943, 69, 113-119.

2   Engel (G.L.), Romano (J.): Delirium, a syndrome of cerebral insufficiency. *J. Chronic Dis.*, 1959, 9, 260-277.

3   Engel (G.L.), Rosenbaum (M.): Delirium. III: Electroencephalographic changes associated with acute alcoholic intoxication. *Arch. Neurol. Psychiatry*, 1945, 53, 44-50.

4   Engel (G.L.), Webb (J.P.), Ferris (E.B.): Quantitative electroencephalographic studies of anoxia in humans: comparison with acute alcoholic intoxication and hypoglycemia. *J. Clin. Invest.*, 1945, 24, 691-697.

5   Folstein (M.F.), Folstein (S.E.), Mc Hugh (P.R.H.): "Mini-mental state". *J. Psychiat. Res.*, 1975, 12, 189-198.

6   Jacobs (J.W.), Bernhard (M.R.), Delgado (A.), Strain (J.J.): Screening for organic mental syndromes in the medically ill. *Annals of Internal Medicine*, 1977, 86, 40-46.

7   Katz (N.M.), Agle (D.P.), De Palma (R.G.) et al.: Delirium in surgical patients under intensive car. *Arch. Surg.*, 1972, 104, 310-313.

8   Kaufman (D.M.), Weinberger (M.), Strain (J.J.), Jacobs (J.W.): Detection of cognitive deficits by a brief mental status examination: the cognitive capacity screening examination, a reappraisal and a review. *General Hospital Psychiatry*, 1979, 1, 3, 247-255.

9   Lipowski (Z.J.): Delirium, clouding of consciousness and confusion. *J. Nerv. Ment. Dis.*, 1967, 145, 227-255.

10 Mattis (S.): The mental status examination for organic mental syndrome in the elderly patient. In: Bellak (L.), Karasu (R.B.) Eds: "The concise handbook of geriatric psychiatry". New-York: Grune and Stratton, 1976, 77-121.

11 Romano (J.), Engel (G.L.): Physiologic and psychologic consideration of delirium. *Med. Clin. North Am.*, 1944, 28, 629-638.

12 Ruesch (J.): Intellectual impairment in head injuries. *Am. J. Psychiatry*, 1944, 100, 480-496.

13 Ruesch (J.): The diagnostic value of disturbances of consciousness. *Dis. Nerv. Syst.*, 1944, 5, 69-83.

14 Ruesch (J.), Moore (B.E.): Measurement of intellectual functions in the acute stage of head injury. *Arch. Neurol. Psychiatry*, 1943, 50, 165-170.

15 Shands (H.C.): An outline of the process of recovery from severe trauma. *Arch. Neurol. Psychiatry*, 1955, 73, 403-409.

16 Talland (G.A.): Deranged memory: a psychonomic study of the amnesia syndrome. New York: Academic Press, 1965.

17 Walls (F.C.), Ruesch (J.): Mental examiners handbook. New York: The Psychological Corporation, 1942.

M | Ib.28

CONFUSION ASSESSMENT SCHEDULE

SPECIFICITY

* * *

TYPE OF INSTRUMENT

Questionnaire
21 items

REFERENCE	Slater (R.), Lipman (A.) · – Staff assessments of confusion and the situation of confused residents in homes for old people. *The Gerontologist,* 1977, vol. 17, n° 6, 523-530.

Language: Original version published in English.
Great Britain

Location: Enclosed in volume two page 51
See ref. biblio n° 34

For all information concerning the instrument write to the author at the following address:

Robert Slater,
Department of Applied Psychology
University of Wales Institute of Science and Technology
Llwyn – J – Grant Rd, Penylan
Cardiff, Wales CF3 7UX, Great Britain

ORIGIN — This is a modified version of a questionnaire suggested by **Slater** and **Roth** in a clinical psychiatry textbook (ref. 33).

PURPOSE — The questionnaire aims to assess the degree of "confusion" amongst a group of subjects designated as confused by those who care for them; the need to avoid such labelling by "carers" is discussed.

POPULATION — Elderly ambulant people who were institutionalized and had reached an advanced stage of senile dementia.

ADMINISTRATION — *Rater:* Non qualified person.

Time required: 10 minutes.

Training: Not necessary

Scoring: Each item scored 0 or 1. Maximum score is 21.

VARIABLES — · Orientation (14 questions).
· Memory (7 questions).

VALIDATION — Carried out on a population of subjects aged from 77 to 84 years resident in old people's homes, using the questionnaire to elaborate their confusion but also drawing upon an estimation of residents' confusion and infirmity made by the staff of the institution. (ref. 34).
· The correlation between the staff's overall assessments of confusion and the questionnaire method of measurement in relation to each of the areas explored (verbal and spatial behaviour) is examined.
· Empirical studies were made of the relationship between the overall staff assessments, the quantitative evaluation of the state of confusion and the social and geographical segregation of the elderly people in the institution.

APPLICATION — **Clinical:** a tentative contribution to diagnosis when a sophisticated evaluation is not feasible.

1   Allport (G.W.): The nature of prejudice. London: Addison-Wesley, 1954.

2   Barrett (A.N.): User requirements in purpose-built local authority residential homes for old people. The notion of domesticity in design. Ph.D. dissertation, Univ. Wales, 1976.

3   Becker (H.S.): Outsiders: studies in the sociology of deviance. New York: Free Press, 1963.

4   Becker (H.S.): Labelling theory reconsidered. In: Rock (P.), Mc Intosh (M.) Eds.: "Deviance and social control". London: Tavistock, 1974.

5   Bromley (D.B.): The psychology of human ageing. Harmondsworth: Penguin Books, 1974.

6   Department of Health and Social Security: A life style for the elderly. London: HMSO, 1976.

7   Department of Health and Social Security and the Welsh Office: The census of residential accomodation: 1970. 1: Residential accommodation for the elderly and for the younger physically handicapped. London: HMSO, 1975.

8   Doust (J.W.), Schneider (R.A.), Talland (G.A.), Walsh (M.A.), Barker (G.B.): Studies of the physiology of awareness: the correlation between intelligence and anoxemia in senile dementia. *Journal of Nervous and Mental Disease*, 1953, 117, 383-397.

9   Erikson (K.T.): Notes on the sociology of deviance. In: Becker (H.S.)Ed.: "The other side". New York: Free Press, 1964.

10 Goffman (E.): Asylums: essays on the social situation of mental patients and other inmates. New York: Doubleday, 1961.

11 Gold (R.L.): Roles in sociological field observations. In: Denzin (N.K.) Ed.: "Sociological methods: a sourcebook". London: Butterworths, 1970.

12 Harris (H.): I sit, therefore I am – a study of madness. *Social Work Today*, 1976, 6, 742-744.

13 Harris (H.), Lipman (A.), Slater (R.): Architectural design: the spatial location and interactions of old people. *Gerontologist*, 1977, 23, 390-400.

14 Henry (J.): Culture against man. Harmondsworth: Penguin Books, 1972.

15 Isaacs (B.), Walkey (F.): The assessment of the mental state of elderly hospital patients using a simple questionnaire. *American Journal of Psychiatry*, 1963, 120, 173-174.

16 Kahn (R.L.), Goldfarb (A.I.), Pollack (M.), Peck (A.): Brief objective measures for the determination of mental status in the aged. *American Journal of Psychiatry*, 1960, 117, 326-329.

17 Kitsuse (J.I.): Societal reaction to deviant behavior. In: Rubington (E.), Weinberg (M.S.). Eds.: "Deviance: The interactionist perspective". New York: Macmillan, 1968.

18 Krech (D.), Crutchfield (R.S.), Ballachey (E.L.): Individual in society. New York: Mc Graw-Hill, 1962.

19 Lemert (E.M.): Human deviance, social problems and social control. Englewood Cliffs, N.J.: Prentice-Hall, 1967.

20 Lipman (A.): Some problems of direct observation in architectural social research. *Architects' Journal*, 1968, 147, 1349-1356.

21 Lipman (A.), Slater (R.): Building high to avoid confusing the elderly confused. *Health and Social Service Journal*, 1976, 56, 1634-1635.

22 Lipman (A.), Slater (R.): Homes for old people: toward a positive environment. *Gerontologist*, 1977, 17, 146-156.

23 Meacher (M.): Taken for a ride, special residential homes for confused old people: a study of separatism in social policy. London: Longman, 1972.

24 Meer (B.), Baker (J.A.): The Stockton geriatric rating scale. *Journal of Gerontology*, 1966, 21, 392-403.

25 Milne (J.S.), Maule (M.M.), Cormack (S.), Williamson (J.): The design and testing of a questionnaire and examination to assess physical and mental health in older people using a staff nurse as the observer. *Journal of Chronic Diseases*, 1972, 25, 385-405.

26 National Council of Social Service: Caring for people: staffing residential homes. London: George Allen and Unwin, 1967.

27 Nie (N.H.), Hull (C.H.), Jenkins (J.G.), Steinbrenner (K.), Bent (D.H.): Statistical package for the social sciences. New York: Mc Graw-Hill, 1975.

28 Pearson (G.): The deviant imagination: psychiatry, social work and social change. London: Macmillan, 1975.

29 Personal Social Services Council: Residential care reviewed. London: Personal Social Services Council, 1977.

30 Plutchik (R.), Conte (H.), Lieberman (M.), Bakur (M.), Grossman (J.), Lehrman (N.): Reliability and validity of a scale for assessing the functioning of geriatric patients. *Journal of the American Geriatrics Society*, 1970, 18, 491-500.

31 Scheff (T.J.): Being mentally ill, a sociological theory. Chicago: Adline, 1966.

32 Shader (R.I.), Harmatz (J.S.), Salzman (C.): A new scale for clinical assessment in geriatric populations: Sandoz-clinical assessment-geriatric (SCAG). *Journal of the American Geriatrics Society*, 1974, 22, 107-113.

33 Slater (E.), Roth (M.): Clinical psychiatry. London: Bailliere, Tindall and Cassell, 1969.

34 Slater (R.), Lipman (A.): Staff assessments of confusion and the situation of confused residents in homes for old people. *The Gerontologist*, 1977, vol. 17, n°. 6, 523-530.

MODIFIED TOOTING BEC QUESTIONNAIRE

SPECIFICITY

| * | * | * |

TYPE OF INSTRUMENT

Questionnaire
16 items

REFERENCE	**Denham (M.J.), Jefferys (P.M.)** · – Routine mental testing in the elderly. *Medicine,* 1978, 1, 1.
	Language: Original version published in English. Translated into French by L. Israël. **Great Britain**
	Location: Enclosed in volume two page 52 See ref. biblio n° 2, 3
	For all information concerning the instrument write to the author at the following address:
	M.J. Denham, Northwick Park Hospital and Clinical Research Centre Watford Road Harrow, Middlesex HA1 3UJ, Great Britain

ORIGIN

Questionnaire adapted from Tooting Bec Hospital test devised by **Doust** et al. (ref. 4).

PURPOSE

To find a short test which is easy and simple to administer, will hold the patient's attention, avoid irritation, but prove to be a useful test of memory, orientation and concentration.

POPULATION

Elderly patients admitted to hospital and questionned within 2-5 days of admission.

ADMINISTRATION

Rater: Physician, psychologist, junior medical staff, unqualified staff.

Time required: 3 minutes.

Training: Not necessary.

Scoring: One mark for each correct answer, giving a maximum score of 16. Empirically, patients can be classified into four groups - severe confusion (0-3), moderate confusion (4-7), mild confusion (8-12), absence of confusion (13-16).

VARIABLES

· Recognition of time, place, persons.
· Knowledge of current events.

VALIDATION

Carried out on elderly patients admitted to an acute geriatric ward at Northwick Park Hospital, these were empirically divided into groups.
  · Non confused patients,
  · Patients mildly confused
  · Patients moderately confused
  · Patients severely confused.
Correlation of results obtained with the presence of incontinence.
Questionnaire not valid in presence of deafness, dysphasia, depression, or in non-British populations.

APPLICATION

Prognosis and future management.

1 Blessed (G.), Tomlinson (B.E.), Roth (M.): The association between quantitative measures of dementia and of senile change in the cerebral grey matter of elderly subjects. *Brit. J. Psychiat.*, 1968, 114, 797.

2 Denham (M.J.), Jefferys (P.M.): Routine mental testing in the elderly. *Modern Geriatrics*, 1972, 2, 275-279.

3 Denham (M.J.), Jefferys (P.M.): Routine mental testing in the elderly. *Medicine*, 1978, 1, 1.

4 Doust (J.W.C.), Schneider (R.A.), Tailand (G.A.) et al.: Studies in physiology of awareness. *J. Nerv. Ment. Dis.*, 1953, 117, 303.

5 Hunt (H.F.): The Hunt Minnesota test of organic brain damage. Minneapolis: University of Minnesota Press, 1943.

6 Isaacs (B.), Walkey (F.A.): Measurement of mental impairment in geriatric practice. *Geront. Clin.*, 1964, 6, 114.

7 Wechsler (D.): The measurement of adult intelligence. 4th ed. Baltimore: Williams and Wilkins, 1958.

ECHELLE D'EFFICIENCE INTELLECTUELLE
INTELLECTUAL EFFICIENCY RATING SCALE

SPECIFICITY

* * *

TYPE OF INSTRUMENT

Psychometric test
5 sub-tests

REFERENCE

Janin (C.), Gaucher (J.), Chapuy (P.) · – Echelle d'efficience intellectuelle de la personne âgée. *La Revue de Gériatrie,* 1978, vol. 3, nº 5, 245-251.

Language: Original version published in French.
France

Location: See ref. biblio nº 4

For all information concerning the instrument write to the author at the following address:

Paul Chapuy,
Service de Gériatrie
Hôpital des Charpennes
C.H.R. de Lyon
27, Grande – rue des Charpennes
69603 Villeurbanne, France

ORIGIN   The sub-tests were inspired by the already known tests of **Benton** (ref. 2), **Bender** (ref. 1), **Wechsler** (ref. 7, 8) and were modified and adapted for an elderly population.

PURPOSE   This test battery was devised in order to enable rapid evaluation of intellectual performances in elderly persons.

POPULATION   All persons over 65 years of age, inpatients or out-patients.

ADMINISTRATION   *Rater:* Physician, psychologist.

Time required: 30 minutes maximum.

Training: Training in scoring psychometric tests

DESCRIPTION   Five tests determining intellectual efficiency:
· Visuo-spatial ability   · General intelligence
· Digit Span   · Arithmetic
· Long and short-term memory

For inpatients the mark obtained from each test may be translated into a standard score by aid of a table published in the reference quoted and this permits construction of a "profile" of intellectual efficiency for each person. The total score in each test or the global score is transformed into an efficiency quotient (E.Q.) and may be converted to a standard score.

VARIABLES   · Visuo-spatial ability   · Attention - concentration
· Short-term and long-term memory   · Logical thought

VALIDATION   **Standardization:** standardization into standard scores was carried out on a population of elderly hospitalized patients. Each class is defined by a minimum and a maximum efficiency quotient (E.Q.) value. Classification ranges from "very poor" with an E.Q. below 73 to "highly superior" with an E.Q. above or equal to 129 (ref. 4).

APPLICATION   This scale may be used for detecting deterioration as well as in research work carried out on hospitalized subjects.
Clinical: Contribution to diagnosis due to organic cerebral disorders.
Research: To be carried out on elderly hospitalized populations.

1 Bender (L.): A visual motor gestalt test and its clinical use. American Orthopsychiatric Association Research Monograph n°. 3, 1938.

2 Benton (A.L.): La signification des tests de rétention visuelle dans le diagnostic clinique. *Revue de Psychologie Appliquée*, 1952, 2, 151-179.

3 Calanca (A.): Les tests mentaux en géronto-psychiatrie. *Annales Médicopsychologiques*, 1964, 122, 21-28.

4 Janin (C.), Gaucher (J.), Chapuy (P.): Echelle d'efficience intellectuelle de la personne âgée. *La Revue de Gériatrie*, 1978, 3, 5, 245-251.

5 Poitrenaud (J.): La "mesure" des déficits intellectuels chez le sujet âgé. *Gazette Médicale de France*, 1968, 75, 16, 3371-3394.

6 Rey (A.): L'examen clinique en psychologie. Paris: P.U.F., 1964, 224 p.

7 Wechsler (D.): Manual for the Wechsler memory scale. New York: Psychological Corporation, 1945.

8 Wechsler (D.): Manual for the Wechsler adult intelligence scale. New York: Psychological Corporation, 1955.

STIMULUS RECOGNITION TEST (S.R.T.)

SPECIFICITY

* * *

TYPE OF INSTRUMENT

Psychometric test
10 items

REFERENCE	**Brink (T.L.), Bryant (J.), Catalano (M.L.), Janakes (C.), Oliveira (C.)** · – Senile confusion: Assessment with a new stimulus recognition test. *Journal of the American Geriatrics Society,* 1979, vol. 27, 3, 126-129.

Language: Published in English.
U.S.A.

Location: See ref. biblio nº 3

For all information concerning the instrument write to the author at the following address:

T.L. Brink,
1044 Sylvan
San Carlos, California 94070, U.S.A.

ORIGIN
The author was inspired by two clinical tests: Mental Status Questionnaire (ref. 14, 15) and the Face Hand Test (ref. 12, 13).

PURPOSE
This clinical test was developed to differentiate demented and non-demented individuals.

POPULATION
All persons over 65 years of age, inpatients or out-patients, of sound speech and hearing.

ADMINISTRATION
Rater: Psychologist.
Time required: 12 minutes.
Training: Short familiarization required.

DESCRIPTION
The instrument consists of 10 trials. At each trial, the subject is presented with a card, the content of which the subject is required to remember. The card changes from one trial to another. The subject is then asked to recognize the original cards from among 4 or 5 similar ones presented successively. The score varies from 0 to 10. Lack of recognition as well as faulty recognitions are counted as failures. If the subject can pass the test he does not have any significant senile dementia.

VARIABLES
Short-term recognition memory.

VALIDATION
When carried out on a population of elderly inpatients, validation has involved the following:
Concurrent validity: with the "Mental Status Questionnaire" and the "Face Hand Test" (ref. 3).
Discriminative validity and sensitivity: between two groups of subjects: the "lucidalert" and the "confused" according to the opinions of the nursing staff (ref. 3).

APPLICATION
Clinical: Screening.
Research: Studies on dementia and memory.

1 Andriola (M.R.): Role of the EEG in evaluating CNS dysfunction. *Geriatrics*, 1978, 33, 2, 59.

2 Brink (T.L.): Brief psychiatric screening of institutionalized aged: a review. *Long Term Care and Health Services Administration Quarterly*, 1980, 6, 253-260.

3 Brink (T.L.), Bryant (J.), Catalano (M.L.), Janakes (C.), Oliveira (C.): Senile confusion: assessment with a new stimulus recognition test. *Journal of the American Geriatrics Society*, 1979, vol. 27, n°. 3, 126-129.

4 Brink (T.L.), Capri (D.), De Neeve (V.), Janakes (C.), Oliveira (C.): Senile confusion: limitations of assessment by mental status questionnaire, face-hand test, and staff ratings. *Journal of the American Geriatrics Society*, 1978, vol. 26, 380-382.

5 Busse (E.W.), Pfeiffer (E.): Mental illness in later life. Washington, DC: American Psychiatric Association, 1973.

6 Cameron (D.E.): Loss of memory. *Postgrad. Med.*, 1966, 45, 202.

7 Craik (F.I.M.), Lockhart (R.S.): Level of processing: a framework for memory research. *J. Verbal Learn. Behavior*, 1972, 11, 671.

8 Dorken (H.): Normal senescent decline and senile dementia. *Med. Services J.*, 1958, 14, 18.

9 Dorken (H.), Kral (V.A.): Psychological investigation of senile dementia. *Geriatrics*, 1951, 6, 151.

10 Ernst (P.), Badash (D.), Beran (B.) et al.: Incidence of mental illness in the aged: unmasking the effects of a diagnosis of chronic brain syndrome. *Journal of the American Geriatrics Society*, 1977, 25, 8, 371-375.

11 Ernst (P.), Beran (B.), Badash (D.) et al.: Treatment of the aged mentally ill: further unmasking of the effects of a diagnosis of chronic brain syndrome. *Journal of the American Geriatrics Society*, 1977, 25, 10, 466-469.

12 Fink (M.), Green (M.), Bender (M.B.): Face-hand test as diagnostic sign of organic mental syndrome. *Neurology*, 1952, 2, 46.

13 Green (M.A.), Fink (M.): Standardization of the face-hand test. *Neurology*, 1954, 4, 211.

14 Kahn (R.L.), Goldfarb (A.I.). Pollack (M.) et al.: Brief objective measures for the determination of mental status in the aged. *American J. Psychiat.*, 1960, 117, 326.

15 Kahn (R.L.), Pollack (M.), Goldfarb (A.I.): Factors related to individual differences in mental status of institutionalized aged. In: Hoch (P.H.), Zubin (J.) Eds: "Psychopathology of aging". New York: Grune and Stratton, 1961.

16 Kinsbourne (M.): Diagnosis of cognitive deficit in the aged. *Postgrad. Med.*, 1971, 50, 191.

17 Liston (E.H.): Occult presenile dementia. *J. Nerv. and Ment. Dis.*, 1977, 164, 263.

18 Orme (J.E.): Intellectual and Rorschach test performances of a group of senile dementia patients and of a group of elderly depressives. *J. Mental Sci.*, 1955, 101, 863.

19 Schaie (K.W.): Age changes in adult intelligence. In: Woodruff (D.S.), Birren (J.E.): "Aging: Scientific perspectives and social issues". New York: D.Van Nostrand, 1975.

20 Schonfeld (D.), Robertson (E.H.): Memory storage and aging. *Canad. J. Psychol.*, 1966, 20, 228-236.

MISPLACED OBJECTS TASK

SPECIFICITY

* * *

TYPE OF INSTRUMENT

Non verbal psychometric test

REFERENCE	**Crook (T.), Ferris (S.), Mac Carthy (M.)** · – The misplaced objects task. A brief test for memory dysfunction in the aged. *Journal of the American Geriatrics Society,* 1979, vol. XXVII, 6, 284-287.
	Language: Original version published in English. **U.S.A.**
	Location: Enclosed in volume two page 25 See ref. biblio № 4
	For all information concerning the instrument write to the author at the following address:
	Thomas Crook, Center on Aging, National Institute of Mental Health 5600 Fischers Lane Rockville, Maryland 20857, U.S.A.

ORIGIN	Test is original.
PURPOSE	To enable screening of memory disorders in aged persons.
POPULATION	All aged persons, inpatients or out-patients.
ADMINISTRATION	*Rater:* Physician, psychologist or non-specialized persons (nursing aides or administrative staff). *Time required:* Two sessions of 3 minutes each, with a break that may last 5 to 30 minutes between sessions. *Training:* No special training necessary.
DESCRIPTION	The subject is asked to find 10 objects which he himself has placed in a house (shown on the plan) divided into 10 parts. The score varies from 0 to 10. One point is given for every object correctly found.
VARIABLES	Recall. Global memory measure.
VALIDATION	Was carried out on an aged population, and involved (ref. 4): concurrent validity calculated in comparison with the discriminative power of the instrument and those of the Guild Memory Scale (ref. 9) for three groups of subjects: young adults, impaired and unimpaired elderly. **Reliability:** Test-retest at one-day interval.
OTHER WORKS cited by author	Facial recognition memory deficits study by Ferris et al. (ref. 8).
APPLICATION	This clinical instrument enables diagnostic and even prognostic assessment in cases of low scores. Screening for memory impairment and also as an outcome measure in severely impaired patients.

1 Botwinick (J.): Cognitive processes in maturity and old age. New York: Springer Publishing Company, 1967, 57-65.

2 Botwinick (J.): Aging and behavior. New York: Springer Publishing Company, 1973, 94-119.

3 Crook (Th.): Psychometric assessment in the aged. In: Raskin (A), Jarvik (L.). Eds.: "Psychopathology and cognitive loss in elderly: Assessment techniques and analyses". New York: Hemisphere Publishing Corporation, 1979.

4 Crook (Th.), Ferris (S.), Mac Carthy (M.): The Misplaced objects task. A brief test for memory dysfunction in the aged. *Journal of the American Geriatrics Society*, 1979, vol. XXVII. n°. 6, 284-287.

5 Crook (Th.), Ferris (S.), Mac Carthy (M.), Rae (D.): Utility of digit recall tasks for assessing memory in the aged. *Journal of Consulting and Clinical Psychology*, 1980, vol. 48, n°. 2, 228-233.

6 Crook (Th.), Ferris (S.), Sathananthan (G.) et al.: The Effect of methylphenidate on test performance in the cognitively impaired aged. *Psychopharmacology*, 1977, 52, 251.

7 Erickson (R.C.), Scott (M.L.): Clinical memory testing. *Psychol. Bull.* 1977., 84, 1130.

8 Ferris (S.), Crook (Th.), Clark (E.), Mac Carthy (M.), Rae (D.): Facial recognition memory deficits in normal aging and senile dementia. *Journal of Gerontology*, 1980, vol. 35, n°. 5, 707-714.

9 Gilbert (J.G.), Levee (R.F.), Catalano (F.L.): A Preliminary report on a new memory scale. *Perceptual and Motor Skills*, 1968, 27, 277.

10 Hulicka (I.M.): Age differences in retention as a function of interference. *J. Gerontol.*, 1967, 2, 1980.

11 Hulicka (I.M.), Weiss (R.L.): Age differences in retention as a function of learning. *J. Consult. Psychol.*, 1965, 29, 125.

12 Lezak (M.D.): Neuropsychological assessment. New York: Oxford University Press, 1976, 344-391.

13 Monge (R.H.), Hultsch (D.): Paired-associate learning as a function of adult age and the lenght of the anticipation and inspection intervals. *J. Gerontol.*, 1971, 26, 157.

14 Raskin (A.), Gershon (S.), Crook (Th.) et al.: The effects of hyperbaric and normobaric oxygen on cognitive impairment in the elderly. *Arch. Gen. Psychiat.*, 1978, 35, 50.

15 Shmavonian (B.M.), Busse (E.W.): The utilization of psychophysiological techniques in the study of the aged. In: Williams (R.H.), Tibbitts (C.), Donahue (W.) Eds: "The process of aging: social and psychological perspectives". New York: Atherton Press, 1963, 160-183.

EXTENDED SCALE FOR DEMENTIA (E.S.D.)

SPECIFICITY

| * | * | * |

TYPE OF INSTRUMENT

Test, 23 sub-tests

REFERENCE	Hersch (E.L.) · – Development and application of the extended scale for dementia. *Journal of the American Geriatrics Society,* 1979, XXVII, 8, 348-354.

Language: Original version published in English.
Canada

Location: Enclosed in volume two page 26
See ref. biblio n̠ 5

For all information concerning the instrument write to the author at the following address:

Edwin Hersch,
London Psychiatric Hospital, Dpt of Education and Research
850 Highbury Avenue
London, Ontario N6A 4H1, Canada

ORIGIN	This instrument was derived from the Mattis Dementia Scale (ref. 3) and the WAIS (ref. 14).
PURPOSE	This instrument was devised to evaluate the degree of dementia and to follow its course both in clinical work and in research.
POPULATION	Demented elderly in or out-patients (especially senile dementia and Alzheimer's disease).
ADMINISTRATION	*Rater:* Psychologist. *Time required:* Approximately one hour. *Training:* One training session necessary.
DESCRIPTION	The test consists of 23 sub-tests, verbal and performance:

1. Responding to commands
2. Digit Span
3. Naming of objects
4. Repetition of syllables
5. Alternating movements
6. Graphomotor activity
7. Cubes
8. Similarities
9. Differences
10. Similarities (multiple choice)
11. Similarities and differences
12. 13. 14. 15. Orientation
16. Information
17. 18. 19. 20. Calculation
21. Assessment of associations
22. 23. Verbal applied memory

The number of items and the score vary depending on the sub-test. The maximum score is 250 points. The lower the score the higher the degree of dementia. An average score in demented subjects is 100 points.

VARIABLES	Cognitive aspects such as: verbal, visual, memory, attention-concentration, and other cognitive skills.
VALIDATION	Carried out on a population of demented hospitalized subjects: **Factor analysis:** only one factor emerges which accounts for a large part of total variance. **Concurrent validity:** correlation with the sub-scale "Confusion - Mental disorganisation" of the "London Psychogeriatric Rating Scale" (ref. 6, 7). **Discriminative sensitivity:** between high and low scores, non-demented subjects. **Reliability:** internal consistency and test-retest reliability at six-week and six-month intervals.
OTHER WORKS cited by author	Research into correlation between test results and E.E.G. or scanner.
APPLICATION	**Clinical:** The test may be used for diagnosis and assessment of functioning, but most of all to follow-up a patient's change over time. **Research:** Drug trials, research in dementia care programmes.

1 Blessed (G.), Tomlinson (B.E.), Roth (M.): The association between quantitative measures of dementia and of senile change in the cerebral grey matter of elderly subjects. *Brit. J. Psychiat.*, 1968, 114, 797.

2 Britton (P.G.), Savage (R.D.): A short form of the WAIS for use with the aged. *Brit. J. Psychiat.*, 1966, 112, 417.

3 Coblentz (J.M.), Mattis (S.), Zingesser (H.) et al.: Presenile dementia. *Arch. Neurol.*, 1973, 29, 299.

4 Fishback (D.B.): Mental status questionnaire for organic brain syndrome, with a new visual counting test. *J. Am. Geriatrics Soc.*, 1977, 25, 167.

5 Hersch (E.L.): Development and application of the extended scale for dementia. *Journal of the American Geriatrics Society*, 1979, vol. XXVII, n°. 8, 348-354.

6 Hersch (E.L.), Csapo (K.G.), Palmer (R.B.): Development of the London psychogeriatric rating scale. *London Psychiat. Hosp. Res. Bull.*, 1978, 1, 3-21.

7 Hersch (E.L.), Kral (V.A.), Palmer (R.B.): Clinical value of the London psychogeriatric rating scale. *Journal of the American Geriatrics Society*, 1978, 26, 348-354.

8 Hie (N.H.), Hull (C.E.), Jenkins (J.G.) et al.: Statistical package for the social sciences. New York: Mc Graw Hill, 1970.

9 Inglis (J.L.): A paired-associate learning test for use with elderly patients. *J. Mental Sci.*, 1959, 105, 440.

10 Kahn (R.L.), Goldfarb (A.I.), Pollack (M.) et al.: Brief objective measures for the determination of mental status in the aged. *Am. J. Psychiat*, 1960, 117, 326.

11 Klingner (A.), Kachanoff (R.), Dastoor (D.P.) et al: A psychogeriatric assessment program. III: Clinical and experimental psychological aspects. *Journal of the American Geriatrics Society*, 1976, 24, 17.

12 Pfeiffer (E.): A short portable mental status questionnaire for the assessment of organic brain deficit in elderly patients. *Journal of the American Geriatrics Society*, 1975, 23, 433.

13 Qureshi (K.N.), Hodkinson (H.M.): Evaluation of a ten-question mental test in the institutionalized elderly. *Age and Ageing*, 1974, 3, 152.

14 Wechsler (D.): Manual for the Wechsler adult intelligence scale. New York: Psychological Corporation, 1955.

KENDRICK BATTERY FOR THE DETECTION OF DEMENTIA IN THE ELDERLY

SPECIFICITY

* * *

TYPE OF INSTRUMENT

Psychometric test
2 sub-tests

REFERENCE	**Kendrick (D.C.), Gibson (A.J.), Moyes (I.C.A.)** · – The revised Kendrick battery: clinical studies. *British Journal of Social and Clinical Psychology,* 1979, 18, 329-340.

Language: Original version published in English. Translated into Spanish.
Great Britain

Location: Enclosed in volume two page 27
See ref. biblio nº 14

For all information concerning the instrument or translation, write to the editor at the following address:

NFER-Nelson Publishing Company Ltd
Darville House
2, Oxford Road East
Windsor, Berkshire SL4 1DF, Great Britain

ORIGIN — Derived from the "Synonym Learning Test" (ref. 7), itself inspired by the Walton Black Test (ref. 22).

PURPOSE — Instrument was developed to screen and assess the course of dementia and at the same time to differentiate it from pseudo-dementia and from depression.

POPULATION — Depressed and demented persons above 55 years of age, living in institution or out-patients.

ADMINISTRATION — *Rater:* General practitioner, psychologist, nurse, social worker and speech therapist.
Time required: 15 minutes.
Training: Half-a-day with regular refresher courses.

DESCRIPTION — This battery is composed of 2 tests:
Object learning: Subject is presented with four cards of different size and content. The four cards contain respectively 10, 15, 20 and 25 objects, 70 in total. Time of presentation is 3 seconds per card.
Digit copying: Numbers in random order and arranged in 10 lines and 10 columns.
There are parallel forms for retesting every subject in order to avoid practice or learning effects. In the first test, one point is given for every correct answer. The total of raw scores is then transformed into a quotient. Scoring in the second test takes into account the correct number and time. Reference is made to tables published in the manual which may be obtained from the above mentioned publisher.

VARIABLES — Short term visual memory. Speed of processing simple information.

VALIDATION — On different populations of the elderly, in good health or suffering from psychiatric or organic disorders, inpatients or out-patients, (ref. 14):
External validity in respect to clinical diagnosis.
Construct validity: factor analyses.
Discriminative sensitivity between healthy subjects and those depressed and demented, in 2 test administrations at a six-week interval, after anti-depressant neuroleptic and electro-convulsant treatment.
Predictive validity for treatment effects.
Reliability: test-retest at 24 hour interval with parallel forms of the objects learning sub-test.
Standardization was carried out (ref. 2).

OTHER WORKS cited by author — Clinical work and research.

APPLICATION — **Clinical:** Diagnosis and prognosis.
Research: Drug trials and, more precisely, assessment of treatment side effects.
Evaluation of cognitive functioning and changes over time within neurological disorders of the C.V.A. type. Screening of population for dementia.

1 Gibson (A.J.), Kendrick (D.C.): The development of a visual learning test to replace the SLT in the Kendrick Battery. *Bulletin of the British Psychological Society*, 1976, 29, 200-201 (Abstract).

2 Gibson (A.J.), Kendrick (D.C.): The Kendrick Battery for the detection of dementia in the elderly. Windsor: NFER Publishing Company; New York: Psychological Corporation, 1979.

3 Gibson (A.J.), Moyes (I.C.A.), Kendrick (D.C.): Cognitive assessment of the elderly long-stay patient. *Brit. J. Psychiat.*, 1980, 137, 551-557.

4 Irving (G.), Robinson (R.A.), McAdam (W.): The validity of some cognitive tests of dementia. *British Journal of Psychiatry*, 1970, 117, 149-156.

5 Kendrick (D.C.): The Assessment of pre-morbid level of intelligence in the elderly patients suffering from diffuse brain pathology. *Psychol. Rep.*, 1964, 15, 88.

6 Kendrick (D.C.): Speed and learning in the diagnosis of diffuse brain – damage in elderly subjects: a Bayesian statistical analysis. *Brit. J. soc. clin. Psychol.*, 1965, 4, 141-148.

7 Kendrick (D.C.): A Cross-validation study of the use of SLT and DCT in screening for diffuse brain pathology in elderly subjects. *Brit. J. Med. Psychol.*, 1967, 40, 173-178.

8 Kendrick (D.C.): The Problem of differentiating dementia from normal ageing and depression. In: Clarke (P.R.F.) Ed: "The Nature and consequences of brain lesions in children and adults". London: BPS Publication, 1968, 28-34.

9 Kendrick (D.C.): The Kendrick Battery of tests: Theoretical assumptions and clinical uses. *Brit. J. soc. clin. Psychol.*, 1972, 11, 373-386.

10 Kendrick (D.C.): Why assess the aged? A Clinical psychologist's view. *Brit. J. Clin. Psychol.*, 1982, 21, 47-54.

11 Kendrick (D.C.): Psychometrics and neurological models: A Reply to Dr Rabbitt: *Brit. J. Clin. Psychol.*, 1982, 21, 61-62.

12 Kendrick (D.C.): Administrative and interpretive problems with the Kendrick Battery for the detection of dementia in the elderly. *Brit. J. Clin. Psychol.*, 1982, 21, 149-150.

13 Kendrick (D.C.), Gibson (A.J.), Moyes (I.C.A.): The Kendrick Battery: Mark II. *Bulletin of the British Psychological Society*, 1978, 31, 177-178.

14 Kendrick (D.C.), Gibson (A.J.), Moyes (I.C.A.): The Revised Kendrick Battery: Clinical studies. *Brit. J. soc. Clin. Psychol.*, 1979, 18, 329-339.

15 Kendrick (D.C.), Moyes (I.C.A.): Activity, depression, medication and performance on the Revised Kendrick Battery. *Brit. J. Soc. Clin. Psychol.*, 1979, 18, 341-350.

16 Kendrick (D.C.), Parboosingh (R.C.), Post (F.): A Synonym learning test for use with elderly psychiatric subjects: a validation study. *Brit. J. Soc. clin. Psychol.*, 1965, 4, 63-71.

17 Kendrick (D.C.), Post (F.): Differences in cognitive status between healthy, psychiatrically ill and diffusely brain-damaged subjects. *Brit. J. Psychiat.*, 1967, 113, 75-81.

18 Maxwell (A.E.): Analysing qualitative data. London: Methuen, 1961.

19 Minghella (Y): 40 Years of ECT. Unpublished Master's Thesis. University of Leeds: Department of Psychiatry Library, 1978.

20 Registrar's Classification of Occupation. London: HMSO, 1970.

21 Tucker (L.H.): A Method for synthesis of factor analytic studies. Dept. of the Army. A.C.O. Personnel Res., Sec. Rep. n°. 984, 1951.

22 Walton (D.), White (J.G.), Black (D.A.), Young (A.S.). The Modified word learning test: a cross validation study. *Brit. J. med. Psychol.*, 1959, 33, 213-220.

GALVESTON ORIENTATION AND AMNESIA TEST (G.O.A.T.)

SPECIFICITY

*	*

TYPE OF INSTRUMENT

Questionnaire
10 items

REFERENCE	**Levin (H.S.), O'Donnell (V.M.), Grossman (R.G.)** · – The Galveston orientation and amnesia test: a practical scale to assess cognition after head injury. *The Journal of Nervous and Mental Disease,* 1979, vol. 167, n⁰ 11, 675-684.
	Language: Original version published in English. **U.S.A.**
	Location: Enclosed in volume two page 53 See ref. biblio n⁰ 22
	For all information concerning the instrument write to the author at the following address:
	Harvey Levin, University of Texas, Medical Branch Division of Neurosurgery Galveston, Texas 77550, U.S.A.

ORIGIN	This instrument was inspired by the previous work of **Pattie** (ref. 26, 27), **Withers** (ref. 35), **Jacobs** (ref. 11), **Libow** (ref. 23), **Plutchik** (ref. 29), **Blessed, Tomlinson** and **Roth** (ref. 4), **Kay** (ref. 19), **Kahn** (ref. 16, 17, 18), **Wilson** (ref. 34), **Folstein** (ref. 8), **Irving** (ref. 10), and **Pfeiffer** (ref. 28).
PURPOSE	Evaluation of cognitive functions during the early stages of recovery after head trauma.
POPULATION	Adults who had sustained head injuries of varying severity, hospitalized and ambulatory. The test was standardized in young adults who had recovered to a normal level of consciousness after a mild head injury.
ADMINISTRATION	*Rater:* Physician, psychologist, nurse. *Time required:* 5 minutes. *Training:* Familiarization with the questionnaire and uniform scoring method. *Scoring:* Varies from 0 to 10 error points on items 1 through 5 and from 1 to 30 on items 6 through 10. The total GOAT score, which is obtained by deducting the sum error points from 100, is an index of the severity of amnesia and disorientation.
VARIABLES	· Temporal orientation · Geographic orientation · Memory for recent events · Anterograde and retrograde amnesia
VALIDATION	Serial administration to 52 young adults with head injuries of varying severity who were evaluated by the Glasgow Coma Scale and computed tomographic scanning during hospitalization. The prognostic significance of scores was evaluated by assessing the outcome (Glasgow Outcome Scale) of 32 of these patients at least 6 months post-injury. The results (ref. 22) showed: **Concurrent validity** with the "Glasgow Coma Scale" and in relation to computed tomographic findings; duration of disorientation and amnesia was longer in patients with bilateral mass lesions or diffuse brain injury as compared to unilateral mass lesions. **Predictive validity** with respect to prognosis, outcome and recovery at least 6 months after injury. High **inter-rater reliability**.
OTHER WORKS cited by author	The instrument was employed in a study of the initial impairment and long term outcome of severe head injuries entered in the pilot phase of the "Coma Data Bank Network" supported by the National Institutes of Health in the United States. The test was also employed in a collaborative study of recovery from mild head injury which was completed at the Comprehensive Central Nervous System Injury Trauma Centers funded by the National Institutes of Health. Administration during hospitalization disclosed similar scores in mild head injures treated in California, New York and Texas. With slight modification the test can also be administered to patients with degenerative dementia.
APPLICATION	**Clinical:** Prognostic information and effects of treatment.

1 Benson (D.F.), Gardner (H.), Meadows (J.C.): Reduplicative paramnesia, *Neurology*, 1967, 26, 147-151.

2 Benson (D.F.), Geschwind (N.): Shrinking retrograde amnesia. *J. Neurol. Neurosurg. Psychiat.*, 1967, 30, 539-544.

3 Benton (A.L.), Van Allen (M.W.), Fogel (M.L.): Temporal orientation in cerebral disease. *J. Nerv. Ment. Dis.*, 1964, 139, 110-119.

4 Blessed (G.), Tomlinson (B.E.), Roth (M.): The association between quantitative measures of dementia and of senile change in the cerebral grey matter of elderly subjects. *Br. J. Psychiatry*, 1968, 114, 797-811.

5 Denny-Brown (D.): Disability arising from closed head injury. *J.A.M.A.*, 1945, 127, 429-436.

6 Field (J.H.A.): A study of the epidemiology of head injury in England and Wales. London: Department of Health and Social Security, 1976.

7 Fisher (C.M.): Concussion amnesia. *Neurology*, 1966, 16, 826-830.

8 Folstein (M.F.), Folstein (S.E.), Mc Hugh (P.R.): "Mini-Mental State": a practical method for grading the cognitive state of patients for the clinician. *J. Psychiat. Res.*, 1975, 12, 189-198.

9 Haglund (R.M.J.), Schuckit (M.A.): A clinical comparison of tests of organicity in elderly patients. *J. Gerontol.*, 1976, 31, 654-659.

10 Irving (G.), Robinson (R.A.), Mc Adam (W.): The validity of some cognitive tests in the diagnosis of dementia. *Br. J. Psychiatry*, 1970, 117, 149-156.

11 Jacobs (J.W.), Bernhard (M.R.), Delgado (A.), Strain (J.J.): Screening for organic mental syndromes in the medically ill. *Ann. Intern. Med.*, 1977, 86, 40-46.

12 Jennett (B.): Assessment of the severity of head injury. *J. Neurol. Neurosurg. Psychiatry*, 1976, 39, 647-655.

13 Jennett (B.), Bond (M.): Assessment of outcome after severe brain damage. *Lancet*, 1975, 1, 480-487.

14 Jennett (B.), Teasdale (G.), Braakman (R.) et al.: Predicting outcome in individual patients after severe head injury. *Lancet*, 1976, 1, 1031-1034.

15 Jennett (B.), Teasdale (G.) Galbraith (S.) et al.: Severe head injuries in three countries. *J. Neurol. Neurosurg. Psychiatry*, 1977, 40, 291-298.

16 Kahn (R.L.), Goldfarb (A.I.), Pollack (M.), Peck (A.): Brief objective measures for the determination of mental status in the aged. *Am. J. Psychiatry*, 1960, 117, 326-328.

17 Kahn (R.L.), Miller (N.E.): Assessment of altered brain function in the aged. In: Storandt (M.), Siegler (I.C.), Elias (M.F.) Eds.: "The clinical psychology of aging". New-York: Plenum Publishing Corp., 1977.

18 Kahn (R.L.), Zarit (S.H.), Hilbert (N.M.), Niederehe (G.): Memory complaint and impairment in the aged. *Arch. Gen. Psychiatry*, 1975, 32, 1569-1573.

19 Kay (D.W.K.): The Epidemiology, and identification of brain deficit in the elderly. In: Eisdorfer (C.), Friedel (R.O.). Eds.: "Cognitive and emotional disturbance in the elderly". Chicago: Year Book Medical Publishers, Inc., 1977.

20 Levin (H.S.), Benton (A.L.): Temporal orientation in patients with brain disease. *Appl. Neurophysiol.*, 1975, 35, 56-60.

21 Levin (H.S.), Grossman (R.G.): Behavioral sequelae of closed head injury: a quantitative study. *Arch. Neurol.*, 1978, 35, 720-727.

22 Levin (H.S.), O'Donnell (V.M.), Grossman (R.G.): The Galveston orientation and amnesia test: a practical scale to assess cognition after head injury. *The Journal of Nervous and Mental Disease*, 1979, vol. 167, n°. 11, 675-684.

23 Libow (L.S.): Senile dementia and "pseudosenility": clinical diagnosis. In: Eisdorfer (C.), Friedel (R.O.), Eds.: "Cognitive and emotional disturbance in the elderly". Chicago: Year Book Medical Publishers, Inc, 1977.

24 Mc Hugh (P.R.), Folstein (M.F.): Psychopathology of dementia: implications for neuropathology. In: Katzman (R.) Ed.: "Congenital and acquired cognitive disorders". New-York: Raven Press, 1979.

25 Overgaard (J.), Hvid-Hansen (O.), Lane (A.M.) et al: Prognosis after head injury based on early clinical examination. *Lancet*, 1973, 2, 631-635.

26 Pattie (A.H.), Gilleard (C.J.): The Clifton assessment schedule. Further validation of a psychogeriatric assessment schedule. *Br. J. Psychiatry*, 1976, 129, 68-72.

27 Pattie (A.H.), Gilleard (C.J.): The two-year predictive validity of the Clifton assessment schedule and the shortened Stockton geriatric rating scale. *Br. J. Psychiatry*, 1978, 133, 457-460.

28 Pfeiffer (E.Λ.): Short portable mental status questionnaire for the assessment of organic brain deficit in elderly patients. *J. Am. Geriatr. Soc.*, 1975, 23, 433-439.

29 Plutchik (R.), Conte (H.), Lieberman (M.): Development of a scale (GIES) for assessment of cognitive and perceptual functioning in geriatric patients. *J. Am. Geriatr. Soc,*, 1971, 19, 614-623.

30 Russell (W.R.): The traumatic amnesias. London: Oxford University Press, 1971.

31 Salzman (C.), Kochansky (G.E.), Shader (R.I.): Rating scales for geriatric psychopharmacology. A review. *Psychopharmacol. Bull.*, 1972, 8, 3-50.

32 Teasdale (G.), Jennett (B.): Assessment of coma and impaired consciousness: a practical scale. *Lancet*, 1974, 2, 81-84.

33 Von Wowern (F.): Post-traumatic amnesia and confusion as an index of severity in head injury. *Acta Neurol. Scand.*, 1966, 42, 373-378.

34 Wilson (L.A.), Brass (W.): Brief assessment of the mental state in geriatric domiciliary practice. The usefulness of the mental status questionnaire. *Age and Ageing*, 1973, 2, 92-101.

35 Withers (E.), Hinton (J.): Three forms of the clinical tests of the sensorium and their reliability. *Br. J. Psychiatry*, 1971, 119, 1-8.

CHECK LIST DIFFERENTIATING PSEUDO-DEMENTIA FROM DEMENTIA

SPECIFICITY

* *

TYPE OF INSTRUMENT

Check - list
22 items

REFERENCE	**Wells (C.E.)** · – Pseudo-dementia. *American Journal of Psychiatry,* 1979, 136, 7, 895-900.

Language: Published in English. Translated into French.
U.S.A.

Location: Enclosed in volume two page 82
See ref. biblio nº 20

For all information concerning the instrument write to the author at the following address:

Charles Wells,
Department of Psychiatry
Vanderbilt University
School of Medicine
Nashville, Tennessee 37232, U.S.A.

ORIGIN

This is an original instrument based on clinical observations of patients with a diagnosis of dementia.

PURPOSE

To make a clinical differentiation of pseudo-dementia from dementia.

POPULATION

Hospitalized patients manifesting dementia type symptoms.

ADMINISTRATION

Rater: Physician.

Time required: 15 minutes.

Training: Neurological training necessary.

Scoring: Yes or no for every item.

VARIABLES

· Clinical course and history
· Complaints and clinical behavior
· Clinical assessment of mental capacities.

VALIDATION

On a group of hospitalized patients (ref. 21):
Concurrent validity with a psychometric test battery and with scanner and E.E.G. results.
External validity in respect of diagnosis, and predictive in respect of evolution.

APPLICATION

This instrument is for clinical use only, allowing separation of dementia from pseudo-dementia. It also enables constitution of homogeneous groups of patients for all types of studies (inclusion in drug trials, in exploitation of epidemiological findings, etc.).

1 American Psychiatric Association: Diagnostic and statistical manual of mental disorders. 2nd ed. Washington, DC: APA, 1968.

2 Duckworth (G.S.), Ross (H.): Diagnostic differences in psychogeriatric patients in Toronto, New York and London. *Can. Med. Assoc. J.*, 1975, 112, 847-851.

3 Folstein (M.F.), Folstein (S.E.), Mc Hugh (P.R.): «Mini-Mental State»: A practical method for grading the cognitive state of patients for the clinician. *J. Psychiat. Res.*, 1975, 12, 189-198.

4 Haward (L.R.C.): Cognition in dementia presenilis. In: Smith (W.L.), Kinsbourne (M.) Eds: "Aging and dementia". New York: Spectrum Publications, 1977.

5 Kiloh (L.G.): Pseudo-dementia. *Acta Psychiat. Scand.*, 1961, 37, 336-351.

6 Liston (E.H., Jr.): Occult presenile dementia *J. Nerv. Ment. Dis.*, 1977, 164, 263-267.

7 Marsden (C.D.), Harrison (M.J.G.): Outcome of investigation of patients with presenile dementia. *Brit. Med. J.*, 1972, 2, 249-252.

8 Mercer (B.), Wapner (W.), Gardner (H.) et al.: A study of confabulation. *Arch. Neurol.*, 1977, 34, 429-433.

9 Nott (P.N.), Fleminger (J.J.): Presenile dementia: the difficulties of early diagnosis. *Acta Psychiat. Scand.*, 1975, 51, 210-217.

10 Post (F.): Dementia, depression and pseudodementia. In: Benson (D.F.), Blumer (D.). Eds: "Psychiatric aspects of neurologic disease". New York: Grune and Stratton, 1975.

11 Rhoads (J.M.): Overwork *J.A.M.A.*, 1977, 237, 2615-2618.

12 Roth (M.): The natural history of mental disorder in old age. *J. Ment. Sci.*, 1955, 101, 281-301.

13 Roth (M.): Mental disorders of the aged: diagnosis and treatment. *Medical World News*, oct. 27, 1975, 35-43.

14 Roth (M.), Myers (D.H.): The diagnosis of dementia. *Br. J. Psychiatry*, special publication 9, 1975, 87-99.

15 Shraberg (D.): The myth of pseudodementia: depression and the aging brain. *Am. J. Psychiatry*, 1978, 135, 601-603.

16 Tomlinson (B.E.), Blessed (G.), Roth (M.): Observations on the brains of non-demented old people. *J. Neurol. Sci.*, 1968, 7, 331-356.

17 Tomlinson (B.E.), Blessed (G.), Roth (M.): Observations on the brains of demented old people. *J. Neurol. Sci.*, 1970, 11, 205-242.

18 Ward (N.G.), Rowlett (D.B.), Burke (P.): Sodium amylobarbitone in the differential diagnosis of confusion. *Am. J. Psychiatry*, 1978, 135, 75-78.

19 Wells (C.E.): Dementia, pseudodementia, and dementia praecox. In: Fann (W.E.), Karacan (J.), Pokorny (A.D.), et al. Eds: "Phenomenology and treatment of schizophrenia": New York: Spectrum Publications, 1977.

20 Wells (C.E.): Pseudodementia. *Am. J. Psychiatry*, 1979, 136, 7, 895-900.

21 Wells (C.E.), Buchanan (B.C.): The clinical use of psychological testing in evaluation in dementia. In: Wells (C.E.) Ed. "Dementia". 2nd ed. Philadephia, PA: Davis Co, 1977.

22 Wells (C.E.), Duncan (G.W.): Danger of overreliance on computerized cranial tomography. *Am. J. Psychiatry*, 1977, 134, 811-813.

ORIENTATION SCALE FOR GERIATRIC PATIENTS

SPECIFICITY

* * *

TYPE OF INSTRUMENT

Questionnaire
10 questions

REFERENCE	**Berg (S.), Svensson (T.)** · – An orientation scale for geriatric patients. *Age and Ageing,* 1980, nº 9, 215-219.

> *Language:* Original version published in Swedish. Translated into English
> **Sweden**
>
> *Location:* English version enclosed in volume two page 54
> See ref. biblio nº 1
>
> *For all information concerning the instrument and the translation, write to the author at the following address:*
>
> Stig Berg,
> Institute of Gerontology
> Brunnsgatan 30
> S-552 55 Jönköping, Sweden

ORIGIN
The orientation scale is inspired by the works of **Kahn et al** (ref. 3), **Lifshitz** (ref. 4), **Pfeiffer** (ref. 5), **Qureshi et al** (ref. 6), **Shapiro et al** (ref. 9), **Roth** (ref. 8), **Stonier** (ref. 10). It consists of 10 questions and is constructed from an initial 20 questions after a factor analysis.

PURPOSE
The scale is intended for geriatric patients and patients suffering from psychogeriatric disorders. The scale differentiates between patients with diagnoses of multi-infarct dementia and dementia of Alzheimer's type and those with no such disorders.

POPULATION
Geriatric and psychogeriatric patients institutionalized for at least 14 days.

ADMINISTRATION
Rater: Physician, nurse, occupational therapist, psychologist.

Time required: 5 minutes.

Training: Not necessary.

Scoring: Correct response gives one point and incorrect no points. A few incorrect responses do not necessarily signify that the subject is disoriented.

VARIABLES
Orientation to time, place and person.

VALIDATION
Was carried out on a geriatric and a psychogeriatric population (ref. 1):
Test-retest reliability and homogeneity.
A factor analysis distinguished a first factor which explained 37% of the total variance.

APPLICATION
Clinical: diagnostic, prognostic.
Research: effects of various therapies.

Ib.37

1 Berg (S.), Svensson (T.): An orientation scale for geriatric patients. *Age and Ageing*, 1980, 9, 215-219.

2 Harman (H.H.): Modern factor analysis. Chicago: University of Chicago Press, 1967.

3 Kahn (R.L.), Goldfarb (A.I.), Pollack (M.), Peck (A.): Brief objective measures for the determination of mental status in the aged. *Am. J. Psychiat.*, 1960, 117, 326-328.

4 Lifshitz (K.): Problems in the quantitative evaluation of patients with psychoses of the senium. *J. Psychol.*, 1960, 49, 295-303.

5 Pfeiffer (E.A.): A Short portable mental status questionnaire for the assessment of organic brain deficit in elderly patients. *J. Am. Geriatrics Soc.*, 1975, 23, 433-441.

6 Qureshi (K.N.), Hodkinson (H.M.): Evaluation of a ten-question mental test in the institutionalized elderly. *Age and Ageing*, 1974, 3, 152-157.

7 Robinson (R.A.): Some problems of clinical trials in elderly people. *Gerontol. Clin.*, 1961, 3, 247-257.

8 Roth (M.), Hopkins (B.): Psychological test performance in patients over 60. I: Senile psychosis and affective disorders of old age. *J. ment. Sci.*, 1953, 99, 439-450.

9 Shapiro (M.B.), Post (F.), Löfving (B.), Inglis (J.): Memory function in psychiatric patients over sixty; some methodological and diagnostic implications. *J. Ment. Sci.*, 1956, 102, 233-246.

10 Stonier (P.D.): Score changes following repeated administration of mental status questionnaire. *Age and Ageing*, 1974, 3, 91-96.

HIERARCHIC DEMENTIA SCALE

SPECIFICITY

| * * * |

TYPE OF INSTRUMENT

Nominal rating scale,
20 sub-scales,
5-10 items each

REFERENCE	**Cole (M.G.), Dastoor (D.)** · – Development of a dementia rating scale: Preliminary communication. *Journal of Clinical and Experimental Gerontology,* 1980, 2, nº 1, 49-63.

Language: Original version published in English.
Canada

Location: Enclosed in volume two page 186
See ref. biblio nº 7

For all information concerning the instrument write to the author at the following address:

Martin G. Cole,
Psychogeriatric Clinic
St. Mary's Hospital,
3830 Avenue Lacombe
Montréal, Québec, H3T 1M5, Canada

ORIGIN
Instrument inspired by neuropsychological and neurological works of: **Luria** (ref. 14), **Constandinides** (ref. 8) and **De Ajuriaguerra** (ref. 1, 8) of the Geneva School, based on the theory of hierarchical stages of cognitive development.

PURPOSE
To measure the intensity and the severity of dementia for clinical and research purposes.

POPULATION
All categories of dementia.

ADMINISTRATION
Rater: Physician, psychologist, nurse.

Time required: 15-30 minutes.

Training: From 5 to 10 hours, depending on the previous training of the examiner.

Scoring: Items are arranged in order of increasing difficulty. One point is awarded for each correct response in the 10 item scales, and two points each in the 5 item scales. It is possible to score both very severe and very mild dementia.

VARIABLES

· Motricity
· Orienting behaviour
· Prefrontal signs
· Disorientation
· Registration
· Recent memory
· Remote memory
· Verbal and written comprehension
· Concentration
· Denomination

· Ideomotor praxis
· Writing
· Graphic praxis
· Reading
· Constructive praxis
· Gnosis
· Ideational praxis
· Looking behaviour
· Calculations
· Similarities

VALIDATION
Studies of **concurrent validity**, test-retest **reliability** and inter-rater reliability carried out on a population of demented patients (multi-infarct dementia and Alzheimer's dementia), using the "Crichton Geriatric Behavioural Rating Scale" and the Blessed Dementia Scale (ref. 7, 18).

APPLICATION
Clinical: contribution to diagnosis and management.
Research: therapeutic trials, prognostic studies.

1 Ajuriaguerra (J. de), Rey Bellet-Muller (M.), Tissot (R.): A propos de quelques problèmes posés par le déficit opératoire de vieillards atteints de démence dégénérative en début d'évolution. *Cortex*, 1964, 1, 103-132.

2 Blessed (G.), Tomlinson (B.E.), Roth (M.): The association between quantitative measures of dementia and of senile change in the cerebral grey matter of elderly subjects. *Brit. J. Psychiat.*, 1968, 114, 797-811.

3 Brun (A), Gustafson (L.): Distribution of cerebral degeneration in Alzheimer's disease: a clinico-pathological study. *Arch. Psychiatr. Nervenkr.*, 1976, 223, 15.

4 Cole (M.G.), Dastoor (D.): Development of a dementia rating scale: I: Some considerations. Proceedings of the 5 th Annual Meeting of the Ontario Psychogeriatric Association, September 1978.

5 Cole (M.G.), Dastoor (D.): Development of a dementia rating scale. II: Determination of hierarchies of function. Proceedings of the 6th Annual Meeting of the Ontario Psychogeriatric Association, September 1979.

6 Cole (M.G.), Dastoor (D.): Development of a dementia rating scale. III: More functional hierarchies. Proceedings of the 7th Annual Meeting of the Ontario Psychogeriatric Association, November 1980.

7 Cole (M.G.), Dastoor (D.): Development of a dementia rating scale. Preliminary communication. *Journal Clinical Experimental Gerontology*, 1980, vol. 2, n°. 1, 49-63.

8 Constantinidis (J.), Richard (J.), Ajuriaguerra (J. de): Dementias with senile plaques and neurofibrillary changes. In: Isaacs (A.D.), Post (F.). Eds: "Studies in Geriatric Psychiatry". London: J. Wiley, 1978.

9 Edwards (A.): On Guttman scale analysis. *Educ. Psychol. Measur.*, 1948, 8, 313.

10 Flavell (J.): The developmental psychology of Jean Piaget. New-York: Van Nostrand, 1963.

11 Goga (J.A.), Hambacher (W.O.): Psychologic and behavioural assessment of geriatric patients: a review. *Journal of the American Geriatrics Society*, 1977, vol. 25, 232.

12 Hubel (D.): The visual cortex of the brain. *Sci. Amer.*, 1963, 209, 54.

13 Lishman (W.A.): Senile and presenile dementias. A report of the MRC Subcommittee. Med. Research Council, 1977.

14 Luria (A.): Higher cortical functions in man. New-York: Basic Books, 1980.

15 Mattis (S.): Mental status examination for organic mental syndrome in the elderly patient. In: Bellak (R.). Ed: "Geriatric psychiatry". New-York: Grune and Stratton, 1976.

16 Perex (F.I.), Gay (J.R.A.), Cooke (N.A.): Neuropsychological aspects of Alzheimer's disease and multi-infarct dementia. In: Nandy (K): "Senile dementia: a biomedical approach". Elsevier North – Holland, Biomedical Press, 1978.

17 Report of the Task Panel on mental health of the elderly. Submitted to the President's commission on Mental Health, 1978.

18 Robinson (R.A.): Some problems of clinical trials in elderly people. *Geront. Clin.*, 1961, 3, 247-257.

BATTERIE DE VIGILANCE EN AMBULATOIRE
VIGILANCE BATTERY FOR OUT-PATIENTS

SPECIFICITY

$*\quad*\quad*$

TYPE OF INSTRUMENT

Psychometric test:
7 sub-tests

REFERENCE	**Israël (L.), Ohlmann (Th.), Chappaz (M.)** · − Batterie d'épreuves psychométriques pour personnes âgées ambulatoires. *Psychologie Médicale,* 1980, tome 12, n⁰ 3, 669-678.

Language: Published in French.
France

Location: Enclosed in volume two page 30
See ref. biblio n⁰ 6

For all information concerning the instrument write to the author at the following address:

Liliane Israël,
Pavillon Chissé, C.H.R.U.
38700 La Tronche
Grenoble, France

ORIGIN — This instrument was done as a parallel version to the Vigilance Battery for Inpatients (Ib. 25). The tests by which the author has been inspired are therefore the same (ref. 8, 9, 10, 11).

PURPOSE — This battery has been designed to assess the same factors as the "Vigilance Battery For Inpatients" but with a more difficult content.

POPULATION — Elderly over 65 years, living in the community.

ADMINISTRATION — *Rater:* Psychologist.

Time required: 15 to 20 minutes according to the subject's speed.

Training: Psychological training is necessary.

DESCRIPTION — Seven short and non-tiring tests

· **4 verbal tests**	· **3 graphic tests**
object ordering	coding
repetition of digits	crossing
memory recall	hole-punching
fluency	

Rating is established from the raw score which is adjusted either to a standard score or a factor score.

VARIABLES — The variables are presented as one general factor: Vigilance, and three group factors:
· Memory
· Fluency
· Psychomotor activities

VALIDATION — Has been investigated on elderly persons living in institutions (ref. 6).
Construct validity, factor analyses of principal components
Standardization (rating scales are normalized on 5 classes)

OTHER WORKS cited by author — Concurrent validity with E.A.C.G. (ref. 3) and two drug trials (ref. 4, 7).

APPLICATION — This instrument enables more precise measurement of individual changes particularly for clinical drug trials for studying efficiency. It can be used together with the "Vigilance Battery for Inpatients" for comparing efficiency of a drug on different populations.

1 Benton (A.L.): La signification des tests de rétention visuelle dans le diagnostic clinique. *Rev. Psych. Appl.*, 1952, 2, 151-179.

2 Israel (L.): Application des techniques psychométriques à l'étude des thérapeutiques à visée cérébrale en milieu gériatrique. Thèse doc. 3ᵉ cycle; UER de psycho; Grenoble, 1977, 157 p.

3 Israel (L.), Georges (D.), Lallemand (A.), Loria (Y.): Echelle d'appréciation clinique et tests psychométriques en gériatrie. Recherche de corrélations. *Thérapie*, 1979, n° 34, 585-590.

4 Israel (L.), Hugonot (R.), Ohlmann (Th.): Efficacité d'une vincamine en ambulatoire. Etude psychométrique en double aveugle. *Revue de Gériatrie*, octobre 1979, tome 4, n° 8, 429.

5 Israel (L.), Ohlmann (Th.): Mise au point et étalonnage d'une batterie d'épreuves psychométriques pour l'examen des personnes âgées. *Gerontology*, 1976, 22, 3, 141-156.

6 Israel (L.), Ohlmann (Th.), Chappaz (M.): Batterie d'épreuves psychométriques pour personnes âgées ambulatoires. *Psychologie Médicale*, 1980, tome 12, n° 3, 669-678.

7 Israel (L.), Ohlmann (Th.), Hugonot (R.): Etude comparative en double insu de l'efficacité d'un anabolisant tissulotrophique dans certaines manifestations du vieillissement cérébral. *Revue de Gériatrie*, mars 1980, tome 5, n° 2, 103-105.

8 Rey (A.): Les troubles de la mémoire et leur examen psychométrique. Bruxelles: Dessart, 1966.

9 Thurstone (L.L.): Primary mental abilities. Paris: Centre de Psychologie Appliquée, 1953.

10 Wechsler (D.): La Mesure de l'intelligence de l'adulte. 4ᵉ ed. Paris: P.U.F., 1973, 291 p.

11 Zazzo (R.): Le test des deux barrages. *Actualités pédagogiques et psychologiques*, 1964, vol. 7, 254.

ECHELLE CLINIQUE D'APTITUDES INTELLECTUELLES
CLINICAL INTELLECTUAL RATING SCALE

SPECIFICITY

* * *

TYPE OF INSTRUMENT

Ordinal rating scale,
9 items, 5 grades

REFERENCE	**Israël (L.), Ohlmann (Th.), Chappaz (M.)** · – Batterie psychométrique à l'usage du médecin généraliste pour apprécier les conduites intellectuelles des personnes âgées. *Psychologie Médicale,* 1980, tome 12, nº 4, 921-938.

Language: Original version published in French.
France

Location: Enclosed in volume two page 111
See ref. biblio nº 5

For all information concerning the instrument write to the author at the following address:

Liliane Israël,
Pavillon Chissé, C.H.R.U.
38700 La Tronche
Grenoble, France

ORIGIN
The items of this original scale have been defined after team discussions.

PURPOSE
It was designed for a quick evaluation of intellectual functioning of the elderly.

POPULATION
Elderly out-patients.

ADMINISTRATION
Rater: General practitioner or psychiatrist.
Time required: 5 minutes.
Training: Not necessary.
Scoring: Total score varies from 9 to 45. If it is less than 15 it is a pathological sign.

VARIABLES
The following variables are assessed:
· Vigilance
· Attention
· General vitality
· Verbal fluency

· Verbal expression
· Tiredness
· Orientation in space
· General memory
· Memory recall

VALIDATION
Factor analysis: 85% of explained variance (ref. 1, 6).
General factor (intellectual dynamism) correlated with memory, awareness and fluency.

OTHER WORKS
cited by author
Numerous drug trials done with general practitioners, a total of 1000 observations (ref. 4).

APPLICATION
Drug trials and clinical assessment.

Ib.40

1   Aubigny (G.), Israël (L.), Ohlmann (Th.): Comparabilité d'une batterie d'épreuves psychométriques et d'une échelle d'évaluation. Communication présentée à Hambourg au XIIe Congrès International de Gérontologie, juillet 1981.

2   Clément (F.): Une épreuve rapide de mesure de l'efficience intellectuelle. *Rev. Psych. Appl.*, 1963, 13, 1, 243-277.

3   Israël (L.), Hugonot (L.), Hugonot (R.): Problèmes posés par les essais médicamenteux effectués avec le concours de médecins praticiens. *Concours Médical*, 24 mars 1979, 101, 2, 2075-78.

4   Israël (L.), Hugonot (R.): Essais médicamenteux en médecine praticienne. Méthodologie et différentes étapes d'une étude nationale effectuée avec le concours de 166 généralistes. *Revue de Gériatrie*, juin 1981, tome 6, n° 6, 263-267.

5   Israël (L.), Ohlmann (Th.), Chappaz (M.): Batterie psychométrique à l'usage du médecin généraliste pour apprécier les conduites intellectuelles des personnes âgées. *Psychologie Médicale*, 1980, tome 12, n° 4, 921-938.

6   Ohlmann (Th.), Israël (L.), Aubigny (G.): Activités cognitives et variables sociobiologiques chez les personnes âgées ambulatoires. Communication présentée à Hambourg, au XIIe Congrès International de Gérontologie, juillet 1981.

7   Wechsler (D.): Echelle clinique de mémoire. Paris: Centre de Psychologie Appliquée, 1976.

8   Wittenborn (J.R.): Wittenborn Psychiatric Rating Scales. New York: Psychological Corporation, 1955.

BATTERIE DE FLUIDITE A L'USAGE DES GENERALISTES
FLUENCY BATTERY FOR GENERAL PRACTITIONERS

SPECIFICITY

* * *

TYPE OF INSTRUMENT

Psychometric test,
5 sub-tests

REFERENCE   Israël (L.), Ohlmann (Th.), Chappaz (M.) · – Batterie psychométrique à l'usage du médecin généraliste pour apprécier les conduites intellectuelles des personnes âgées. *Psychologie Médicale,* 1980, tome 12, nᵒ 4, 921-938.

Language: Published in French.
France

Location: Enclosed in volume two page 31
See ref. biblio nᵒ 7

For all information concerning the instrument write to the author at the following address:

Liliane Israël,
Pavillon Chissé, C.H.R.U.
38700 La Tronche
Grenoble, France

ORIGIN   A number of sub-tests are inspired by existing tests in the literature and adapted for the elderly (ref. 1, 2, 8, 9, 10, 11, 12, 13, 14). Others have been created by the author (ref. 6).

PURPOSE   This battery has been specially designed to be administered by general practitioners in out-patient clinics. It allows the assessment of effects of vasoactive drugs on intellectual fluency measured through associative speed and mental operations.

POPULATION   Elderly patients over 60 years living in the community consulting general practitioners.

ADMINISTRATION   *Rater:* Physician, psychologist, secretary, etc...
Time required: 15-25 minutes according to individual speed.
Training: 1 session of 2-3 hours.

DESCRIPTION   Five short and non-tiring tests
· matched pictures **(L. Israel)**   · mental control **(Wittenborn)**
· playing cards **(L. Israel)**   · letter and word fluency **(Thurstone)**
· perception **(Witkin)**
Rating is established from raw scores which are adjusted to standardized scores and factor scores.

VARIABLES   One general factor, fluency and 2 group factors: memory and attention.

VALIDATION   Was done on the out-patient population living at home or in residential institutions (ref. 7).
Construct validity (75% of explained variance)
Standardization by subgroups not yet published

OTHER WORKS cited by author   Three multicentre drug trials on 970 patients examined by 166 general practitioners (ref. 5).

APPLICATION   Drug trials, clinical examination (ref. 3).

1 Benton (A.L.): La signification des tests de rétention visuelle dans le diagnostic clinique. *Rev. Psychol. Appl.* 1952, 2, 151-179.

2 Clément (F.): Une épreuve rapide de mesure de l'efficience intellectuelle. *Rev. Psychol. Appl.*, 1963, 13, 1, 243-277.

3 Israel (L.): Application of psychometric techniques to the study of treatment affecting brain functioning. In: "Drugs studies in CVD and PVD": proceedings of the international symposium, Geneva, May 25-26 1981. Paris: Pergamon Press, 1982, 89-95.

4 Israel (L.), Hugonot (L.), Hugonot (R.): Problèmes posés par les essais médicamenteux effectués avec le concours de médecins praticiens. *Concours Médical*, 24 mars 1979, 101, 2, 2075-2078.

5 Israel (L.), Hugonot (R.): Essais médicamenteux en médecine praticienne. Méthodologie et différentes étapes d'une étude nationale effectuée avec le concours de 166 généralistes. *Revue de Gériatrie*, Juin 1981, tome 6, n° 6, 263-267.

6 Israel (L.), Ohlmann (Th.), Chappaz (M.): Batterie d'épreuves psychométriques pour personnes âgées ambulatoires. *Psychologie Médicale*, 1980, tome 12, n° 3.

7 Israel (L.), Ohlmann (Th.), Chappaz (M.): Batterie psychométrique à l'usage du médecin généraliste pour apprécier les conduites intellectuelles des personnes âgées. *Psychologie Médicale*, 1980, tome 12, n° 4, 921-938.

8 Lhermitte (J.), Signoret (J.L.): Analyse neuropsychologique et différenciation des syndromes amnésiques. *Revue Neurologique*, 1972, 126, 3, 161-177.

9 Rey (A.): Les troubles de la mémoire et leur examen psychométrique. Bruxelles: Dessart, 1966.

10 Thurstone (L.L.): Primary mental abilities. Paris: Centre de Psychologie Appliquée, 1953.

11 Wechsler (D.): Echelle clinique de mémoire. Paris: Centre de Psychologie Appliquée, 1976.

12 Witkin (H.A.), Oltman (P.K.), Cox (P.W.), Ehrlichman (E.), Hamm (R.M.), Rinaler (R.W.): Field dependence-independence and psychological differentiation, a bibliography through 1972. Princeton: E.T.S., 1973.

13 Wittenborn (J.R.): Wittenborn psychiatric rating scales. New York: Psychological Corporation, 1955.

14 Zazzo (R.): Le test des deux barrages. *Actualités pédagogiques et psychologiques*, 1964, vol. 7, 254.

BATTERIE DE MEMOIRE EN AMBULATOIRE
MEMORY BATTERY FOR OUT-PATIENTS

SPECIFICITY

* * *

TYPE OF INSTRUMENT

Psychometric test,
7 sub-tests

REFERENCE | **Israël (L.), Ohlmann (Th.)** · − Structure factorielle de la mémoire appréciée à travers une batterie d'épreuves psychologiques chez des personnes âgées ambulatoires: son application aux essais cliniques contrôlés. *Encéphale,* 1980, 6, 181-195.

Language: Published in French.
France

Location: Enclosed in volume two page 32
See ref. biblio n⁰ 12

For all information concerning the instrument write to the author at the following address:

Liliane Israël,
Pavillon Chissé, C.H.R.U.
38700 La Tronche
Grenoble, France

ORIGIN | Some of these sub-tests were inspired by previously existing tests in the literature which have been adapted for use with the elderly (ref. 1, 4, 13, 14, 15, 16). Others were designed and created by the author (ref. 5).

PURPOSE | This memory test has been designed for two purposes: fundamental and applied research. The aim was to assess factor structure of memory and to measure effects of drugs and other kinds of therapies.

POPULATION | Elderly over 65 years, living at home or in homes for the elderly.

ADMINISTRATION | *Rater:* Psychologist.

Time required: 10-20 minutes.

Training: Psychological training is necessary.

DESCRIPTION | Battery consists of 7 short and non-tiring tests:
· Recall **(Rey)**   · Memorizing a story **(Barbizet)**
· Digit span **(Wechsler)**   · Matched pictures **(Israel)**
· Fluency **(Jung)**   · Learning words **(Rey)**
· Mental control **(Wechsler)**
Rating is established from raw scores which are standardized or adjusted to factor scores.

VARIABLES | The factor structure resulting from this research has one general factor and three specific ones. The general factor is global memory (61,25% of explained variance). The group factors are:
· immediate memory (16,70% of explained variance)
· learning (12,78% of explained variance)
· fluency (9,77% of explained variance)

VALIDATION | **Construct validity** through factor analysis by principal components (explained variance 72%) has been demonstrated on a population of retired people over 65 years (ref. 10, 11).
A standardized scaling has been made into 5 or 7 classes.

OTHER WORKS cited by author | Drug trials or clinical examination (ref. 7, 8, 9).

APPLICATION | **Clinical:** to distinguish normal from pathological ageing.
Research: can be used in drug trials to determine the specific effect of a drug which is supposed to improve memory. With this battery, the impact on attention can be differentiated from the impact on learning and fluency.

1 Barbizet (J.): Epreuves pour l'étude clinique de la mémoire. *Sem. Hôp. Paris*, 1963, 20, 993-995.

2 Barbizet (J.): Le Problème du codage cérébral, son rôle dans les mécanismes de la mémoire. *Ann. Méd. Psych.*, 1964, 1, 1.

3 Barbizet (J.): Pathologie de la mémoire. Paris: P.U.F., 1970.

4 Benton (A.): Manuel du test de rétention visuelle. Paris: Centre de Psychologie Appliquée, 1960.

5 Israel (L.): Recherche et mise au point d'une batterie d'épreuves psychologiques pour l'examen de la mémoire des personnes âgées. *Gerontology*, 1976, 22, 3, 157-186.

6 Israel (L.): Memory disorders as criteria of dependency in old people: evaluation and measurement. In: Munnichs (J.M.A.), Van den Heuvel (W.J.A.) Eds: "Dependency or interdependency in old age». The Hague: Martinus Nijhoff, 1976, 75.

7 Israel (L.): A novel method for drug trials using a rating scale for measuring the memory activity of old people. Communication présentée au XIe Congrès International de Gérontologie, Tokyo, 1978.

8 Israel (L.): Mémoire et méthodes d'évaluation. *Concours Médical*, 11 juillet 1981, suppl. au n° 28, 54-61.

9 Israel (L.): Application of psychometric techiques to the study of treatment affecting brain functioning. In: "Drugs studies in CVD and PVD": proceedings of the international symposium, Geneva, May 25-26 1981. Paris: Pergamon Press, 1982, 89-95.

10 Israel (L.), Doret (J.), Hugonot (R.): Les troubles de la mémoire chez les personnes âgées: sondage effectué auprès d'une population de 782 retraités de la ville de Grenoble. *Revue de Gériatrie Médicale*, nov. 1979, tome 4, n° 9, 455.

11 Israel (L.), Hugonot (R.): Activité du duxil gouttes sur la mémoire des personnes âgées. Appréciation objective par des tests psychométriques. Communication présentée au Symposium Duxil, Paris, 25 janvier 1980.

12 Israel (L.), Ohlmann (Th.): Structure factorielle de la mémoire appréciée à travers une batterie d'épreuves psychologiques chez des personnes âgées ambulatoires: son application aux essais cliniques contrôlés. *L'Encéphale*, 1980, VI, 181-195.

13 Marie (J.), Andrey (B.): L'analyse scientifique des déficits mnésiques. Grenoble: P.U.G., 1974.

14 Rey (A.): Les troubles de la mémoire et leur examen psychométrique. Bruxelles: Dessart, 1966.

15 Rey (A.): L'examen clinique en psychologie. 2ᵉ édition. Paris: P.U.F., 1964.

16 Wechsier (D.): Echelle clinique de la mémoire. Paris: Centre de Psychologie Appliquée, 1945.

17 Wechsler (D.): La mesure de l'intelligence de l'adulte. 4ᵉ ed. Paris: P.U.F., 1973, 291 p.

EXAMEN PSYCHOLOGIQUE POUR PERSONNES AGEES HOSPITALISEES
PSYCHOLOGICAL EXAMINATION FOR ELDERLY INPATIENTS

SPECIFICITY

* * *

TYPE OF INSTRUMENT

Psychometric test:
7 sub-tests

REFERENCE	Instrument not published.
	Language: Original version in French. **France**
	Location: Enclosed in volume two page 33
	For all information concerning the instrument write to the author at the following address:
	Liliane **Israël,** Pavillon Chissé, C.H.R.U. 38700 La Tronche Grenoble, France

ORIGIN

This test battery is a parallel version to "Vigilance Battery" (Ib 25) for the elderly in an institution but on a less difficult content. The tests inspiring the author are classical tests from the literature: **Zazzo** (ref. 6), **Clement** (ref. 1), **Wechsler** (ref. 5), **Rey** (ref. 3), **Thurstone** (ref. 4).

PURPOSE

This battery of tests has been designed with the clinical purpose to assess the severity of mental deterioration in the elderly population.

POPULATION

Elderly over 65 years, hospitalized in geriatric hospitals, short term and long term stay unit.

ADMINISTRATION

Rater: Psychologist.

Time required: 20-25 minutes according to the speed of the subject.

Training: Psychological training is necessary.

DESCRIPTION

This battery of tests is composed of 7 short and non tiring tests adapted for the elderly:
· Picture ordering (ref. 2)   · **Rey's** test of memory (ref. 3)
· Hidden object by L. **Israel,** (ref. 2)   · Coding by **Clement** (ref. 1)
· Digit span by **Wechsler,** (ref. 5)   · Crossing by **Zazzo** (ref. 6)
· Verbal fluency by **Thurstone** (ref. 4)
Rating is established from raw scores which are transformed into standard or factor scores.

VARIABLES

Three specific factors:
· Memory
· Fluency
· Psychomotor activity

Two indices:
· Efficiency
· Precision

VALIDATION

Factor analysis of the second level has determined three specific factors but not a general factor. Standardization into normalized scales of 5 and 7 classes is unpublished.

OTHER WORKS
cited by author

Clinical examination, multicentre studies in 10 towns (Bordeaux, Clermont-Ferrand, Lille, Nice, Grenoble, Rennes, Rueil, Strasbourg, Toulouse et Louviers).

APPLICATION

This instrument should be used for clinical purposes for differentiating levels of mental deterioration. **It is not recommended for use in drug trials.**

1 Clément (F.): Une épreuve rapide de mesure de l'efficience intellectuelle. *Revue de Psychologie Appliquée*, 1963, 13, 1, 243-277.

2 Israel (L.), Ohlmann (Th.): Mise au point et étalonnage d'une batterie d'épreuves psychométriques pour l'examen des personnes âgées. *Gerontology*, 1976, Vol. 22, 3, 141-156.

3 Rey (A.): Les troubles de la mémoire et leur examen psychométrique. Bruxelles: Dessart, 1966.

4 Thurstone (L.L.): Primary mental abilities. Paris: Centre de Psychologie Appliquée, 1953.

5 Wechsler (D.): La mesure de l'intelligence de l'adulte. 4ᵉ éd. Paris: P.U.F., 1973, 291 p.

6 Zazzo (R.): Le test des deux barrages. *Actualités pédagogiques et psychologiques*, 1964, vol. 7, 254.

GUILD MEMORY TEST

SPECIFICITY

* *

TYPE OF INSTRUMENT

Psychometric test:
8 sub-tests

REFERENCE **Gilbert (J.G.), Levee (R.F.), Catalano (F.L.)** · – Guild Memory Test Manual. Bloomfield: Unico National Mental Health Research Foundation, 1981.

Language: Original version published in English.
U.S.A.

Location: Enclosed in volume two page 34
See ref. biblio nº 6

For all information concerning the instrument write to the publisher at the following address:

Unico National Mental Health Research Foundation
72, Burroughs Place
Bloomfield, New Jersey 07003, U.S.A.

ORIGIN Test inspired by the work of **Babcock** (ref. 1), **Benton** (ref. 2), **Wechsler** (ref. 7 and 8).

PURPOSE Test conceived with the goal of differentiating the various aspects of memory and using it conjointly with the Wechsler Adult Intelligence Scale.

POPULATION Aged persons ambulatory or institutionalized, and without severe physical or mental disorders.

ADMINISTRATION *Rater:* Psychologist.

Time required: 20 to 30 minutes.

Training: Practice in psychometric tests

DESCRIPTION I . Test comprises 8 sub-tests:
· Immediate and delayed recall of two texts read by the examiner
· Paired associates: immediate and delayed recall.
· Digits forward and reversed.
· Association of numerical symbols to geometric figures.
II. There are two parallel forms, A and B

Scoring: The scoring varies according to the sub-test. The raw scores can be transformed into standard scores.

VARIABLES Six memory variables:
Verbal contents: · Immediate memory
· Delayed recall
· Immediate memory and concentration
· Immediate recall of paired associates
· Delayed recall of paired associates.
Non-verbal contents: Non-verbal memory.

VALIDATION Used on voluntary aged persons not presenting important psychiatric or physical problems; they have included (ref. 3):
Concurrent validity with the Wechsler Memory Scale
Reliability: split-half and concordance between the two parallel forms;
Standardization takes account of age and intellectual level as measured by the WAIS vocabulary for both the young and aged adult (ref. 6).

APPLICATION **Clinical:** Instrument permits the evaluation of memory capacities of normal subjects and a diagnostic differential between the memory problems on healthy, aged subjects, patients suffering from organic cerebral difficulties and by those with psychiatric problems.
Research: Works on memory.

1 Babcock (H.): An experiment in the measurement of mental deterioration. *Arch. Psych.,* 1930, 18, 117, 1-105.

2 Benton (A.L.): The revised visual retention test. New York: Psychological Corporation, 1955.

3 Crook (Th.), Gilbert (J.): Operationalizing memory impairment for elderly persons: the Guild memory test. *Psychological Reports*, 1980, 47, 1315-1318.

4 Gilbert (J.G.), Levee (R.F.): Patterns of declining memory. *Journal of Gerontology*, 1971, 26, 70-75.

5 Gilbert (J.G.), Levee (R.F.), Catalano (F.L.): A preliminary report on a new memory scale. *Perceptual and Motor Skills*, 1968, 27, 277-278.

6 Gilbert (J.G.), Levee (R.F.), Catalano (F.L.): Guild memory test: Manual. Bloomfied: Unico National Mental Health Research Foundation, 1981.

7 Wechsler (D.A.): A standardized memory scale for clinical use. *Journal of Psychology*, 1945, 19, 87-95.

8 Wechsler (D.A.): Manual for Wechsler adult intelligence scale. New York: Psychological Corporation, 1955.

SHOPPING LIST TASK

SPECIFICITY

$*$ $*$ $*$

TYPE OF INSTRUMENT

Psychometric test
10 items - 5 trials

REFERENCE	**Mc Carthy (M.), Ferris (S.H.), Clark (E.), Crook (T.)** · – Acquisition and retention of categorized material in normal aging and senile dementia. *Experimental Aging Research,* 1981, vol. 7, n° 2, 127-135.

Language: Original version published in English.
U.S.A.

Location: See ref. biblio n° 16

For all information concerning the instrument write to the author at the following address:

Martin Mac Carthy,
Columbia University Center for Geriatrics and Gerontology
and Long Term Care Gerontology Center
100 Haven Avenue, Tower 3 – 29th Floor
New York, N.Y.. 10032, U.S.A.

ORIGIN — This is a verbal test inspired by a critical review of works dealing with memory disorders of elderly persons, (ref. 1, 3, 7, 9, 13, 14, 18, 21).

PURPOSE — This instrument was conceived with the aim of studying the assessment of memory disorders of subjects suffering from senile dementia and non-deteriorated aged persons.

POPULATION — All aged in-patients or out-patients complaining of memory disorders.

ADMINISTRATION — *Rater:* Psychologist, physician.
Time required: 10 minutes.
Training: Knowledge of the test.

DESCRIPTION — The test consists of a list of ten words related to grocery products (milk, eggs, apples, sugar, and butter). Each word is projected on a screen for 3 seconds. After the ten words have been projected, the subject recalls verbally those of them that he can remember.

The instrument consists of five trials. Fifteen minutes after the last trial a recall test of a different nature is administered. In case of failure, a recognition test with imposed words is carried out. Successful recognition points a deficiency at the level of recall. Failure in recognition indicates a deficiency at the level of recording or retention.

Scoring: Scoring is based on the number of correctly recalled items. Learning is considered as successful if the subject has recalled correctly the list of words after two consecutive trials.

VARIABLES — The instrument assesses: verbal learning, retention, immediate or delayed recall.

VALIDATION — **Norms** of distribution (median and standard deviation) concerning the sub-test of deferred recall are given for three groups of subjects (young and elderly normal adults and senile demented) in terms of their learning performance (ref. 16).

APPLICATION — **Clinical:** This instrument makes it possible to detect elderly with significant memory disorders.

1 Botwinick (J.), Storandt (M.): Memory related functions and age. Springfied, Illinois: Charles C. Thomas, 1974.

2 Craik (F.I.M.): Age differences in recognition memory. *Quarterly Journal of Experimental Psychology*, 1971, 23, 316-323.

3 Craik (F.I.M.): Age differences in human memory. In: Birren (J.E.), Schaie (K.W.) Eds: "Handbook of the psychology of aging". New York: Van Nostrand Reinhold Company, 1977.

4 Crook (T.), Ferris (S.H.), McCarthy (M.): The misplaced objects task: a brief test for memory dysfunction in the aged. *Journal of the American Geriatrics Society*, 1979, 27, 284-287.

5 Crook (T.), Ferris (S.H.), McCarthy (M.), Rae (D.): The utility of digit recall tasks for assessing memory in the aged. *Journal of Consulting and Clinical Psychology*, 1980, 48, 228-233.

6 Crook (T.), Gilbert (J.G.), Ferris (S.H.): Operationalizing memory impairment for elderly persons: The Guild memory test. *Psychological Reports*, 1980, 47, 1315-1318.

7 Erber (J.I.): Age differences in recognition memory. *Journal of Gerontology*, 1974, 29, 177-181.

8 Ferris (S.H.), Crook (T.), Clark (E.), Mc Carthy (M.), Rae (D.): Facial recognition memory deficits in normal aging and senile dementia. *Journal of Gerontology*, 1980, 35, 707-714.

9 Fozard (J.L.), Waugh (N.C.): Proactive inhibition of prompted items. *Psychonomic Science*, 1969, 17, 67-68.

10 Gilbert (J.G.), Levee (R.F.): Patterns of declining memory. *Journal of Gerontology*, 1971, 26, 70-75.

11 Gilbert (J.G.), Levee (R.F.), Catalano (F.L.): A preliminary report on a new memory scale. *Perceptual and Motor Skills*, 1968, 27, 277-278.

12 Gordon (S.K.), Clark (W.C.): Application of signal detection theory to prose recall and recognition in elderly and young adults. *Journal of Gerontology*, 1974, 29, 64-72.

13 Gordon (S.K.), Clark (W.C.): Adult age differences in word and nonsense syllabe recognition memory and response criterion. *Journal of Gerontology*, 1974, 29, 659-665.

14 Harwood (E.), Naylor (G.F.K.): Recall and recognition memory in elderly and young subjects. *Australian Journal of psychology*, 1969, 21, 251-257.

15 Loftus (E.F.), Cole (W.): Retrieving attributes and name information from semantic memory. *Journal of Experimental Psychology*, 1974, 104, 1116-1122.

16 McCarthy (M.), Ferris (S.H.), Clark (E.), Crook (T.): Acquisition and retention of categorized material in normal aging and senile dementia. *Experimental Aging Research*, 1981, vol. 7, n° 2, 127-135.

17 McNulty (J.A.), Caird (W.): Memory loss with age: retrieval or storage? *Psychological Reports*, 1966, 19, 229-230.

18 Schoenfield (D.), Robertson (B.A.): Memory storage and aging. *Canadian Journal of Psychology*, 1966, 20, 228-236.

19 Siegel (S.): Non-parametric methods for the behavioral sciences. New York: Mc Graw-Hill, 1956.

20 Tulving (E.): Episodic and semantic memory. In: Tulving (E.), Donaldson (W.) Eds: "Organization of memory". New York: Academic Press, 1972.

21 Warrington (E.K.), Silberstein (M.): Questionnaire technique for investigating verbal memory. *Quarterly Journal of Experimental Psychology*, 1970, 22, 508-512.

MEMORY ACTIVITY SCALE

SPECIFICITY

* *

TYPE OF INSTRUMENT

Performance
psychometric test:
14 sub-tests

REFERENCE	**Loiseau (P.), Signoret (J.L.), Strube (E.), Broustet (D.), Dartigues (J.F.)** · – Nouveaux procédés d'appréciation des troubles de la mémoire chez les épileptiques. *Revue Neurologique,* 1982, 138, 387-400.

Signoret (J.L.), Whitelem (A.) · – Memory battery scale. *I.N.S. Bulletin,* 1979, 2, 26.

Language: Original version in French. Translated into English by the author.
France

Location: Enclosed in volume two page 36
See above references

For all information concerning the instrument write to the author at the following address:

Jean-Louis Signoret,
Clinique Neurologique et Neuropsychologique
Hôpital de la Salpêtrière
47, Boulevard de l'Hôpital
75651 Paris Cedex 13, France

ORIGIN
This original test ranks among a series of works oriented towards differentiation of memory syndromes.

PURPOSE
This test was devised to estimate memory efficiency, learning and recall, in verbal and visual modalities.

POPULATION
All persons capable of understanding instructions.

ADMINISTRATION
Rater: Psychologist, physician.

Time required: 45 minutes.

DESCRIPTION
The test consists of two independent parts, each one linking two modalities of administration verbal and visual one.
The first part deals with registration and retention and is composed of ten sub-tests: "Acquisition" (4), "Recall" (2), "Retention" (4). The second part comprises two types of learning: serial and associative and is sub-divided into four sub-tests: Serial learning (2) and Associative learning.
Scoring: four types of scores may be established for each modality and for the total test.
· Memory: total score obtained from the first part of test.
· Forgetting: weighted difference between scores obtained from "acquisition" and "retention".
· Learning: total score obtained from the second part of test.
· Memory efficiency: total score.

VARIABLES
The test concerns memory capacity.

VALIDATION
The norms of distribution, means and standard deviations are indicated for three groups of subjects: normal adults, adults suffering from amnesia syndrome and adults suffering from Alzheimer's disease.

APPLICATION
Evaluation of memory efficiency in the context of clinical examination.

BILAN D'EVALUATION DU SYNDROME DEMENTIEL
EVALUATION OF THE DEMENTIA SYNDROME

SPECIFICITY

* * *

TYPE OF INSTRUMENT

Compound instrument
Questionnaire, test

REFERENCE	Instrument not published.

Language: Original version published in French (ref. 15).
France

Location: Enclosed in volume two page 187
See ref. biblio nº 15

For all infomation concerning the instrument write to the following address:

Liliane Israël,
Pavillon Chissé, C.H.R.U.
38700 La Tronche
Grenoble, France

Claudine Arnaud Montani,
Pavillon Elisée Chatin C.H.R.U.
38700 La Tronche
Grenoble, France

ORIGIN
This instrument is based upon theoretical basis described by **J. Ajuriaguerra** and his collaborators concerning disturbance of cognitive functions and more specifically the notions of structural analysis, involution, homogeneity and non-homogeneity, and the principle of transfer of learning (ref. 1 to 10).

PURPOSE
This instrument of a general evaluation of the dementia syndrome was established to assess the effects of a psychomotor rehabilitation of demented patients and to estimate the nature and intensity of the instrumental functioning disturbance.

POPULATION
Aged people, in or out-patient with a dementia syndrome.

ADMINISTRATION
Rater: Psychologist, physician, occupational therapist.

Time required: 20 to 30 min depending on the patient's capacity.

Training: Clinical training is necessary as well as a good knowledge of the guidelines developed by J. Ajuriaguerra and the School of Geneva.

Scoring: Clinical assessment is principally focused on the mechanisms applied. It is very important to consider above all the patient's whole mental approach to understand how and why he either failed or was successful in the tests.

DESCRIPTION
This evaluation includes twenty tests inspired by psychometry or by genetic psychology. Their content concerns the examination of:

Memory
· Long term memory
· Short term memory
· Topographic memory
· Learning of construction

Operational functioning:
· Conservation field
· Relations field
· Classes field

Visual Gnosies

Spatial Representation and Structuration

VALIDATION
It concerns a non-standardized clinical estimation in relation to each particular case, which is for the moment at an experimental phase.

APPLICATION
Clinical: General status: These evaluations provide information on the nature and intensity of the dementia syndrome, on the neurological and sensorial status as well as the cognitive activities underlying the instrumental functions.
Care planning
Evaluation of changes.
Research: Experimental or epidemiological studies.

1 Ajuriaguerra (J. de), Boehme (M.), Richard (J.), Sinclair (J.), Tissot (R.): Désintégration des notions de temps dans les démences dégénératives du grand âge. *Encéphale*, 1967, 5, 385-438.

2 Ajuriaguerra (J. de), Cordeiro (D.), Steeb (U.), Fot (K.), Tissot (R.), Richard (J.): A propos de la désintégration des capacités d'anticipation des déments dégénératifs du grand âge. *Neuropsychologia*, 1969, 7, 301-311.

3 Ajuriaguerra (J. de), Gainotti (J.), Tissot (R.): Le comportement des déments de grand âge face à l'échec ou à un risque d'échec. *J. de Psych. Norm. et Path.*, 1969, 3, 319-346.

4 Ajuriaguerra (J. de), Kluser (J.P.), Velghe (J.), Tissot (R.): Praxies idéatoires et permanence de l'objet. Quelques aspects de leur désintégration conjointe dans les syndromes démentiels du grand âge. *Psychiat. Neurol.*, 1965, 150, 306-319.

5 Ajuriaguerra (J. de), Muller (M.), Tissot (R.): A propos de quelques problèmes posés par l'apraxie dans les démences. *Encéphale*, 1960, 5, 375-401.

6 Ajuriaguerra (J. de), Rego (A.), Richard (J.), Tissot (R.): Psychologie et psychométrie du vieillard. *Confront. Psychiat.*, 1970, 5, 27-37.

7 Ajuriaguerra (J. de), Rego (A.), Tissot (R.), Richard (J.): De quelques aspects des troubles de l'habillage dans les démences tardives dégénératives ou à lésions vasculaires diffuses. *Ann. Psychol.*, 1967, 2, 189-218.

8 Ajuriaguerra (J. de), Rey-Bellet-Muller (M.), Tissot (R.): A propos de quelques problèmes posés par le déficit opératoire des vieillards atteints de démence dégénérative en début d'évolution. *Cortex*, 1964, 1, 103-132 et 232-256.

9 Ajuriaguerra (J. de), Richard (J.), Rodriguez (R.), Tissot (R.): Quelques aspects de la désintégration des praxies idéomotrices dans les démences du grand âge. *Cortex*, 1966, II, 438-462.

10 Ajuriaguerra (J. de), Steeb (U.), Richard (J.), Tissot (R.): Processus d'induction dans les démences dégénératives du grand âge. *Encéphale*, 1970, 3, 239-268.

11 Andrey (B.): Les praxies grapho-motrices. *Bulletin de Psychol Scol.*, 1969, 6, 111-131.

12 Barbizet (J.): Epreuves pour l'étude clinique de la mémoire. *Sem. Hôpit.*, 1963, 19, 663 et 20, 993-995.

13 Barbizet (J.): Pathologie de la mémoire. Paris: P.U.F., 1970.

14 Barbizet (J.), Grison (B.): Etude des fonctions supérieures. *Concours Médical*, 1970, 3, 529-534.

15 Israel (L.), Arnaud (C.), Boutrelle (J.), Hugonot (R.): Bilans d'évaluation des effets d'une rééducation psychomotrice sur des sujets âgés atteints de démence. *Encéphale*, 1979, 5, 269-284.

16 Longeot (F.): L'échelle de développement de la pensée logique. Issy-Les-Moulineaux: Editions Scientifiques et Psychotechniques, 1974.

17 Marie (J.), Andrey (B.): L'analyse scientifique des déficits mnésiques. Grenoble: P.U.G., 1974.

18 Piaget (J.): La construction du réel chez l'enfant. *Actualités Pédagogiques et Psychologiques*, 1973.

19 Piaget (J.), Inhelder (B.): La représentation de l'espace chez l'enfant. *Opus*, 1972.

20 Rey (A.): Les troubles de la mémoire et leur examen psychométrique. Bruxelles: Dessart, 1966.

21 Richard (J.): Quelques aspects de la désintégration des fonctions supérieures, du système nerveux central dans les démences tardives. *Médecine et Hygiène*, 1964, 22, 411-412.

22 Richard (J.): Désintégration de la notion de temps dans les démences dégénératives du grand âge. 3e Symposium de Bel-Air (septembre 1967), 1968, 29, 12.

23 Wechsler (D.): Etude clinique de la mémoire. Paris: Centre de Psychologie Appliquée, 1945-1960.

24 Wechsler (D.): La mesure de l'intelligence de l'adulte. 4e édition. Paris: P.U.F., 1973.

BEHAVIOR

Ic.1	Nurses' Observation Scale for Inpatient Evaluation	HONIGFELD	1965
Ic.2	Discharge Readiness Inventory (*)	HOGARTY	1966
Ic.3	Archétype Test à 9 éléments	DURAND	1967
Ic.4	Short Scale for the Assessment of Mental Health	SAVAGE	1967
Ic.5	Patient Activity Check-List (*)	AUMACK	1969
Ic.6	V.I.R.O. Orientation Scale (*)	KASTENBAUM	1972
Ic.7	Adult Personality Rating Schedule (*)	KLEBAN - BRODY	1972
Ic.8	Senior Apperception Technique (*)	BELLAK	1973
Ic.9	Behavior Rating Scale	WILLIAMS	1973
Ic.10	Present State Examination	WING - SARTORIUS	1973
Ic.11	D - Test (*)	FERM	1974
Ic.12	Geriatric Mental State Schedule	COPELAND	1976
Ic.13	Hypochondriasis Scale Institutional Geriatric	BRINK	1978
Ic.14	Short Psychiatric Evaluation Schedule	PFEIFFER	1979
Ic.15	Survey Psychiatric Assessment Schedule	BOND	1980
Ic.16	Evaluation Clinique de la Personnalité (*)	ISRAEL	1980
Ic.17	M. Test (*)	MEZZENA	1981
Ic.18	Behaviour and Mood Disturbance Scale (*)	GREENE	1982

(*) Instruments which can be classified as "Mental Social"

NURSES' OBSERVATION SCALE FOR INPATIENT EVALUATION (N.O.S.I.E.)

SPECIFICITY

** Rating scale of 80 items
* Rating scale of 30 items

TYPE OF INSTRUMENT

Ordinal rating scale
with 5 grades
2 versions:
80 and 30 items

REFERENCE **Honigfeld (G.), Klett (C.J.)** · – The nurses' observation scale for inpatient evaluation. A new scale for measuring improvement in chronic schizophrenia. *Journal of Clinical Psychology,* 1965, 21, 65-71.

Language: Original version published in English. Translated into French by Pichot et al. Version with 30 items (ref. 7). There are translations in German, Spanish, Italian and Swedish.
U.S.A.

Location: Nosie 30 enclosed in volume two page 112
See ref. biblio nᵒ 4

For all information concerning the instrument write to the author at the following address:

Gilbert Honigfeld
Sandoz Inc.
Route 10 – East Hannover
New Jersey U.S.A.

ORIGIN Most of the 100 initial items have been drawn from previous scales (ref. 1, 2, 6, 9). Their formulation was clarified and modified to allow a scoring based on observations, and adjusted to a 5 point evaluation. A certain number of items are original, 20 items were omitted for insufficient inter-rater reliability or because of a bias in distribution of scores (the NOSIE 80).
The NOSIE 30 is derived directly from the NOSIE 80. Only the items most sensitive to therapeutic effects analysis were retained from the factor analysis.

PURPOSE To make a sufficiently sensitive scale to measure changes resulting from therapy in aged schizophrenic patients. The authors have made an abbreviated scale of 30 items (NOSIE) in order to get a brief scale to extend the limits posed by the age of the population concerned, and exclude the items that were the least sensitive to change.

POPULATION NOSIE 80: aged hospitalized schizophrenic patients.
NOSIE 30: adult hospitalized patients with chronic schizophrenia.

ADMINISTRATION *Rater:* Nurse, nurse's aide. The author recommends two independent evaluations for each patient.

Time required: 20 minutes.

Training: Familiarization with the scoring system.

Scoring: Is based on a 3 day consecutive observation of the patient. All the items are assessed according to a frequency scale of 0 (never) to 4 (always), 15 items are scored in reverse order (0 = 4,1 = 3). One can calculate the factor scores by adding up the scores of items belonging to a factor. As patients were subjected to two evaluations, the mark for each item ranges from 0 to 8. For the NOSIE 30 there is a global score. Taking into account the frequency of relatively asymptomatic clinical pictures as well as disorders of communication, the instrument is not a scale of symptoms and is more suited to the observation of behaviour, especially in its interpersonal aspects, than to provide data such as might result from a psychiatric interview.

VARIABLES NOSIE 80: 7 factors

I   Social competence
II Social interests
III Personal neatness
IV Cooperation
V   Irritability
VI Manifest psychosis
VII Psychotic depression

NOSIE 30: 6 factors

I   Social competence
II Social interests
III Personal neatness
IV Irritability
V   Manifest psychosis
VI Retardation

VALIDATION

NOSIE 80: Hospitalized male chronic schizophrenic patients, aged 55-69 not administered any psychotropic drugs for at least 28 days, comprising:

Factor analysis, calling for the exclusion of 19 items whose loading was inferior to 40 yielded the above 7 factors.

Sensitivity and discriminative validity: study of efficiency of three drugs and a placebo.

Inter-rater reliability: two raters.

The **norms** for the factor scores were established as cumulative percentage frequencies beginning with a population whose average age was 66.

NOSIE 30: Hospitalized male chronic schizophrenic patients aged 26-74 (mean age 52,4) comprising (ref. 4):

Factor analysis on the intercorrelations matrix using as variables differences between before-and-after treatment scores. The results give 6 above mentioned factors.

Sensitivity and discriminative validity: study of therapeutic effectiveness reflected by 6 factor scores and a total score.

The authors give a scaling for 6 factor scores and a total score by raw score and percentile.

APPLICATION

Clinical research with elderly patients, chronic schizophrenic patients, drug trials.

Ic.1

BIBLIOGRAPHY

1 Aumach (L.): A social adjustment behavior rating scale. *J. Clin. Psychol.*, 1962, 18, 436-441.

2 Burdock (E.I.), Hakerem (G.), Hardesty (A.S.), Zubin (J.): A ward behavior rating scale for mental hospital patients. *J. Clin. Psychol.*, 1960, 16, 246-247.

3 Honigfeld (G.), Gillis (R.D.), Klett (C.J.): Nosie-30: a treatment-sensitive ward behavior scale. *Psychological Reports*, 1966, 19, 180-182.

4 Honigfeld (G.), Klett (C.J.): The nurses' observation scale for inpatient evaluation: a new scale for measuring improvement in chronic schizophrenia. *Journal of Clinical Psychology*, 1965, 21, 65-71.

5 Honigfeld (G.), Rosenblum (M.P.), Blumenthal (I.J.), Lambert (H.L.), Roberts (A.J.): Behavioral improvement in the older schizophrenic patient: drug and social therapies. *J. Amer. Geriatrics Society*, 1965, vol. 13, n°. 1, 57-72.

6 Lorr (M.), O'Connor (J.P.), Stafford (J.W.): A psychotic reaction profile. *J. Clin. Psychol.*, 1960, 16, 241-245.

7 Pichot (P.), Samuel Lajeunesse (B.), Blanc (J.), Galopin (D.), Selva (G.): Une échelle d'observation du comportement en salle des malades mentaux hospitalisés: la Nosie-30. *Revue de Psychologie Appliquée*, 1969, vol. 19, n°. 1, 35-43.

8 Rashkis (H.A.): The research community. *Arch. Gen. Psychiat.*, 1961, 5, 578-586.

9 Shatin (L.), Freed (E.X.): A behavioral rating scale for mental patients. *J. Ment. Sci.*, 1955, 101, 644-653.

DISCHARGE READINESS INVENTORY

SPECIFICITY

* *

TYPE OF INSTRUMENT

Ordinal rating scale
45 items, 9 grades

REFERENCE	**Hogarty (G.E.)** · – Discharge readiness: the components of casework judgment. *Social Casework,* 1966, 47, 165-171.
	Language: Original version published in English. **U.S.A.**
	Location: Enclosed in volume two page 113 See ref. biblio n° 5

ORIGIN   Original test based on clinical experience of social workers in psychiatric institutions.

PURPOSE   Test developed for social workers with the aim of evaluating the suitability of chronic psychiatric patients for discharge based entirely on clinical considerations.

POPULATION   Chronic mental patients placed in hospitals, young or old.

ADMINISTRATION *Rater:* Social worker.

Time required: 30 minutes.

Training: Clinical experience in psychiatry and knowledge of the test.

VARIABLES   Four aspects are considered:
· Psycho-social adequacy
· Belligerence
· Community adjustment potential
· Manifest psychopathology.

VALIDATION   **Face validity** was studied (ref. 5).
Inter-rater reliability was verified (ref. 5).

APPLICATION   The instrument is intended for clinical use by social workers allowing them to evaluate the possibility for chronic psychiatric cases with schizophrenia to leave hospital. It can also serve in the field of research and interviews.

Ic.2

1 Adelson (D.): Social factors in the placement of the chronic schizophrenic patient. Paper presented at the annual meeting of the American Orthopsychiatric Association, Los Angeles, March 1962.

2 Casey (J.F.) et al.: Combined drug therapy of chronic schizophrenics. *American Journal of Psychiatry*, may 1961, vol. 117, 1002.

3 Doehne (E.F.) et al.: Rehabilitative potential in "chronic" mental patients. *Archives of General Psychiatry*, march 1965, vol. 12, 241-244.

4 Hogarty (G.E.): The discharge readiness inventory: validity as an outcome measure in the treatment of chronic schizophrenia. Paper read before the Study Group on Psychopharmacology and Social Therapy. Fifth annual meeting of the American College of Neuropsychopharmacology, San Juan, PR, December 1966.

5 Hogarty (G.E.): Discharge readiness: the components of a casework judgment. *Social Casework*, march 1966, 47, 165-171.

6 Hogarty (G.E.): Hospital differences in the release of discharge ready chronic schizophrenics. *Archives of General Psychiatry*, march 1968, vol. 18, 367-372.

7 Lorr (M.) et al.: Syndromes of psychosis. New York: Macmillan Co, 1963, 26-29.

8 NIMH-PSC: Collaborative study on drug treatment in chronic schizophrenia. Printed copy. Washington, DC, April 1965.

9 Slear (M.G.): Psychiatric patients: clinically improved but socially disabled. *Social Work*, April 1959, vol. 4, 64-71.

ARCHETYPE TEST A 9 ELEMENTS (A.T. 9)

ARCHETYPE TEST OF 9 ELEMENTS

SPECIFICITY

* *

TYPE OF INSTRUMENT

Projective test
Drawing, narration
and questionnaire,
27 responses

REFERENCE	**Durand (Y.)** · – Eléments d'utilisation pratique et théorique du test AT 9. *Annales du Centre d'Enseignement Supérieur de Chambéry,* 1967, n° 5, 133-172.

Language: Original version published in French. Translations in Portuguese (in Brazil) and English.
France

Location: Enclosed in volume two page 40
See ref. biblio n° 3

For all information concerning the instrument or translations, write to the author at the following address:

Yves Durand,
Centre de Recherche et d'Applications
Psychosociologiques – (CRAPS)
Université de Savoie
33, rue des Fleurs
73000 Chambéry, France

ORIGIN	Original instrument inspired by the works by **Gilbert Durand** (ref. 1) on the functioning of imagination as a defence mechanism against anxiety.
PURPOSE	Initially, the instrument was conceived for experimental purposes to verify the theory by G. Durand on the functioning of imagination. It was later transformed into a clinically applicable test.
POPULATION	Populations of all ages, in or out-patients.
ADMINISTRATION	*Rater:* Psychiatrist or well trained psychologist.
	Time required: An hour to an hour and a half.
	Training: Knowledge of the thesis and the author's work are necessary.
DESCRIPTION	The whole comprises a drawing, a story, a questionnaire composed of six questions and a summary table requiring 27 answers.

DESCRIPTION The point is to compose in 30 min. a drawing comprising a fall, a sword, a refuge, a devouring monster, something cyclical (that turns around, reproduces itself or progresses), a character (person), water, an animal and fire. The evaluation is qualitative. There is no score.

The subject's subconscience is revealed in the drawing by looking the way in which anxiety towards the fall and the monster is portrayed, in addition to the organisation of defences against anxiety. The narration translates the attempt to rationalize the subconscience. It is analysed through its form (power of construction) and its contents (link between different elements). The narration and drawing are compared with information supplied by the questionnaire. The questionnaire and the general synthesis provide evidence of resources represented by the imagination as a mean of combatting anxiety, as well as the degree of internal cohesion of the different levels of personality.

VARIABLES	Structure of imagination, neuroses, psychoses, psychosomatic disorders.
VALIDATION	**Construct validity** with the theory which gives rise to the test. Categories of replies: structure of the drawing, type of images, functions and symbols.
	Other validation studies are under way.
OTHER WORKS cited by author	Several doctoral theses dissertations dedicated to the study of psychopathological syndromes have been carried out with the aid of AT 9.
APPLICATION	**Research:** Studies applied either to exploration of the symbolic sphere of imagination functioning or to deterioration of that functioning.
	Clinical: Diagnostic and prognostic. Psychotherapeutic.

1   Durand (G.): Les structures anthropologiques de l'I-
maginaire. Paris: Bordas, 1969.

2   Durand (Y.): Structures de l'Imaginaire et comportement. *Les Cahiers Internationaux de Symbolisme*,
1964, n°. 4, 61-80.

3   Durand (Y.): Eléments d'utilisation pratique et théorique du test A.T.9. *Annales du Centre d'Enseignement
Supérieur de Chambéry*, 1967, n°. 5, 133-172.

4   Durand (Y.): Eléments d'étude expérimentale de la
fonction symbolique. *Annales du Centre d'Enseignement Supérieur de Chambéry*, 1969, n°. 7, 131-166.

5   Durand (Y.): La formulation expérimentale de l'Imaginaire et ses modèles. *Circé*, 1969, n°. 1, 151-248.

6   Durand (Y.): L'archétype du refuge: son étude expérimentale et clinique. *Circé*, 1970, n°. 2, 175-277.

7   Durand (Y.): Symbolisation et structures de l'Imaginaire. Les Etudes Philosophiques. Paris: Presses Universitaires de France, 1971.

8   Durand (Y.): Introduction au mythodrame. *Annales
du Centre de Recherches sur l'imaginaire*, 1976.

9   Durand (Y.): L'exploration expérimentale de l'Imaginaire: élaboration d'une méthode de recherche psychologique et sociologique: l'A.T.9. Thèse pour le
Doctorat d'Etat ès-Lettres et Sciences Humaines.
Grenoble: Université des Sciences Sociales, 1981.

10 Durand (Y.), Morenon (J.): L'Imaginaire de l'alcoo-
lisme. Paris: Les Editions Universitaires, 1972.

11 Durand (Y.), Schnetzler (J.P.): Une méthode d'étude
des structures imaginaires: le test A.T.9. Comptes ren-
dus du Congrès de Psychiatrie et de Neurologie de
Langue Française. Paris: Masson, 1966, 294-303.

SHORT SCALE FOR ASSESSMENT OF MENTAL HEALTH

SPECIFICITY

* * *

TYPE OF INSTRUMENT

Check list with 15 items, scored Yes-No

REFERENCE	**Savage (R.D.), Britton (P.G.)** · – A short scale for the assessment of mental health in the community aged. *British Journal of Psychiatry,* 1967, 113, 521-523.

Language: Original version published in English.
U.S.A.

Location: Enclosed in volume two page 84
See ref. biblio n° 25

For all information concerning the instrument write to the author at the following address:

R.D. Savage,
Psychology Section
School of Social Inquiry
Murdoch University
Murdoch, Western Australia 6150

ORIGIN   Psychological measure derived from a statistical analysis of **Hathaway** and **McKinley's** "Minnesota Multiphasic Personality Inventory" (ref. 11) on a random sample of community subjects above 70 years of age. The 15 items most highly correlated with the psychiatric diagnosis and the MMPI general factor of Mental Health, were selected for the new short scale.

PURPOSE   The evaluation of general mental health, to identify existing psychopathological problems in a quick, simple yet valid and reliable way.

POPULATION   All aged persons, hospitalized or in the community.

ADMINISTRATION   *Rater:* Physician, psychologist, nurse, social worker.

Time required: 5 minutes.

Training: Necessary.

Scoring: Questions are read out to the subject, not presented in written form. Responses are of a yes-no nature. The pathological response, according to the items, is scored and is indicated on the test sheet in capital letters. Above a total score of 6, the subject's behavior is considered as pathological. Authors recommend the use in conjuction with the "Wechsler Adult Intelligence Scale" (ref. 22, 23, 30).

VARIABLES   Cover different areas: anxiety about health and state of health felt by subject, somatic symptoms, sleep, activities, etc.

VALIDATION   Carried out on 2 randomly selected populations of aged ambulatory community resident persons who had all undergone psychiatric assessment, at the end of which they were classified as "normal" or "abnormal", they comprised studies of (ref. 25, 28):
Empirical validity with regard to psychiatric clinical diagnosis.
Validity, reliability and **standardization** data, presenting means, standard deviations and standard errors for normal and abnormal aged subjects.

OTHER WORKS
cited by author   Research on the impairment of intellectual functioning and learning ability and the study of personality and adjustment of aged persons.

APPLICATION   **Clinical:** preliminary investigation of psychological abnormality, prognosis.
Research: therapeutic intervention.

1 Bolton (N.), Britton (P.G.), Savage (R.D.): Some normative data on the Wechsler adult intelligence scale and its indices in an aged population. *J. Clin. Psychol.*, 1966, 22, 2, 184-188.

2 Bolton (N.), Savage (R.D.): Neuroticism and extraversion in elderly normal subjects and psychiatric patients, some normative data. *Brit. J. Psychiat.*, 1971, 118, 473-474.

3 Bolton (N.), Savage (R.D.), Roth (M.): The modified word learning test and the aged psychiatric patient. *Brit. J. Psychiat.*, 1967, 113, 1139-1140.

4 Britton (P.G.), Bergmann (K.), Kay (D.W.K.), Savage (R.D.): Mental state, cognitive functioning, physical health and social class in the community aged. *J. Gerontol.*, 1967, 22, 4, 1, 517-521.

5 Britton (P.G.), Savage (R.D.): A short form of the WAIS for use with the aged. *Brit. J. Psychiat.*, 1966, 112, 417-418.

6 Britton (P.G.), Savage (R.D.): Some normative data on a community aged population on the MMPI. *Brit. J. Psychiat.*, 1966, 112, 941-943.

7 Britton (P.G.), Savage (R.D.): The factorial structure of the WAIS on an aged sample. *J. Gerontol.*, 1968, 23, 2, 183-186.

8 Britton (P.G.), Savage (R.D.): The factor structure of the MMPI in an aged population. *J. Genet. Psychol.*, 1969, 114, 13-17.

9 Dixon (J.C.): Cognitive structure in senile conditions with some suggestions for developing a brief screening test of mental status. *J. Gerontol.*, 1965, 20, 41-49.

10 Hall (E.H.), Savage (R.D.), Bolton (N.), Blessed (G.), Pidwell (D.): Intellect, mental illness and survival in the aged: a longitudinal investigation. *J. Gerontol.*, 1972, 27, 2, 237-244.

11 Hathaway (S.R.), Mc Kinley (J.C.): The Minnesota multiphasic personality inventory manual. Revised. New York: The Psychological Corporation, 1951.

12 Kay (D.W.K.), Beamish (P.), Roth (M.): Old age mental disorders in Newcastle – upon – Tyne. Part I: a study of prevalence. *Brit J. Psychiat.*, 1964, 110, 146-158.

13 Kay (D.W.K.), Beamish (P.), Roth (M.): Old age mental disorders in Newcastle – upon – Tyne. Part II: a study of possible social and medical causes. *Brit. J. Psychiat.*, 1964, 110, 668-682.

14 Savage (R.D.): Intellect and mental illness. *Durham Research Rev.*, 1964, 15, 145-151.

15 Savage (R.D.): Psychometric assessment in the aged. Some recent advances in cognitive and personality measurement. R.M.P.A. Conference, Newcastle, october 20, 1966.

16 Savage (R.D.): The measurement and structure of intellect in the aged. Paper. Nat. Soc. Res. Ageing. London, 1970.

17 Savage (R.D.): Intellectual assessment. In: Mittler (P.) Ed.: "The psychological assessment of mental and physical handicaps". London: Methuen, 1970.

18 Savage (R.D.): Psychometric assessment and clinical diagnosis in the aged. In: Kay (D.W.K.), Walk (A.) Eds: "Recent developments in psychogeriatrics". London: R.M.P.A., 1971.

19 Savage (R.D.): Old age. In: Eysenck (H.J.) Ed.: "Handbook of abnormal psychology". 2nd edition. London: Pitman Med. Pub., 1973.

20 Savage (R.D.): Psychometric techniques with the aged. In: Howells (J.G.) Ed.: "Modern perspectives in psychogeriatrics". Edinburgh: Oliver and Boyd, 1974.

21 Savage (R.D.): Intellect and personality in the aged. In: Smith (W.L.) Ed.: "Ageing and dementia", 1976.

22 Savage (R.D.): Intellectual impairment in the elderly. Paper presented at the Geigy Symposium on Psychogeriatrics, may 1978. Brisbane: University of Queensland, 1978.

23 Savage (R.D.): Intellect, personality and adjustment in the aged. In: Lynn (R.) Ed.: "Dimensions of personality". Oxford: Pergamon Press, 1981.

24 Savage (R.D.), Bolton (N.): A factor analysis of learning impairment and intellectual deterioration in the elderly. *J. Genet. Psychol.*, 1968, 113, 117-182.

25 Savage (R.D.), Britton (P.G.): A short scale for the measurement of mental health in the aged community. *Brit. J. Psychiat.*, 1967, 113, 521-523.

26 Savage (R.D.), Britton (P.G.), Bolton (N.), Hall (E.H.): Intellectual functioning in the aged. An advanced original text. Methuen, 1973.

27 Savage (R.D.), Britton (P.G.), O'Connor (D.), George (S.), Hall (E.H.): A developmental study of intellectual functioning in the community aged. *J. Genet. Psychol.*, 1972, 121, 163-167.

28 Savage (R.D.), Gaber (L.B.), Britton (P.G.), Bolton (N.): Personality and adjustment in the aged. Advanced original text. Academic Press, 1977.

29 Savage (R.D.), Hall (E.H.): A performance learning measure for the aged. *Br. J. Psychiat.*, 1973, 122, 721-723.

30 Wechsler (D.): Manual for the Wechsler adult intelligence scale. New York: Psychological Corporation, 1955.

PATIENT ACTIVITY CHECK-LIST

SPECIFICITY

> *

TYPE OF INSTRUMENT

> Check list, 24 items
> Scored Yes-No

REFERENCE	**Aumack (L.)** · – The patient activity check-list: an instrument and an approach for measuring behavior. *Journal of Clinical Psychology,* 1969, 25, 134-137.
	Language: Original version published in English. **U.S.A.**
	Location: Enclosed in volume two page 85 See ref. biblio nº 3

ORIGIN

Inspired by works of **Higgs** on the behavior of schizophrenics (ref. 5).

PURPOSE

To review activities of hospitalized psychiatric patients in order to measure their improvement, but avoiding the bias due to subjectivity of an observer, frequently involved in treatment.

POPULATION

Hospitalized psychiatric patients.

ADMINISTRATION

Rater: All members of the nursing team.

Time required: Very short.

Training: Rapid familiarization with the instrument.

Scoring: Yes - No.

VARIABLES

24 items ranging from inappropriate and disturbed behavior, withdrawal, to active appropriate behavior.

VALIDATION

With hospitalized psychiatric patients, covering:
External validity in relation to clinical observations
Predictive validity for changes resulting from alteration in the physical and social environment and regrouping by personal affinities.
Discriminative sensitivity between open and closed-ward patients.
Inter-rater reliability between 2 psychologists.
Test-retest after a ten-week interval, stability during the day for three repeated scorings.
Split-half.

OTHER WORKS
cited by author

Studies of correlation with age (ref. 2).

APPLICATION

Clinical and sociological studies within a hospital.

1 Alsobrook (J.M.): Health – engendering aides for psychiatric patients: implications for therapeutic milieu. Paper read at American Psychological Association, Washington, DC, 1967.

2 Aumack (L.): Social psychological research in a mental hospital setting. Technical report n°. 67-2. Danville, Illinois: Veterans Administration Hospital. 1967.

3 Aumack (L.): The patient activity check-list: an instrument and an approach for measuring behavior. *J. Clin. Psychol.*, 1969, 25, 134-137.

4 De Vries (D.L.): Effects of environmental change and of participation on the behavior of mental patients. Unpublished Master's thesis. University of Illinois, 1967.

5 Higgs (W.J.): The effects of an environmental change upon behavior of schizophrenics. Unpublished Master's thesis. University of Illinois, 1964.

6 Jackson (J.): Structural characteristics of norms. In: Steiner (I.D.), Fishbein (M.) Eds.: "Current studies in social psychology". New York: Holt, Rinehart and Winston, 1965.

7 Lorr (M.): Rating scales, behavior inventories and drugs. In: Uhr (L.), Miller (J.G.) Eds: «Drugs and behavior». New York: John Wiley and Sons, 1960, 519-539.

8 Lyerly (S.B.), Abbott (P.S.): Handbook of psychiatric rating scales. Public Health Service Publication n°. 1495. Bethesda, Maryland: National Institute of Mental Health, 1966.

9 McGrath (J.E.): A methodology for design of a criterion system for social psychological research in a mental hospital setting. Research Report n°. 66-2. Danville, Illinois: Veterans Administration Hospital, 1967.

VIRO ORIENTATION SCALE

SPECIFICITY

* * *

TYPE OF INSTRUMENT

Nominal rating scale
4 grades

REFERENCE	**Kastenbaum (R.), Sherwood (S.)** · − VIRO: a scale for assessing the interview behavior of elderly people. In: Kent (D.P.), Kastenbaum (R.), Sherwood (S.) Eds.: "Research planning and action for the elderly: the power and potential of social science". New York: Behavioral publications, 1972, 166-200.
	Language: Original version published in English. **U.S.A.**
	Location: Enclosed in volume two page 115 See ref. biblio nº 16

ORIGIN

The instrument is the result of clinical experience of the authors and critical reflections by numerous investigators and practitioners on the necessity to consider as an dependent variable the behavior of an aged subject during psychiatric interview (ref. 1, 2, 3, 4, 5, 6, 8, 10, 11, 12, 13, 15, 17, 18, 19, 21, 22, 23, 24, 25, 27, 29, 31, 32, 33).

PURPOSE

To evaluate psycho-motor behavior, cognitive functions and quality of contact with an aged subject, as well as changes in behavior during the interview.

POPULATION

Aged in and out-patients.

ADMINISTRATION

Rater: Physician, psychologist, nursing personnel, social worker.

Time required: Five minutes.

Training: Knowledge of the instrument requires several training sessions.

Scoring: Ranging from 0 to 3.
0 is the point considered socially negative, 3 is positive. Factor scores allowing a profile of the behavior of the subject, can be calculated.
Note: The items are presented in IBM punch card format.

VARIABLES

· **V** igour
· **I** ntactness
· **R** elationships
· **O** rientation

VALIDATION

Inter-rater **reliability** and inter-factor correlations have been calculated (ref. 16).

APPLICATION

Clinical: Screening (especially for dependency)
Contribution to diagnosis
Prognosis on the likely course of an aged subject in adaptation to daily life.
Research: Drug trials
Training in behavioral observation.

1 Armitage (P.), Blendis (L.M.), Smyllie (H.C.): The measurement of observer disagreement in the recording of signs. *Journal of the Royal Statistical Social Series A*, 1966, 129, 98-109.

2 Bales (R.F.), Hare (A.P.): Diagnostic use of the interaction profile. *Journal of Social Psychology*, 1965, 67 (second half), 239-258.

3 Benny (M.), Riesman (D.), Star (S.A.): Age and sex in the interview. *American Journal of Sociology*, 1957, 62, 143-152.

4 Buehler (J.S.): Two experiments in psychiatric interrater reliability. *Journal of Health and Human Behavior*, 1966, 7, 192-202.

5 Caplow (T.): The dynamics of information interviewing. *American Journal of Sociology*, 1957, 62, 165-171.

6 Dexter (L.A.): Role relationships and conceptions of neutrality in interviewing. *American Journal of Sociology*, 1957, 62, 143-152.

7 Donahue (W.): Relationship of age of perceivers to their social perceptions. *The Gerontologist*, 1965, 5, 241-245, 276-277.

8 Fletcher (C.M.), Oldman (P.D.): Diagnosis in group research. In: Witts (L.J.) Ed.: "Medical surveys and clinical trials". London: Oxford University Press, 1964.

9 Goldfarb (A.I.): The evaluation of geriatric patients following treatment. In: Hoch (P.H.), Zubin (J.). Eds.: «Evaluation of psychiatric treatment». New York: Grune and Stratton, 1964.

10 Haley (J.): Strategies of psychotherapy. New York: Grune and Stratton, 1963.

11 Hunt (W.A.), Schwartz (M.L.): Reliability of clinical judgments as a function of range of pathology. *Journal of Abnormal Psychology*, 1965, 70, 32-33.

12 Hyman (H.H.), Cobb (W.J.), Feldman (J.J.), Hart (C.W.), Stember (C.H.): Interviewing in social research. Chicago: University of Chicago Press, 1954.

13 Kastenbaum (R.): Multiple personality in later life. A developmental interpretation. *The Gerontologist*, 1964, 4, 68-71.

14 Kastenbaum (R.): Engrossment and perspective in later life: A developmental-field approach. In: Kastenbaum (R.) Ed.: "Contributions to the psychobiology of aging". New-York: Springer, 1965.

15 Kastenbaum (R.): Developmental-field theory and the aged person's inner experience. *The Gerontologist*, 1966, 6, 10-13.

16 Kastenbaum (R.), Sherwood (S.): VIRO: a scale for assessing the interview behavior of elderly people. In: Kent (D.P.), Kastenbaum (R.), Sherwood (S.) Eds: "Research planning and action for the elderly: the power and potential of social science". New-York: Behavioral Publications, 1972, 166-200.

17 Katz (D.): Do interviewers bias polls? *Public Opinion Quarterly*, 1942, 6, 248-268.

18 Kincaid (H.V.), Bright (M.): Interviewing and business elite. *American Journal of Sociology*, 1958, 63, 304-311.

19 Lenski (G.E.), Leggett (J.C.): Caste, class and deference in the research interview. *American Journal of Sociology*, 1960, 65, 463-467.

20 Parl (B.): Basic statistics. Garden City, N.Y.: Doubleday, 1967.

21 Rice (S.A.): Contagious bias in the interview: A methodological note. *American Journal of Sociology*, 1930, 35, 420-423.

22 Robinson (D.), Rohde (S.): Two experiments with an anti-semitism poll. *Journal of Abnormal and Social Psychology*, 1946, 41, 136-144.

23 Robinson (W.S.): The statistical measurement of agreement. *American Sociological Review*, 1957, 22, 17-25.

24 Robinson (W.S.): The geometric interpretation of agreement. *American Sociological Review*, 1959, 24, 338-345.

25 Rosenthal (R.): On the social psychology of the psychological experiment. *American Scientist*, 1963, 51, 268-283.

26 Runyon (R.P.), Haber (A.): Fundamentals of behavioral statistics. Reading, Mass: Addison-Wesley Publishing, 1968.

27 Schafer (R.): Clinical application of psychological tests. New York: International Universities Press, 1950.

28 Sherwood (S.): A demonstration program in a home for the aged: observation research and practice. In: Duke University Council on Gerontology: Proceedings of Seminars 1965-1969. Durham, NC: Duke University, Regional Center for the Study of Aging, 1969.

29 Slater (P.E.), Kastenbaum (R.): Paradoxical effects of drugs: Some personality and ethnic correlates. *Journal of the American Geriatrics Association*, 1966, 14, 1016-1034.

30 Spiegel (M.R.): Theory and problems of statistics. New-York: Schaum Publishing, 1961.

31 Spitzer (R.L.), Cohen (J.), Fleiss (J.L.), Endicott (J.): Quantification of agreement in psychiatric diagnosis. *Archives of General Psychiatry*, 1967, 17, 83-87.

32 Sullivan (H.S.): The psychiatric interview. New-York: Norton, 1954.

33 Vidich (A.J.): Participant observation and the collection and interpretation of data. *American Journal of Sociology*, 1955, 60, 354.

ADULT PERSONALITY RATING SCHEDULE (A.P.R.S.)

SPECIFICITY

* * *

TYPE OF INSTRUMENT

Ordinal rating scale 50 items, 5 grades

REFERENCE	**Kleban (M.H.), Brody (E.M.)** · – Prediction of improvement in mentally impaired aged: personality ratings by social workers. *Journal of Gerontology,* 1972, vol. 27, nº 1, 69-76.
	
	Language: Original version published in English.
	   U.S.A.
	
	Location: Enclosed in volume two page 116
	   See ref. biblio nº 4
	
	For all information concerning the instrument write to the author at the following address:
	
	   Morton Kleban,
	   Philadelphia Geriatric Center,
	   5301 Old York Road,
	   Philadelphia, Pennsylvania 19141, U.S.A.

ORIGIN

The scale is of double origin: works by **Brody** (ref. 1, 2) and discussions among the members of the nursing team of the Geriatric Center of Philadelphia with regard to a project concerning individual treatment applied in case of incapacities of the elderly ("excess disabilities": difference found between observed functional incapacity and determined physical impairment).

PURPOSE

The scale was conceived for experimental purposes in order to evaluate the personality at two different periods of life and thus predict the evolution of deteriorated patients according to their previous personality.

POPULATION

Deteriorated elderly.

ADMINISTRATION

Rater: Social worker. Those closest to the subject.

Time required: 15 to 30 minutes.

Training: Not necessary.

Scoring: The scale has 5 grades: very low, low, medium, high and very high. When the evaluation of personality was done by immediate relatives, the method of averaging scores from different raters, was used.

VARIABLES

The following aspects of personality are assessed by this scale:
· Attitudes towards others and activities.
· Aggressiveness, negativism
· Emotional investment
· Social integration
· Anxiety

VALIDATION

With a deteriorated female population over 80 years of age and control group, covering (ref. 4): Correlation between an evaluation of personality in middle age and the present day in order to determine its continuity.
Two **factor analyses** were done by the principal components method and by varimax: one based on the evaluation of middle-age personality, the other on present personality. The correlation between the results on these two occasions was calculated.
Predictive validity for progress under treatment evaluated by the nursing team on a 7 point scale. The predictive validity of each of the factors taken separately was analysed on a group of patients and a control group.

OTHER WORKS
cited by author

Study of results of a double scoring by the immediate relatives on one hand and by social workers on the other, of predictive validity and inter-rater reliability (ref. 5).

APPLICATION

Study of the course of personality constants of an adult person growing old.
Prognosis for deterioration.

Ic.7

1 Brody (E.M.); Individualized treatment of mentally-impaired aged. NIMH Grant 15.047, 1966 (mimeo).

2 Brody (E.M.), Kleban (M.H.), Lawton (M.P.), Silverman (H.A.): Excess disabilities of mentally impaired aged: impact of individualized treatment. *Gerontologist*, 1971, 11, 124-132.

3 Kahn (R.S.): Comments. In: "Proceedings of the York House Institute on the mentally impaired aged". Philadelphia: Philadelphia Geriatric Center, 1965.

4 Kleban (M.H.), Brody (E.M.): Prediction of improvement in mentally impaired aged: personality ratings by social workers. *Journal of Gerontology*, 1972, 27, 1, 69-76.

5 Kleban (M.H.), Brody (E.M.), Lawton (M.P.): Personality traits in the mentally-impaired aged and their relationship to improvements in current functioning. *Gerontologist*, 1971, 11, 134-140.

6 Noyes (A.P.), Kalb (L.C.): Modern clinical psychiatry. Philadelphia: W.B. Saunders, 1958.

SENIOR APPERCEPTION TECHNIQUE (S.A.T.)

SPECIFICITY

TYPE OF INSTRUMENT

* * *

Projective test:
16 blanks

REFERENCE	**Bellak (L.), Bellak (S.S.)** · – Manual for the Senior Apperception Technique. Larchmont, New York: C. P.S., 1973.
	Language: English. **U.S.A.**
	Location: See ref. biblio nº 1

ORIGIN

The instrument was inspired by the T.A.T. of **Murray** (ref. 3) and G.A.T. of **Wolk** (ref. 4).

PURPOSE

The instrument was designed to arouse the reactions of the elderly to unstructured material and so to lead them to project themselves by attributing to someone else their own wishes, desires, fears and behavior.

POPULATION

Elderly out-patients.

ADMINISTRATION

Rater: Qualified psychologist.

Time required: Maximum five minutes per blank.

Training: Training in projective techniques.

Scoring: Essentially qualitative. Norms for the duration of stories have been applied on small samples. There is no need to use all the cards.

VARIABLES

Facing daily life situations.

DESCRIPTION

The respondent is asked to tell a story with a development and an end in which each card represents the beginning of the story. The last card represents a person in the mood of dreaming, and he is asked to tell his dream.

VALIDATION

The work of Kahanna (ref. 2) demonstrates the utility of S.A.T. blanks with an aged population.

APPLICATION

Essentially clinical, to get to know the view of life of aged people.

1 Bellak (L.), Bellak (S.S.): Manual for the Senior Apperception Technique. Larchmont, New York: C.P.S., 1973.

2 Kahana (B.): "Use of projective techniques in personality assessment of the aged". In: Storandt (M.), Siegler (I.C.), Elias (M.F.) Eds: "Clinical psychology of aging". New York: Plenum Press, 1978.

3 Murray (H.A.): Thematic Apperception Test Manual. Cambridge: Harvard University Press, 1943.

4 Wolk (R.L.), Rustin (S.), Seiden (R.A.): A custom made projective technique for the aged: The Gerontological Apperception Test. *Journal of the Long Island Consultation Center*, 1966, n°. 4, 7-17.

BEHAVIOR RATING SCALE

SPECIFICITY

* * *

TYPE OF INSTRUMENT

Analogic rating scale
from 0-10, 50 items

REFERENCE	**Williams (J.R.)** · – Preliminary studies aimed at increasing the reliability of a behavior rating scale for use with geriatric and infirm patients. *Journal of Gerontology,* 1973, 28, 4, 510-515.

Language: Original version published in English. Translated into French by L. Israel. **U.S.A.**

Location: Enclosed in volume two page 118
See ref. biblio n° 13

For all information concerning the instrument write to the author at the following address:

Joseph Williams,
115 West Third Street
Manteno, Illinois 60950, U.S.A.

ORIGIN — Scale designed in Kankakee State Hospital.

PURPOSE — To survey present status and degree of change in physical, mental and social behavior of aged and infirm subjects.

POPULATION — Hospitalized geriatric and infirm patients.

ADMINISTRATION — *Rater:* Employee personnel.

Time required: 30 min. approximately.

Training: Necessary for better reliability.

Scoring: Each of 10 categories of behavior is defined by 5 specific items of behavior; each item is scored (0, 1, 2) which permits expression of each category on a scale of 0-10. The perfect score is thus 100.

VARIABLES — The 10 variables or categories are:
· Mental alertness
· Upkeep in personal appearance
· Favourableness of attitude
· Degree of security or calm
· Involvement in useful activity
· Undertaking of responsibility
· Response to "real" stimuli
· Appropriateness of speech
· Adaptability
· Self-confidence

VALIDATION — Behavior categories selected on the basis of their similarity to both factorially resolved traits of significance and experienced employee observations of what were thought to be significant items. Reliability measurement: four controlled studies of inter-rater agreement (ref. 13). Also related studies (ref. 12, 14, 15, 16, 17, 18).

APPLICATION — Can be used as a clinical instrument to evaluate the physical, mental and social behavior before and after various therapeutic regimens and to serve as a type of evidence for discharge or modification in treatment procedure.

1 Cattell (R.B.), Stice (G.F.): Handbook for the 16 personality factor questionnaire. Champaign, Ill: Institute For Personality and Ability Testing, 1953.

2 Guilford (J.P.): Psychometric methods. New-York: Mc Graw-Hill, 1936.

3 Hackerman (N.): The future of graduate education, if any. *Science*, 1972, 175, 475.

4 Hase (H.C.), Goldberg (L.R.): Comparative validity of different strategies of constructing personality inventory scales. *Psychological Bulletin*, 1967, 67, 231-248.

5 Levine (D.): Psychiatric rating scales, platonic true scores and scientific method. *Psychological Bulletin*, 1969, 71, 274-275.

6 Lorr (M.), O'Connor (J.P.), Stafford (J.W.): The Psychotic reaction profile. Beverly Hills: Western Psychological Services, 1961.

7 Mc Donald (J.R.): Are the data worth gathering? *Science*, 1972, 176, 1377.

8 Stevens (S.S.): Adaptation level vs. the relativity of judgment. *American Journal of Psychology*, 1958, 71, 633-646.

9 Stone (L.A.): Magnitude estimation and numerical category scale evaluations of category scale adjectival stimuli on three clinical judgmental continua. *Journal of Clinical Psychology*, 1970, 26, 24-27.

10 Williams (J.R.): The definition and measurement of conflict in terms of P-technique: a test of validity. Unpublished PhD dissertation, Univ. of Illinois, 1958.

11 Williams (J.R.): A test of the validity of P-technique in the measurement of internal conflict. *Journal of Personality*, 1959, 27, 418-437.

12 Williams (J.R.): The use of "likability" ratings and ability scores in the prediction of school achievement. *Journal of Educational Research*, 1963, 57, 90-92.

13 Williams (J.R.): Preliminary studies aimed at increasing the reliability of a behavior rating scale for use with geriatric and infirm patients. *Journal of Gerontology*, 1973, vol. 28, n°. 4, 510-515.

14 Williams (J.R.), Csalany (L.), Misevic (G.): Drug therapy with and without group discussion: effects of various regimens on the behavior of geriatric patients in a mental hospital. *Journal of the American Geriatrics Society*, 1967, 15, 34-40.

15 Williams (J.R.), Dewitt (W.R.), Hurt (R.W.): Ability, likability, and motivation of students as they relate to prediction of achievement. *Journal of Educational Research*, 1971, 65, 155-158.

16 Williams (J.R.), Knecht (W.W.): Teachers' ratings of high school students on "likability" and their relation to measures of ability and achievement. *Journal of Educational Research*, 1962, 56, 152-155.

17 Williams (J.R.), Kriauciunas (R.), Rodriquez (A.): Physical, mental and social rehabilitation of elderly and infirm patients. *Hospital and Community Psychiatry*, 1970, 21, 130-132.

18 Williams (J.R.), Ziemer (C.): Objective observations and comments relative to the application of the Scope results of Kankakee state hospital. Unpublished report, 1970.

19 Wittenborn (J.R.): Wittenborn psychiatric rating scales. New-York: Psychological Corporation, 1955.

PRESENT STATE EXAMINATION (P.S.E.)

SPECIFICITY

*

TYPE OF INSTRUMENT

| Questionnaire, |
| 20 items |

REFERENCE	**Wing (J.K.), Cooper (J.E.), Sartorius (N.)** · – Measurement and classification of psychiatric symptoms: An instruction manual for the P.S.E. and CATEGO program. London: Cambridge University Press, 1974.
	Language: Original version published in English. Translations in over 30 languages. **Great Britain**
	Location: See ref. biblio n⁰ 43
	For all information concerning the instrument or translations, write to the author at the following address:
	John Wing, MRC Social Psychiatry Unit Institute of Psychiatry de Crespigny Park, London SE5 8AF, Great Britain

ORIGIN	Clinical observations.
PURPOSE	To provide a reliable description of the symptoms present at examination and during the previous month, a brief description of syndromes during previous episodes, a listing of possible factors of diagnostic significance, and a standard classification.
POPULATION	Can be used with inpatients (except for dementia), other patient groups, and population samples.
ADMINISTRATION	*Rater:* Psychiatrist (full PSE) Trained lay interviewers (first 40 items)
	Time required: 45-60 minutes.
	Training: One week training course essential. Good clinical experience necessary for full interview.

VARIABLES   20 sections:

1. Introduction	10. Obsessions
2. Health, worrying, tension	11. Depersonalisation
3. Autonomic anxiety	12. Others perceptual disorders
4. Thinking, concentration	13. Thought insertion, etc.
5. Depressed mood	14. Hallucinations
6. Self and others	15. Delusions
7. Appetite, sleep, retardation	16. Sensorium
8. Irritability	17. Insight
9. Expansive mood	18-20. Behaviour, affect, speech

VALIDATION	International Pilot study of Schizophrenia (Ref. 47). US-UK Diagnostic Project (Ref. 11), General population samples (Ref. 44).
APPLICATION	**Research:** · Epidemiological studies · Therapeutic trials · Nosological research **Clinical:** · Description of mental state · Prognostic studies · Training of psychiatrists.

1 Bartko (J.J.), Gulbinat (W.) Eds.: Multivariate statistical methodologies used in the international pilot study of schizophrenia. Washington, D.C.: National Institute of Mental Health, 1980.

2 Bartko (J.J.), Kramer (M.), Williams (K.): Some multivariate statistical techniques: report from the IPSS. USA: Division of Biometry, NIMH, 1975.

3 Carpenter (W.T.) et al.: Another view of schizophrenic subtypes: report from the IPSS. *Arch. Gen. Psychiatry*, 1976, 33, 508-516.

4 Carpenter (W.T.), Bartko (J.J.), Strauss (J.S.), Hawk (A.B.): Signs and symptoms as predictors of outcome: report from the IPSS. *Am. J. Psychiatry*, 1978, 135, 8, 940.

5 Carpenter (W.T.), Strauss (J.S.): Cross-cultural evaluation of Schneider's first – rank symptoms of schizophrenia: a report from the IPSS. *Am. J. Psychiatry*, 1974, 121, 682.

6 Cranach (M. Von), Cooper (J.E.): Changes in rating behaviour during the learning of a standardized psychiatric interview. *Psychological Medicine*, nov. 1972, vol. 2. n°. 4, 373-380.

7 Jablensky (A.), Sartorius (N.): Culture and Schizophrenia. In: "Proceedings of symposium on schizophrenia: biological and behavioural aspects", Amsterdam, 1974. Amsterdam: H. van Praag, 1975, 99-124.

8 Jablensky (A.), Sartorius (N.): Schizophrenia succeeded by affective illness: catamnesic study and statistical enquiry. *Psychological Medicine*, 1977, 7, 619-634.

9 Jablensky (A.): Schwarz (R.), Tomov (T.): WHO collaborative study on impairments and disabilities associated with schizophrenia disorders. A preliminary communication: objectives and methods. In: «Epidemiological research as basis for the organization of extramural psychiatry»: proceedings of the second European Symposium on Social Psychiatry. *Acta Psychiatrica Scandinavica*, 1980, Suppl. 285, vol. 62.

10 Kabesova (L.), Skoda (C.): Predictors of the outcome of the two years course of the IPSS WHO Prague subsample, closing report of a research. *Archives of the PRI Prague*, Appendix 14, p. 34.

11 Kendel (R.E.), Everitt (B.), Cooper (J.E.), Sartorius (N.), David (M.E.): The reliability of the "Present State Examination". *Social Psychiatry*, 1968, 3, 123-129.

12 Leff (J.P.): Culture and the differentiation of emotional stress. *Brit. J. Psychiatry*, 1973, 121, 329.

13 Leff (J.P.): Transcultural influences on psychiatrists' rating of verbally expressed emotion. *Brit. J. Psychiatry*, 1974, 125, 336.

14 Leff (J.P.): International variations in the diagnosis of psychiatric illness. *Brit. J. Psychiatry*, 1977, 131, 329.

15 Lin (T.): Reducing variability in international research. *Social Psychiatry*, 1969, 47, 47.

16 Lorr (M.), Klett (C.J.), McNair (D.M.), Lasky (J.): Inpatient multidimensional psychiatric scale: manual. Palo Alto: Consulting Psychologists Press, 1963.

17 Luria (R.E.), Mc Hugh (P.R.): Reliability and clinical utility of the "Wing" Present State Examination. *Arch. Gen. Psychiatry*, 1974, vol. 30, 866-871.

18 Predictors of the two years course of the WHO IPSS Prague subsample (abstract). *Cs. Psychiat.*, 1976, 71, 4, 263.

19 Psychiatric diagnosis, classification and statistics: functional psychoses, with special emphasis on schizophrenia, report of a seminar. London, 1965.

20 Research on specific mental disorders: IPSS. Meeting of investigators. Geneva, 1965.

21 Research on specific mental disorders: IPSS. Meeting of investigators. Geneva, 1966.

22 Research on specific mental disorders: IPSS. Meeting of investigators. Geneva, 1967.

23 Sartorius (N.): The cross-national standardization of psychiatry diagnosis and classification. In: Pflanz (M.), Schach (E.) Eds.: "Cross national sociomedical research: concepts, methods, practice". Stuttgart: G. Thieme Publishers, 1976.

24 Sartorius (N.), Brooke (E.), Lin (T.): Reliability of psychiatric assessment in international research. In: Hare (E.H.), Wing (J.K.) Eds: "Psychiatric epidemiology: proceedings of the international symposium held Aberdeen University", 1969. London: Oxford University Press, 1970.

25 Sartorius (N.), Jablensky (A.), Shapiro (R.): The WHO international pilot study of schizophrenia. Preliminary communication. *Psychological Medicine*, 1977, 2, 422.

26 Sartorius (N.), Jablensky (A.), Shapiro (R.): Two-year follow-up of the patients included in the WHO international pilot study of schizophrenia. Preliminary communication. *Psychological Medicine*, 1977, 7, 529-541.

27 Sartorius (N.), Jablensky (A.), Shapiro (R.): Cross – cultural differences in the short-term prognosis of schizophrenic psychoses. *Schizophrenia Bulletin*, 1979, vol. 4, 102-113.

28 Sartorius (N.), Jablensky (A.), Strömgren (E.), Shapiro (R.): Validity of diagnostic concepts across cultures: preliminary report from the IPSS. In: Cromsell (W), Matthyse. Eds.: "Nature of schizophrenia". New York: John Wiley and sons, 1978.

29 Sartorius (N.), Shapiro (R.), Barrett (K.): International pilot study of schizophrenia: preliminary communication. *Psychological Medicine*, 1972, 2, 422.

30 Sartorius (N.), Shapiro (R.), Jablensky (A.): The international pilot study of schizophrenia. *Schizophrenia Bulletin*, 1974, n. 11, 21.

31 Schizophrenia: a multi-national study. Summary of the initial phase of the IPSS. *P.H.P.*, 1975, n°. 63.

32 Shepard (M), Brooke (E), Cooper (J.E.), Lin (T.Y.): An experimental approach to psychiatric diagnosis. *Acta Psychiat. Scand.*, 1968, Suppl. 201.

33 Skoda (C.), et al.: Diagnostic agreement of groups of Czechoslovak and an international group of psychiatrists presented with discrete sequences of information on patients. A report from the IPSS. *Socijalna Psihijatria*, 1976, 3, 265.

34 Skoda (C.), Baudis (P.), Matesova (A.), Kabesova (L.), Skodova (M.): First admissions of depressive phase of affective psychoses in Prague, 1963-1972. *Cs.Psychiat.*, 1977. 73.

35 Skoda (C.), Dostal (T.), Kabesova (L.), Syrova (M.), Skodova (M.): Different diagnostic discriminative value of microsyndromes. Report from the IPSS WHO. *Cs. Psychiat.*, 1976, 72, 88-97.

36 Skoda (C.), Husak (I.), Janough (J.), et al: Computer written standardized present state examination and its diagnostic informativeness. *Cs. Psychiat.*, 1971, 67, 352.

37 Skoda (C.), Syrova (M.), Kabesova (L.), Reigrova (J.): Predictors of a five-year course impairment of social functions. Report from the WHO IPSS, 1977.

38 Spitzer (R.L.), Fleiss (J.L.), Burdock (E.I.), Hardesty (A.S.): The mental status schedule: rationale, reliability and validity. *Comprehensive Psychiatry*, 1964, 5, 384.

39 Wing (J.K.): Preliminary communication. A technique for studying psychiatric morbidity in in-patient and out-patient series and in general population samples. *Psychological Medicine*, 1976, 6, 665-671.

40 Wing (J.K.): Methodological issues in psychiatric case-identification. *Psychological Medicine*, 1980, 10, 5-10.

41 Wing (J.K.): Innovations in social psychiatry. *Psychological Medicine*, 1980, 10, 219-230.

42 Wing (J.K.), Birley (J.L.T.), Cooper (J.E.), Graham (P.), Isaacs (A.D.): Reliability of a procedure for measuring and classifying "present psychiatric state". *Brit. J. Psychiat.*, 1967, 113, 499-515.

43 Wing (J.K.), Cooper (J.E.), Sartorius (N): The measurement and classification of psychiatric symptoms: an instruction manual for the PSE and CATEGO program. London: Cambridge University Press, 1974.

44 Wing (J.K.), Nixon (J.M.), Mann (S.A.), Leff (J.P.): Reliability of the PSE (ninth edition) used in a population survey. *Psychological Medicine*, 1977, 7, 505-516.

45 Wittenborn (J.R.): Wittenborn psychiatric rating scales. New York: Psychological Corporation, 1955.

46 World Health Organization: International Pilot Study of Schizophrenia. Vol. 1. WHO Offset publication, 1974, n°. 2.

47 World Health Organization: International Pilot Study of Schizophrenia: meeting of an advisory group. Geneva: WHO, 1975.

48 World Health Organization: Schizophrenia: an international follow-up study. Geneva: WHO; Chichester: John Wiley and Sons, 1979.

D - TEST

SPECIFICITY

* * *

TYPE OF INSTRUMENT

Rating Scale
13 items and
6 levels

REFERENCE	**Ferm (L.)** · – Behavioural activities in demented geriatric patients: a study based on evaluations made by nursing staff members on patients' scores on a simple psychometric test. *Gerontologia Clinica,* 1974, 16, 185-194.

Language: Original version in Finnish. Abbreviated version in English.
Finland

Location: Enclosed in volume two page 121
See ref. biblio nº 2

For all information concerning the instrument write to the author at the following address:

Liisa Ferm,
Koskelan Sairaskoti,
Käpyläntie 11,
00600 Helsinki 60, Finland

ORIGIN
This instrument was initially comprised of 62 items but has been reduced to 13 in an abridged version. The construction of the test was based on work by **Isaacs** and **Walkey** (ref. 6), **Grauer** (ref. 4), **Kahn** (ref. 7), **Pfeiffer** (ref. 8), **Inglis** (ref. 5) and **Wechsler** (ref. 11).

PURPOSE
The instrument was constructed in order to compare the level of dementia and its correlates in overt behavior.

POPULATION
Psychogeriatric in and out-patients.

ADMINISTRATION
Rater: Psychologist for the full length version. Health care personnel and physicians for the abridged version.
Time required: 30 minutes.
Training: Knowledge of mental tests.
Scoring: 6 levels.

VARIABLES
· Memory
· Concentration
· Communication
· Recognition of persons
· Cooperation

· Toilet
· Dressing
· Mobility
· Sleeping
· Continence
· Agitation

VALIDATION
On a population of psychogeriatric patients a test analysis was done (ref. 2, 3) concerning:
Empirical validity
Predictive validity
Inter-rater reliability
Test-retest reliability

OTHER WORKS
cited by author
Internal consistency. Further item analyses under way.

APPLICATION
Clinical work:
Differential diagnoses
Diagnosing the degree of dementia
Judicial matters concerning the client.

Research:
Epidemiological studies
Rehabilitation
Indication of placement.

1 Ajuriaguerra (J. de), Tissot (R.): Some aspects of psychoneurologic disintegration in senile dementia. In: Müller, Ciompi: "Senile dementia". Bern: Huber, 1968.

2 Ferm (L.): Behavioural activities in demented geriatric patients: study based on evaluations made by nursing staff members and on patients'scores on a simple psychometric test. *Gerontologia Clinica*, 1974, 16, 185-194.

3 Ferm (L.): Changes of intellectual functioning and nursing dependency in institutionalized old people. In: "Societas Gerontologica Fennica Yearbook Geron". 1976, XXI, 64-71.

4 Grauer (H.), Birnbom (F.): A geriatric functional rating scale to determine the need for institutional care. *Journal of the American Geriatrics Society*, 1975, 10. 472-476.

5 Inglis (J.): A paired-associate learning test for use with the elderly psychiatric patients. *J. Ment. Sci.*, 1964, 105, 440-443.

6 Isaacs (B.), Walkey (F.A.): The measurement of mental impairment in geriatric practice. *Geront. Clin.*, 1964, 6, 114-123.

7 Kahn (R.), Goldfarb (A.I.), Pollack (M.) et al.: Brief objective measures for the determination of mental status in the aged. *Am. J. Psychiat.*, 1960, 117, 326.

8 Pfeiffer (E.): A short portable mental status questionnaire for the assessment of organic brain deficit in elderly patients. *Journal of the American Geriatrics Society*, 1975, 10, 433-441.

9 Silver (C.P.): Simple methods of testing ability in geriatric patients. *Geront. Clin.*, 1972, 14, 110-122.

10 Slater (E.), Roth (M.): Clinical psychiatry. London: Bailliere, Tindall and Cassel, 1969.

11 Wechsler (D.): The measurement and appraisal of adult intelligence. Baltimore: Williams and Wilkins, 1958.

12 Wilson (L.A.), Brass (W.): Brief assessment of the mental state in geriatric domiciliary practice. The usefulness of the mental status questionnaire. *Age and Ageing*, 1973, 2, 92-101.

GERIATRIC MENTAL STATE SCHEDULE

SPECIFICITY

* * *

TYPE OF INSTRUMENT

Questionnaire,
600 items

REFERENCE	**Copeland (J.R.M.), Kelleher (M.J.), Kellett (J. M.), Gourlay (A.J.), Gurland (B.J.), Fleiss (J.L.), Sharpe (L.)** · – A semi-structured clinical interview for the assessment of diagnosis and mental state in the elderly: the Geriatric Mental State Schedule. I: Development and reliability. *Psychological Medicine,* 1976, 6, 439-449.

Gurland (B.J.), Fleiss (J.L.), Goldberg (K.), Sharpe (L.), Copeland (J.R.M.), Kelleher (M.J.), Kellett (J.M.) · – A semi-structured clinical interview for the assessment of diagnosis and mental state in the elderly: the Geriatric Mental State Schedule. II: A factor analysis. *Psychological Medicine,* 1976, 6, 451-459.

Language: Original version published in English. Translations in Danish, German, Duch, French.
Great Britain

Location: See ref. biblio n̊ 9 and 17

For all information concerning the instrument or translations write to the author at the following address:

John Copeland,
University Dept. of Psychiatry
Royal Liverpool Hospital, P.O. Box 147
Liverpool L 69 3 BX, Great Britain

ORIGIN
The interview is based on a factor analysis of the Combined Mental State Schedule which contained items adapted from the Present State Examination developed by **Wing** et al (ref. 29), and the Present State Schedule by **Spitzer** et al (ref. 26).
Practically the whole of the "Mental State Questionnaire" (ref. 19) and the "Face Hand Test" (ref. 14) have been included. 209 new items were added specially for elderly persons and changes made both in the content (cognitive functions, taking into account both organic and sensory deficits) and in the form of the interview (the clarity and conciseness of statements).

PURPOSE
Assessment, specially for diagnosis, of the mental state of elderly subjects. In the form of a semi-structural interview, this instrument allows the gathering of reliable and standardized information for the purposes of research.

POPULATION
Essentially for elderly patients admitted to hospital. Has also been used successfully on community subjects (short version).

ADMINISTRATION
Rater: Psychiatrist, psychologist, nurse, social worker.

Time required: 30-40 minutes.

Training: 10 to 20 interviews with patients followed by a discussion of rating with a trained interviewer are recommended.

Scoring: The semistructured interview deals with the mental state of the subject during the previous month and contains about 200 questions from which 600 items are rated.
Instructions for the rating of items are included in the schedule.

VARIABLES
Psychiatric symptoms: 21 factors.
Depression, anxiety, impaired memory, retarded speech, hypomania, somatic concerns, observed belligerence, reported belligerence, obsessions, drug-alcohol dependence, cortical dysfunction, disorientation, lack of insight, depersonalization-derealization, paranoid delusion, subjective experience of disordered thought, visual hallucination, auditory hallucination, abnormal motor movements, non-social speech, incomprehensibility.

VALIDATION

Performed on a hospital and community sample in New York and London (ref. 9 and 17).
Factor analysis revealed the 21 factors mentioned above.
Construct validity differentiated the results of the factor analysis of diagnostic groups (Depression/organic pathology).
External validity, a clinical classification of mood disorders and dementia by comparison with outcome over several months, also by a projected clinical diagnosis based on memory disturbance and by comparison of data gathered from clinical, physical, social, biochemical and radiological examinations.
Concurrent validity by psychometric tests concerned specially with organic diagnoses.
Inter-rater reliability with 3 experienced psychiatrists, interviewers. Interview observers: test-retest.

OTHER WORKS
cited by author

Short form adapted for early detection but not for studies of prevalence.
A computerised diagnostic system Agecat is in course of preparation.

APPLICATION

Research: Nosological research (concerned with the definition of exclusive symptom categories) and comparison of symptom profiles, research into prognosis.
Studies of change after treatment. Epidemiological studies.

Ic.12   BIBLIOGRAPHY

1 Cohen (J.): A coefficient of agreement for nominal scales. *Educational and Psychological Measurement*, 1960, 20, 37-46.

2 Cohen (J.): Weighted kappa: nominal scale agreement with provision for scaled disagreement or partial credit. *Psychological Bulletin*, 1968, 70, 213-220.

3 Cooper (J.E.), Kendall (R.E.), Gurland (B.J.), Sharpe (L.), Copeland (J.R.M.), Simon (R.): Psychiatric diagnosis in New York and London. London: Oxford University Press, 1972.

4 Copeland (J.R.M.), Evaluation of diagnostic methods: international comparison. In: Post (F.) Ed.: "Studies in geriatric psychiatry". New York: John Wiley and sons, 1979, 191-209.

5 Copeland (J.R.M.), Kelleher (M.J.), Duckworth (G.), Smith (A.): Reliability of psychiatric assessment in older patients. *International Journal of Aging and Human Development*, 1976, 7, 313-322.

6 Copeland (J.R.M.), Kelleher (M.J.), Kellett (J.M.), Barron (G.), Cowan (D.W.), Gourlay (A.J.): Evaluation of a psychogeriatric service: the distinction between psychogeriatric and geriatric patients. *British Journal of Psychiatry*, 1975, 126, 21-29.

7 Copeland (J.R.M.), Kelleher (M.J.), Kellett (J.M.), Gourlay (A.J.), Barron (G.), Cowan (D.W.), De Gruchy (J.), Gurland (B.J.), Sharpe (L.), Simon (R.), Kuriansky (J.B.), Stiller (P.): Diagnostic differences in psychogeriatric patients in New York and London. *Canadian Psychiatric Association Journal*, 1974, 19, 267-271.

8 Copeland (J.R.M.), Kelleher (M.J.), Kellett (J.M.), Gourlay (A.J.), Cowan (D.W.), Barron (G.), De Gruchy (J.), Gurland (B.J.), Sharpe (L.), Simon (R.), Kuriansky (J.B.), Stiller (P.): Cross-national study of diagnosis of the mental disorders: a comparison of the diagnoses of elderly psychiatric patients admitted to mental hospitals serving Queens County, New York, and the former borough of Camberwell, London. *British Journal of Psychiatry*, 1975, 126, 11-20.

9 Copeland (J.R.M.), Kelleher (M.J.), Kellett (J.M.), Gourlay (A.J.), Gurland (B.J.), Fleiss (J.L.), Sharpe (L.): A semi-structured clinical interview for the assessment of diagnosis and mental state in the elderly: the geriatric mental state schedule. I: development and reliability. *Psychological Medicine*, 1976, 6, 439-449.

10 Cowan (D.W.), Copeland (J.R.M.), Kelleher (M.J.), Kellett (J.M.), Gourlay (A.J.), Smith (A.), Barron (G.), De Gruchy (J.), Kuriansky (J.), Gurland (B.J.), Sharpe (L.), Stiller (P.), Simon (R.): Cross-national study of the diagnosis of the mental disorders:a comparative psychometric assessment of elderly patients admitted to mental hospitals serving Queens County, New York and the former borough of Camberwell, London, *British Journal of Psychiatry*, 1975, 126, 560-570.

11 Duckworth (G.S.), Ross (H.): Diagnostic differences in psychogeriatric patients in Toronto, New York, and London, England. *Canadian Medical Association Journal*, 1975, 112, 847-850.

12 Fleiss (J.L.), Gurland (B.J.), Cooper (J.E.): Some contributions to the measurement of psychopathology. *British Journal of Psychiatry*, 1971, 119, 647-656.

13 Fleiss (J.L.), Gurland (B.J.), Des Roche (P.): Distinctions between organic brain syndrome and functional psychiatric disorders: based on the Geriatric Mental State Interview. *International Journal of Aging and Human Development*, 1976, 7, 323-330.

14 Goldfarb (A.I.): The evaluation of geriatric patients following treatment. In: Hoch (P.), Zubin (J.) Eds: "The evaluation of psychiatric treatment". New York: Grune and Stratton, 1964.

15 Gurland (B.J.): The comparative-frequency and types of depression in various adult age groups. *Journal of Gerontology*, 1976, 31, 283-292.

16 Gurland (B.J.), Copeland (J.R.M.), Sharpe (L.), Kelleher (M.): The geriatric mental status interview (GMS). *Int'l Aging and Human Development*, 1976, vol. 7, n°. 4, 303-311.

17 Gurland (B.J.), Fleiss (J.L.), Goldberg (K.), Sharpe (L.), Copeland (J.R.M.); Kelleher (M.J.), Kellett (J.M.): A semi-structured clinical interview for the assessment of diagnosis and mental state in the elderly: the geriatric mental state schedule. II: a factor analysis. *Psychological Medicine*, 1976, 6, 451-459.

18 Gurland (B.J.), Kuriansky (J.B.), Sharpe (L.), Simon (R.), Stiller (P.), Copeland (J.R.M.), Kelleher (M.J.), Kellett (J.M.), Gourlay (A.J.), Cowan (D.W.), Barron (G.): A comparison of the outcome of hospitalization of geriatric patients in public psychiatric wards in New York and London. *Canadian Psychiatric Association Journal*, 1976, 21, 6, 421-431.

19 Kahn (R.L.), Goldfarb (A.I.), Pollack (M.), Peck (M.), Peck (A.): Brief objective measures for the determination of mental status in the aged. *American Journal of Psychiatry*. 1960, 117, 326-328.

20 Kelleher (M.J.), Copeland (J.R.M.), Gurland (B.J.), Sharpe (L.):Assessment of the older psychiatric inpatient. *International Journal of Aging and Human Development*, 1976, 7, 295-302.

21 Kellett (J.M.), Copeland (J.R.M.), Kelleher (M.J.): Information leading to accurate diagnosis in the elderly. *British Journal of Psychiatry*, 1975, 12, 423-430.

22 Kendell (R.E.), Everitt (B.), Cooper (J.E.), Sartorius (N.), David (M.E.): The reliability of the present state examination. *Social Psychiatry*, 1968, 3, 123-129.

23 Leff (J.P.), Wing (J.K.): Trial of maintenance therapy in schizophrenia. *British Medical Journal*, 1971, III, 599-604.

24 Lipsedge (M.S.), Rees (L.W.), Pike (D.J.): A double-blind comparison of dothiepin and amitriptyline for the treatment of depression with anxiety. *Psychopharmacologia*, 1971, 19, 153-162.

25 Spitzer (R.L.), Endicott (J.): Diagno: a computer program for psychiatric diagnosis utilizing the differential diagnostic procedure. *Archives of General Psychiatry*, 1968, 18, 746-756.

26 Spitzer (R.L.), Fleiss (J.L.), Burdock (E.I.), Hardesty (A.S.): The mental status schedule: rationale, reliability and validity. *Comprehensive Psychiatry*, 1964, 5, 384-395.

27 Wing (J.K.), Birley (J.L.T.), Cooper (J.E.), Graham (P.), Isaacs (A.D.): Reliability of a procedure for measuring present psychiatric state. *British Journal of Psychiatry*, 1967, 113, 499-515.

28 Wing (J.K.), Cooper (J.E.), Sartorius (N.): The measurement and classification of psychiatric symptoms. London: Cambridge University Press, 1970.

29 Wing (J.K.), Cooper (J.E.), Sartorius (N.): Present state examination. Ninth edition of interview schedule. London: Cambridge University Press, may 1973.

30 World Health Organization: Schizophrenia: report on an international pilot study. Geneva: World Health Organization, 1972.

HYPOCHONDRIASIS SCALE INSTITUTIONAL GERIATRIC (H.S.I.G.)

SPECIFICITY

* * *

TYPE OF INSTRUMENT

Check list, 6 items
scored Yes-No

REFERENCE	**Brink (T.L.), Belanger (J.), Bryant (J.), Capri (D.), Janakes (C.), Jasculca (S.), Oliveira (C.)** · – Hypochondriasis in an institutional geriatric population: construction of a scale (H.S.I.G.). *Journal of the American Geriatrics Society,* 1978, vol. 26, 12, 557-559.

Language: Original version published in English. Translation in Spanish.
U.S.A.

Location: Enclosed in volume two page 86
See ref. biblio nº 4

For all information concerning the instrument or translation, write to the author at the following address:

T.L. Brink,
1044 Sylvan,
San Carlos, California 94070, U.S.A.

ORIGIN
The instrument began with 27 questions taken from the MMPI and the scale by **Pilowski** (ref. 13) given to a population divided into hypochondriacs, confused and quarrelsome paranoids. The only 6 items differentiating the hypochondriacs significantly from other patients have been retained and adapted for aged subjects (ref. 3, 4, 5, 6, 9).

PURPOSE
Evaluation of hypochondrical attitudes, necessary but not sufficient for the diagnosis of hypochondria in resident elderly suffering from multiple organic disorders.

POPULATION
All aged persons.

ADMINISTRATION
Rater: Physician. (The experience has, however, proved that the rater's function does not influence the scores). Administered in writing or orally.

Time required: 1 minute.

Training: Familiarization with the items particularly concerning the scoring of answers to questions 5 and 6.
Scoring: On the score sheet the answer indicating a hypochondriacal attitude ("H") is indicated. Each such answer contributes a supplementary point. The global score varies from 0-6.

VARIABLES
Hypochondriasis.

VALIDATION
With psychiatric aged patients, covering (ref. 6):
Validity and discriminating **sensitivity** between hypochondriacs and those who are not affected. (A few false positives, but no false negatives).
Study of **correlation** with the measure of depression by Zung's scale or the author's scale of geriatric depression, with the measure of dementia by the "Face Hand Test", and the "Stimulus Recognition Test", with a self-administration of memory and with the "Social Readjustment Rating Scale" evaluating the situational stress factors.

APPLICATION
Clinical: Contribution to diagnosis.
Research: When hypochondria is a variable to be evaluated among others.

1 Alarcon (R. de): Earlier diagnosis of the depressions of the aged. *Rev. Med. Univ. Navarra*, 1968, 12, 193.

2 Biran (S.): Die Hypochondrie und der Sammelbegriff des eingebildeten Krankseins. *Acta Psychotherap. and Psychosom.*, 1963, 11, 343.

3 Brink (T.L.): Self-ratings of memory versus psychometric ratings of memory and hypochondriasis. *Journal of the American Geriatrics Society*, 1981, 29, 537-538.

4 Brink (T.L.), Belanger (J.), Bryant (J.), Capri (D.), Janakes (C.), Jasculca (S.), Oliveira (C.): Hypochondriasis in an institutional geriatric population: construction of a scale (HSIG). *Journal of the American Geriatrics Society*, 1978, vol. 26, nº. 12, 557-559.

5 Brink (T.L.), Capri (D.), De Neeve (V.), Janakes (C.), Oliveira (C.): Hypochondriasis and paranoia: similar delusional systems in an institutionalized geriatric population. *Journal of Nervous and Mental Disease*, 1979, 167, 224-228.

6 Brink (T.L.), Janakes (C.), Martinez (N.): Geriatric hypochondriasis: situational factors. *Journal of the American Geriatrics Society*, 1981, vol. 29, nº. 1, 37-39.

7 Busse (E.W.): Hypochondriasis in the elderly: a reaction to social stress. *Journal of the American Geriatrics Society*, 1976, 24, 145.

8 Fenyon (F.E.): Hypochondriasis: a clinical study. *Brit. J. Psychiat.*, 1964, 110, 478

9 Fenyon (F.E.): Hypochondriasis: a survey of some historical, clinical and social aspects. *Brit. J. Med. Psychol.*, 1965, 38, 117.

10 Grof (P.), Saxema (B.), Cantor (R.) et al.: Doxepin versus amitriptyline in depression. *Current Therap. Res.*, 1974, 16, 470.

11 Muzio (M.), Cichetti (V.), Gabrielli (F.): Sulpiride in the treatment of psychoneurosis. *Rev. Psichiat.*, 1973, 8, 252.

12 Pfeiffer (E.): The use of drugs which influence behavior in the elderly. In: "Drugs and the elderly". Los Angeles: University of Southern California Press, 1975, 33-51.

13 Pilowski (I.): Dimensions of hypochondriasis. *Brit. J. Psychiat.*, 1967, 113, 89.

14 Sullivan (H.S.): Clinical studies in psychiatry. New York: Norton, 1940.

15 Sullivan (H.S.): Conceptions of modern psychiatry. New York: Norton, 1940.

16 Sullivan (H.S.): The interpersonal theory of psychiatry. New York: Norton, 1953.

17 Walsh (A.C.): Hypochondriasis associated with organic brain syndrome: a new approach to therapy. *Journal of the American Geriatrics Society*, 1976, 24, 430.

SHORT PSYCHIATRIC EVALUATION SCHEDULE

SPECIFICITY

$* \quad * \quad *$

TYPE OF INSTRUMENT

Check list
15 questions
scored Yes-No

REFERENCE	**Pfeiffer (E.)** · – A short psychiatric evaluation schedule: a new 15-item monotonic scale indicative of functional psychiatric disorder. In: "Brain function in old age": Bayer-Symposium VII. Springer Verlag, 1979, 228-236.

Language: Original version published in English.
U.S.A.

Location: Enclosed in volume two page 87
See ref. biblio. nº 8

For all information concerning the instrument write to the author at the following address:

Eric Pfeiffer,
Medical Center
Suncoast Gerontology Center
Box 50
12901 North 30th Street
Tampa, Florida 33612, U.S.A.

ORIGIN

The questionnaire was inspired by several instruments: M.M.P.I. (ref. 5), Mini-mult by **Kincanon** (ref. 6) and that by **Savage** and **Britton** (ref. 9). The selection of the 15 retained items was based on case of response, ability to simplify formulation and power to discriminate psychopathology.

PURPOSE

To measure in a simple and rapid way the presence and extent of functional psychiatric symptomatology, without trying to formulate a diagnosis, which would require a much more complex instrument.

POPULATION

All aged persons out-or inpatients.

ADMINISTRATION

Rater: Physician, psychologist, nurse, social worker.

Time required: 7 minutes

Training: Brief instructions explaining scoring.

Scoring: Each question demands an answer of the Yes-No type. The total score varies from 0-15. From 0-3 the subject can be considered as normal. From 6-15 the presence of pathology is quite certain, 4 and 5 correspond to an intermediate state.

VARIABLES

The following psychiatric aspects are assessed:
· Depression
· Hypochondria
· Anxiety
· Dissatisfaction
· Anti-social behavior

VALIDATION

On population of 1.000 aged people covering:
Concurrent validity in relation to "Mini-Mult" (Ref. 6)
Discriminative sensitivity between groups differing on Mini-mult scores of morbidity
Study of a percentage of questionnaires completed by a given population, in relation to age, sex, role, level of education, to determine the practical utility of the instrument by comparing it with other scales and test.

APPLICATION

Clinical:
· Assessment of functional disorders
· Prognosis

Research:
· Drug trials
· Studies and research in psycho-geriatrics.

1 Busse (E.W.), Pfeiffer (E.): Behavior and adaptation in late life. 2nd ed. Boston: Little, Brown and Co., 1977.

2 Donnelly (J.): Personal communication, 1975.

3 Fillenbaum (G.G.), Pfeiffer (E.): The Mini-Mult: a cautionary note. *J. Consult. Clin. Psychol.*, 1976, 44, 698-703.

4 Haglund (R.M.J.), Schuckit (M.A.): A clinical comparison of tests of organicity in elderly patients. *Gerontology*, 1976, 31, 654-659.

5 Hathaway (S.R.), Mc Kinley (J.C.): The Minnesota multiphasic personality inventory manual. Revised ed. New York: The Psychological Corporation, 1951.

6 Kincannon (J.C.): Prediction of the standard MMPI scale scores from 71 items: the Mini-Mult. *J. Consult. Clin. Psychol.*, 1968, 32, 319-325.

7 Pfeiffer (E.): A short portable mental status questionnaire for the assessment of organic brain deficit in elderly patients. *J. Am. Geriatr. Soc.*, 1975, 23, 433-441.

8 Pfeiffer (E.): A short psychiatric evaluation schedule: a new 15-item monotonic scale indicative of functional psychiatric disorder. In: "Brain function in old age": Bayer-Symposium VII. Springer-Verlag, 1979, 228-236.

9 Savage (R.D.), Britton (P.G.): A short scale for the assessment of mental health in the community aged. *Br. J. Psychiatry*, 1967, 113, 521-523.

10 Woodberry (M.): Item analysis for potential information content, computer program. Unpublished. Duke University, 1974.

SURVEY PSYCHIATRIC ASSESSMENT SCHEDULE (S.P.A.S.)

SPECIFICITY

* * *

TYPE OF INSTRUMENT

Questionnaire and
check-list 51 items

REFERENCE	**Bond (J.), Brooks (P.), Carstairs (V.), Giles (L.)** · – The reliability of a survey psychiatric assessment schedule for the elderly. *British Journal of Psychiatry*, 1980, 137, 148-162.
	Bond (J.), Carstairs (V.). – Services for the Elderly. Scottish Health Service Studies nº 42. Edinburgh: Scottish Home and Health Department, 1982.
	
	Language: Original version published in English.
	      Great Britain
	
	Location: Enclosed in volume two page 193
	      See ref. biblio. nº 4 and 5
	
	For all information concerning the instrument write to the author at the following address:
	
	      John Bond,
	      The University of Newcastle-upon-Tyne
	      Health Care Research Unit
	      21 Claremont Place
	      Newcastle-upon-Tyne NE2 4AA, Great Britain

ORIGIN

This instrument was derived from the Geriatric Screening Schedule (Copeland, et. al., unpublished) which is itself a shortened version of the Geriatric Mental State Schedule (ref. 14). The instrument excludes observation or judgement of the fieldworker in the estimation of the severity of psychiatric symptoms.

PURPOSE

The purpose of the instrument is to measure the prevalence of organic psychiatric disorders, affective disorders and psychoneuroses and schizophrenia or paranoid disorders. It was developed for use in a survey of the service requirements of an elderly population which was undertaken in Scotland in 1976.

POPULATION

The instrument was designed for use with people aged 65 or over living in private households and institutions.

ADMINISTRATION

Rater: Physician, psychologist, nurse, social worker or trained research worker.

Time required: 10-25 minutes

Training: Non-psychiatric users require training with the instrument.

Scoring: Individual items are scored according to respondent's answers. Three groups of items are summed to provide an overall score. They vary from 0 to 12 for organic disorders; 0 to 65 for affective disorders and psychoneuroses; and 0 to 10 for schizophrenia and paranoid disorders.

VARIABLES

Three groups of items: · organic disorders (item 1-11)
                         · affective disorders and psychoneuroses (item 12-41)
                         · Schizophrenia and paranoid disorders (item 42-51)

VALIDATION

The validation of the instrument was undertaken in a population of people aged 65 or over. Respondents were recruited from five sources: psychiatric hospital, geriatric hospital, residential home, psychogeriatric day hospital and from a general practitioner's list (ref. 4). The severity of diagnosis was established by a psychiatrist. The following cutting points for indicating severity from each of the global scores was determined for half the sample and tested on the other half:

1. Absence of organic disorder: 9-12   2. Absence of affective disorders or psychoneuroses: 0-10
   Moderate organic disorder: 7-8   Presence of affective disorders or psychoneuroses: 11-65
   Severe organic disorder: 0-6   3. All positive responses indicate the possibility of schizophrenia or paranoid disorder.

OTHER WORKS
cited by author

Studies of presence of psychiatric diseases in a population of 5000 old people (ref. 4).

APPLICATION

Epidemiological studies, prevalence studies, longitudinal studies.

1 Berg (R.L.), Browning (F.E.), Hill (J.G.), Wenkert (W.): Assessing the health care needs of the aged. *Health Services Research*, 1970, 36-59.

2 Bergmann (K.), Gaber (L.B.), Foster (E.M.): The development of an instrument for early ascertainment of psychiatric disorder in elderly community residents: a pilot study. In: Degwitz (R.), Radebold (H.), Schulte (P.W.) Eds: "Geronto-Psychiatrie, 4, Janessen Symposen". Dusseldorf, 1975, 84-119.

3 Blessed (G.), Tomlinson (B.E.), Roth (M.): The association between quantitative measures of dementia and of senile change in cerebral grey matter of elderly subjects. *British Journal of Psychiatry*, 1968, 114, 797-811.

4 Bond (J.), Brooks (P.), Carstairs (V.), Giles (L.): The reliability of a survey psychiatric assessment schedule for the elderly. *British Journal of Psychiatry*, 1980, 137, 148-162.

5 Bond (J.), Carstairs (V.): Services for the elderly. Scottish Health Service Studies, n° 42. Edinburgh: Scottish Home and Health Department, 1982.

6 Bremer (J.): A social psychiatric investigation of a small community in northern Norway. *Acta Psychiatrica Scandinavica*, Supplement 62, 1951.

7 Brodman (K.), Erdmann (A.J.), Irving (L.), Wolfe (H.G.): The Cornell medical index: an adjunct to medical interview. *Journal of the American Medical Association*, 1949, 140, 530-534.

8 Brown (A.C.), Fry (J.): The Cornell medical index health questionnaire in the identification of neurotic patients in general practice. *Journal of Psychosomatic Research*, 1962, 6, 185-190.

9 Carpenter (W.T.), Sacks (M.H.), Strauss (J.S.), Bartko (J.J.), Rayner (J.): Evaluating signs and symptoms: comparison of structured interview and clinical approaches. *British Journal of Psychiatry*, 1976, 128, 397-403.

10 Cohen (J.): A coefficient of agreement for nominal scales. *Educational and Psychological Measurement*, 1960, 20, 37-46.

11 Cole (N.J.), Branch (C.H.), Shaw (O.M.): Mental illness: a survey assessment of community rates, attitudes and adjustments. *Archives of Neurology and Psychiatry*, 1957, 77, 393-398.

12 Cooper (J.E.), Copeland (J.R.M.), Brown (G.W.), Harris (T.), Gourlay (A.J.): Further studies on interviewer training and inter-rater reliability of the present state examination (PSE). *Psychological Medicine*, 1977, 7, 517-523.

13 Copeland (J.R.M.), Kelleher (M.J.), Kellett (J.M.), Gourlay (A.J.), Cowan (D.W.), Barron (G.), De Gruchy (J.), Gurland (B.J.), Sharpe (L.), Simon (R.), Kuriansky (J.), Stiller (P.): Cross-national study of diagnosis of the mental disorders: a comparison of the diagnoses of elderly psychiatric patients admitted to mental hospitals serving Queens County, New York and the former borough of Camberwell, London. *British Journal of Psychiatry*, 1975, 126, 11-20.

14 Copeland (J.R.M.), Kelleher (M.J.), Kellett (J.M.), Gourlay (A.J.), Gurland (B.J.), Fleiss (J.L.), Sharpe (L.): A semi-structured clinical interview for the assessment of diagnosis of mental state in the elderly: the geriatric mental state schedule. I: Development and reliability. *Psychological Medicine*, 1976, 6, 439-449.

15 Essen–Möller (E.): Individual traits and morbidity in a Swedish rural population. *Acta Psychiatrica Scandinavica*, Supplement 100, 1956.

16 Goldberg (D.P.): The detection of psychiatric illness by questionnaire. Oxford University Press, 1972.

17 Goldberg (D.P.), Cooper (B.), Eastwood (M.R.), Kedward (H.B.), Shepherd (M.):A standardized psychiatric interview for use in community surveys. *British Journal of Preventive and Social Medicine*, 1970, 24, 18-23.

18 Gruenberg (E.M.): A mental health survey of older people. New York: Utica, 1961.

19 Gurland (B.J.), Fleiss (J.L.), Goldberg (K.), Sharpe (L.), Copeland (J.R.M.), Kelleher (M.J.), Kellett (J.M.): A semi-structured clinical interview for the assessment of diagnosis and mental state in the elderly: the geriatric mental state schedule: II: a factor analysis. *Psychological Medicine*, 1976, 6, 451-459.

20 Gurland (B.J.), Kuriansky (J.), et al.: The comprehensive assessment and referral evaluation (CARE): rationale development and reliability. *International Journal of Aging and Human Development*, 1977, 8, 9-42.

21 Hodkinson (H.M.): Evaluation of a mental test score for assessment of mental impairment in the elderly. *Age and Ageing*, 1972, 1, 233-238.

22 Ingham (J.G.), Rawnsley (K.), Hughes (D.): Psychiatric disorder and its declaration in contrasting areas of South Wales. *Psychological Medicine*, 1972, 117, 149-156.

23 Irving (G.), Robinson (R.A.), Mc Adam (W.): The validity of some cognitive tests in the diagnosis of dementia. *British Journal of Psychiatry*, 1970, 117, 149-156.

24 Isaacs (B.), Akhtar (A.J.): The set test: a rapid test of mental function in old people. *Age and Ageing*, 1972, 1, 222-226.

25 Isaacs (B.), Walkey (F.A.): Measurement of mental impairment in geriatric practice. *Gerontologia Clinica*, 1964, vol. 6, 114-123.

26 Kahn (R.L.), Goldfarb (A.I.), Pollack (M.), Peck (A.): Brief objective measures for the determination of mental status in the aged. *American Journal of Psychiatry*, 1960, 117, 326-328.

27 Kane (R.A.), Kane (R.L.),: Assessing the elderly. A practical guide to measurement. Lexington: Lexington Books, 1981.

28 Kay (D.W.K.), Beamish (P.), Roth (M.): Old age mental disorders in Newcastle-upon-Tyne. I. *British Journal of Psychiatry*, 1964, 110, 145-158.

29 Kendell (R.E.), Everett (B.), Cooper (S.R.), Sartorius (N.), David (M.E.): The reliability of the present state examination. *Social Psychiatry*, 1968, 3, 123-128.

30 Leighton (D.C.), Harding (J.S.), Macklin (D.B.), Mac Millan (A.M.), Leighton (A.H.): The character of danger. New York: Basic Books, 1963.

31 Ley (P.): Acute psychiatric patients. In: Mittler (P.). "The Psychological assessment of mental and physical handicap". London: Methuen, 1970.

32 Maxwell (A.E.): Analysing qualitative data. London: Methuen, 1961.

33 Meer (B.), Baker (J.A.): The Stockton geriatric rating scale. *Journal of Gerontology*, 1966, vol. 21, 392-403.

34 Milne (J.S.), Maule (M.M.), Cormack (S.), Williamson (J.): The design and testing of a questionnaire and examination to assess physical and mental health in older people using staff nurse as observer. *Journal of Chronic Diseases*, 1972, 25, 385-405.

35 Nielson (J.): Geronto-psychiatric period-prevalence investigation in a geographically delimited population. *Acta Psychiatrica Scandinavica*, 1963, 38, 307-330.

36 Player (D.A.), Irving (G.), Robinson (R.A.): Psychiatric, psychological and social findings in a pilot community health survey. *Health Bulletin*, 1971, 29, 104-107.

37 Powell (C.), Crombie (A.): The Kilsyth questionnaire: a method of screening elderly people at home. *Age and Ageing*, 1974, 3, 23-28.

38 Rawnsley (K.): Congruence of independent measures of psychiatric morbidity. *Journal of Psychosomatic Research*, 1967, 10, 84-93.

39 Robinson (R.A.): Assessment scales in a psycho-geriatric unit. In: Stocker (G.) et al.. Eds.: "Assessment in cerebrovascular insufficiency". Stuttgart: Georg Thieme Verlag, 1971.

40 Spitzer (R.L.), Fleiss (J.L.): A re-analysis of the reliability of psychiatric diagnosis. *British Journal of Psychiatry*, 1974, 125, 341-347.

41 Srole (L.), Langner (T.S.), Michael (S.T.), Opler (M.K.), Rennie (T.A.C.): Mental health in the metropolis – the midtown Manhattan study. vol. 1. New York: Mc Graw-Hill, 1962.

42 Stonier (P.D.): Score changes following repeated administration of mental status questionnaire. *Age and Ageing*, 1974, vol. 3, 91-96.

43 Taylor (H.G.), Bloom (L.M.): Cross-validation and methodological extension of the Stockton geriatric rating scale. *Journal of Gerontology*, 1974, vol. 29, n°. 2, 190-193.

44 Wilson (L.A.), Brass (W.): Brief assessment of the mental state in geriatric domiciliary practice. The usefulness of the mental status questionnaire. *Age and Ageing*, 1973, 2, 92-101.

45 Wilson (L.A.), Grant (K.), Witney (P.M.), Kerridge (D.F.): Mental state of elderly hospital patients related to occupational therapists assessment of activities of daily living. *Gerontologia Clinica*, 1973, vol. 15, 197-202.

46 Wing (J.K.), Birley (J.L.T.), Cooper (J.E.), Graham (P.), Isaacs (A.D.): Reliability of a procedure for measuring and classifying present psychiatric state. *British Journal of Psychiatry*, 1967, 113, 499-515.

EVALUATION CLINIQUE DE LA PERSONNALITE
CLINICAL EVALUATION OF PERSONALITY

SPECIFICITY

* * *

TYPE OF INSTRUMENT

Ordinal rating scale
5 grades,
26 bipolar items

REFERENCE	**Israël (L.), Ohlmann (Th.), Hugonot (L.), Drouet d'Aubigny (G.)** · − Echelle clinique d'évaluation de la personnalité. Validation par analyse factorielle en gériatrie. *L'Encéphale*, 1980, VI, 81-91.

Language: Published in French. Translated into English but not validated.
France

Location: Enclosed in volume two page 122
See ref. biblio. nº 3

For all information concerning the instrument write to the author at the following address:

Liliane Israël,
Pavillon Chissé, C.H.R.U.
38700 La Tronche,
Grenoble, France

ORIGIN
This instrument is a synthesis of numerous scales published in the literature (ref. 1, 2, 4, 5, 6, 7, 8, 9, 10, 12, 13, 14, 15, 16, 17). The 49 items which were more frequently used were reduced to 26 items after factor analysis (ref. 3).

PURPOSE
To assess an individual personality and its changes under the impact of external agents, like drugs, environment etc.

POPULATION
Elderly over 65 years, living at home or in homes for the elderly

ADMINISTRATION
Rater: Psychologist or physician

Time required: 10 minutes

Training: Necessary for non-verbal communication and handling patients

Characteristics: a glossary which allows a precise definition of all 26 items with the purpose to eliminate misunderstanding of the specific semantic connotation.

Scoring: Minimum rating is 1 and maximum is 5, the total score varies from 26 to 130. When the score decreases, it means that there is an improvement and when the score increases it means that there is a worsening.

VARIABLES
One general factor "mental health" and 9 group factors:

Social adaptation:
Social ease
Adaptability
Receptivity
Psychopathic tendencies

Emotional aspects:
Emotional maturity
Inhibition
Depression
Well-being
Guilt

VALIDATION
Validity: **Factor analysis** of Facord type computed from correlations between items expressed in Kendall's π (59% of explained variance) resulted in the previous experimental scale of 40 items being reduced to 26 (ref. 3).
Inter-rater reliability with two raters (ref. 3).

OTHER WORKS
cited by author
Psychotropic drug trials and clinical examination.

APPLICATION
This scale allows a clinical diagnosis of mental disorders through a structural assessment of personality which could be complementary to the dynamic assessment realised through a projective test. It is mainly used in drug trials for psychotropic drugs and in all psychological researches in which personality has an important role.

1 Hamilton (M.): General problems of psychiatric rating scales especially for depression. In: Pichot (P.) Ed: "Psychological measurements in psychopharmacology. Mod. Probl. Pharmacopsychiat.". Basel: Karger, 1974, 7, 125-138.

2 Heimann (H.), Bodon-Schrod (H.), Schmocker (A.M.), Bobon (D.P.): Auto-évaluation de l'humeur par une liste d'adjectifs, la "Befindlichkeits Skala" de Zerssen. L'Encéphale, 1975, 1, 2, 165-183.

3 Israel (L.), Ohlmann (Th.), Hugonot (L.), Drouet d'Aubigny (G.): Echelle clinique d'évaluation de la personnalité. Validation par analyse factorielle en gériatrie. L'Encéphale, 1980, 6, 81-91.

4 Kahn (R.), Goldfard (A.), Pollack (M.), Peck (A.): Brief objective measures for the determination of mental status in the aged. Am. J. Psychiatry, 1960, 117, 326-328.

5 Lawton (M.P.): The Philadelphia Geriatric Center Morale Scale: a revision. J. of Gerontology, 1975, 30, 85-89.

6 Lawton (M.P.), Brody (E.): Assessment of older people: self-maintaining and instrumental activities of daily living. Gerontologist, 1969, 9, 179-186.

7 Lorr (M.): Rating scales and checklists for the evaluation of psychopathology. Psychol. Bull., 1954, 51, 119-127.

8 Lubin (B.): Adjective checklists for measurement of depression. Arch. Gen. Psychiatry, 1965, 12, 57-62.

9 Lucero (R.J.), Meyer (B.T.): A Behaviour rating scale suitable for use in mental hospitals. J. Clin. Psychol, 1951, 7, 250-259.

10 Meer (B.), Baker (J.A.): The Stockton Geriatric Rating Scale. J. of Gerontology, 1966, 21, 392-403.

11 Nuttin (J.): La structure de la personnalité. Paris: P.U.F., 1968, 280p.

12 Osgood (C.E.): Semantic differential technique in the comparative study of cultures. Amer. Anthrop, 1964, 66, 171-200.

13 Osgood (C.E.): Cross-cultural comparability in attitude measurement via multilingual semantic differentials. In: "Reading in attitude theory and measurement". New York: Martin Fishkein, John Wiley, 1967, 108-116.

14 Wyatt (R.J.), Jupfer (D.J.): A fourteen symptom behavior and mood rating scale for longitudinal patient evaluation by nurses. Psychol. Rep., 1963, 23, 1331-1334.

15 Zerssen (D. von), Strain (F.), Schwarz (D.): Evaluation of depressive states especially in longitudinal studies. In: Pichot (P.) Ed: "Psychological measurements in psychopharmacology". Basel: Karger, 1974, 189-202.

16 Zung (W.W.): Depression in the normal aged. Psychosomatics, 1967, 8, 287.

17 Zung (W.W.K.): The measurement of affects: depression and anxiety. In: Pichot (P.) Ed: "Psychological measurements in psychopharmacology". Basel: Karger, 1974, 170-188.

M. TEST

SPECIFICITY

*

TYPE OF INSTRUMENT

Projective test

REFERENCE	**Mezzena (G.), Fassio (M.), Gallo (I.), Graziano (C.), Lacava (R.), Mazzone (M.), Panero (A.), Veronese-Morosini (M.)** · − M. Test: un contributo all'esplorazione dello stile di vita. *Quaderno della Rivista di Psicologia Individuale*, 1981, nº 5.

Language: Original version published in Italian.
Italy

Location: See ref. biblio nº 1

For all information concerning the instrument write to the publisher at the following address:

Libreria Internazionale Cortina,
Corso Marconi, 34/A
10125 Torino, Italy

ORIGIN

This projective test is inspired in its form of administration by the T.A.T. by **Murray** (ref. 2), by the Psychodiagnostic test of **Rorschach** (ref. 3) from which it borrowed the system of scoring and interpretation by Adlers' psychoanalytical concepts.

PURPOSE

The instrument is developed for clinical use and is intended to evaluate "the life style" or rather the modalities of existence of a person in the interaction with the environment.

POPULATION

Adults of all ages, hospitalized or not, including day-care centres.

DESCRIPTION

Beginning with unstructured photographic material, the respondent is asked to say what he imagines to be represented by the doll's different position. Through his story the subject projects his own attitudes, feelings, opinions and preoccupations. This ambiguous material representing the different positions of one and the same person allows him to reveal his preoccupations and the deeply set traits of his personality. The answers are collected and qualitatively evaluated according to their contents.

ADMINISTRATION

Rater: Physician, psychologist, psychoanalyst.

Time required: minimum 20 minutes

Training: Knowledge of projective techniques is necessary.

Scoring: In a summary table one marks the answers registered according to qualitative categories and the system of quotation scoring in the handbook (ref. 1).

VARIABLES

Personality scoring as a motivator of behaviour and more particularly "life style":

· Social feeling	· Destructive activity
· Call for help	· Passivity absenteeism
· Exhibitionism	· Joy
· Need for approval	· Sadness
· Aggressiveness	· Sexuality
· Violence	· Playing
· Constructive activity	· Tension

VALIDATION

In progress.

APPLICATION

Clinical: Psychodiagnostic evaluation.
Research: Drug trials

1 Mezzena (G.), Fassio (M.), Gallo (I.), Graziano (C.), Lacava (R.), Mazzone (M.), Panero (A.), Veronese-Morosini (M.): M. Test: un contributo all'esplorazione dello stile di vita. *Quaderno della Rivista di Psicologia Individuale*, 1981, n°. 5.

2 Murray (H.A.): Thematic Apperception Test manual. Cambridge: Harvard University Press, 1943.

3 Rorschach (H.): Psychodiagnostic. Méthode et résultats d'une expérience diagnostique de perception. Interprétation libre de formes fortuites. 5e éd. française. Paris: Presses Universitaires de France, 1976.

BEHAVIOUR AND MOOD DISTURBANCE SCALE

SPECIFICITY

* * *

TYPE OF INSTRUMENT

Ordinal rating scale
31 items, 5 grades

REFERENCE	**Greene (J.G.), Smith (R.), Gardiner (M.), Timbury (G.C.)** · – Measuring behavioural distur- bance of elderly demented patients in the community and its effects on relatives: a factor analytic study. *Age and Ageing,* 1982, 11, 121-126.

        Language: Original version in English.
                           Great Britain

        Location: Enclosed in volume two page 124
                           See ref. biblio n⁰ 4

        For all information concerning the instrument write to the author at the following address:

               John Greene,
               Department of Psychology
               Gartnavel Royal Hospital
               1055 Great Western Road
               Glasgow G12 OXH, Great Britain

ORIGIN	The existing literature (ref. 1, 2, 6, 7, 8, 9, 10).
PURPOSE	To enable relatives to make a standard assessment of the mood and behaviour disturbance shown by elderly demented persons living at home. It can also be used as a research instrument.
POPULATION	Demented elderly persons living at home.
ADMINISTRATION	*Rater:* Relatives living with or caring for the elderly person in the community
	Time required: 15 to 20 minutes
	Training: Not required
	Scoring: Each item rated 0 to 4 according to severity
VARIABLES	· Apathetic-Withdrawn Behaviour · Active-Disturbed Behaviour · Mood Disturbance
VALIDATION	Scale developed by means of a factor analysis and a test-retest reliability study carried out on relati- ves' ratings of the behaviour of a group of elderly demented persons (ref. 4).
OTHER WORKS cited by author	Longitudinal study of therapeutic programme being carried out in a day hospital for elderly de- mented patients (ref. 5).
APPLICATION	· Prognosis · Placement and management of patients (day hospital, long stay care, return to home). · Assessment of therapy and intervention. · Any research projects being carried out on elderly demented persons living in the community.

1 Bergmann (K.): How to keep the family supportive. *Geriatr. Med.*, 1979, 23, 53-57.

2 Bergmann (K.), Foster (E.M.), Justice (A.W.), Matthews (V.): Management of the elderly demented patient in the community. *Brit. J. Psychiat.*, 1978, 132, 441-449.

3 Greene (J.G.), Smith (R.), Gardiner (M.): Evaluating reality orientation with psychogeriatric day hospital patients. In: Taylor (R.), Gilmore (A.) Eds.: "Recent trends in social gerontology". Gower Publishing Co., 1982.

4 Greene (J.G.), Smith (R.), Gardiner (M.), Timbury (G.C.): Measuring behavioural disturbance of elderly demented patients in the community and its effects on relatives: a factor analytic study. *Age and Ageing*, 1982, 11, 121-126.

5 Greene (J.G.), Timbury (G.C.): A geriatric psychiatry day hospital service: a five-year review. *Age and Ageing*, 1979, 8, 49-53.

6 Gurel (L.), Linn (M.W.), Linn (B.S.): Physical and mental impairment of function evaluation in the aged: The PAMIE Scale. *J. Gerontol.*, 1972, 1, 83-90.

7 Lawton (M.P.), Brody (E.M.): Assessment of older people: self-maintaining and instrumental activities of daily living. *Gerontologist*, 1969, 9, 179-186.

8 Meer (B.), Baker (J.): The Stockton geriatric rating scale. *J. Gerontol.*, 1966, 21, 372-403.

9 Pattie (A.H.), Gilleard (C.): Manual of the Clifton assessment procedures for the elderly. Sevenoaks, Kent: Hodder and Stoughton, 1979.

10 Wilkinson (I.A.), Graham-White (J.): Psychogeriatric dependency rating scales (P.G.D.R.S.): A method of assessment for use by nurses. *Br. J. Psychiat.*, 1980, 137, 558-565.

MENTAL SOCIAL

SELF PERCEPTION QUESTIONNAIRE

SPECIFICITY

$$* \quad * \quad *$$

TYPE OF INSTRUMENT

Questionnaire
Self-adminstered
110 questions

REFERENCE	**Preston (C.), Gudiksen (K.S.).** – A measure of self-perception among older people. *Journal of Gerontology*, 1966, 21, 63-71

Language: Original version published in English.
U.S.A.

Location: Enclosed in volume two page 55
See ref. biblio nº 7

For all information concerning the instrument write to the author at the following address:

Caroline Preston,
Department of Psychiatry
University Hospital RP-10
Seattle, Washington 98195, U.S.A.

ORIGIN The authors were prompted to undertake the study because of the **Sytman** thesis (ref. 8), of the theoretical concepts of **Miyamoto,** (ref. 6) and of non-directive interviews with 120 subjects.

PURPOSE The questionnaire was developed for the purpose of assessing how older persons perceived themselves and their environment. The instrument also allows the detection of signs of depression (slightly elevated scores)

POPULATION All elderly able to understand the questions.

ADMINISTRATION Self administration

Time required: About an hour

Training: Not necessary

Scoring: True-false

VARIABLES This questionnaire assesses the following variables:
· Measure of attitudes
  Perception of self and others
  Family relationships
· Current interests and past experiences
· Intellectual activities and mood.

OTHER WORKS
cited by author 242 subjects over 65 years of age and of different socio-economic characteristcs were examined.

APPLICATION Prognosis of behavior.

II.1

1 Edwards (A.L.): The social desirability variable in personality assessment and research. New York: Dryden, 1957, 108 p.

2 Edwards (A.L.): Experimental design in psychological research. New York: Rinehart and Co, 1960, 398 p.

3 Kogan (W.S.), Fordyce (W.E.): The control of social desirability: a comparison of three different Q sorts and a check-list, all composed of the same item. *J. Consult. Psychol.*, 1962, 26, 26-30.

4 Kramer (C.): Extension of multiple range tests to group means with unequal numbers of replications. *Biometrics*, 1956, 12, 307, 310.

5 La Forge (R.), Suczek (R.F.): The interpersonal dimensions of personality. III: An interpersonal checklist. *J. Pers.*, 1955, 24, 95-112.

6 Miyamoto (F.S.): Social aspects of aging. *The Bulletin Fr. Steilacoom Wash.*, 1964, 8, 132-138.

7 Preston (C.E.), Gudiksen (K.S.): A measure of self-perception among older people. *J. Geront.*, 1966, 21, n°. 1, 63-71.

8 Sytman (A.L.): Psycho-social changes associated with aging. Unpublished thesis, Univ. Washington, Seattle, 1963, 34 p.

SOCIAL DYSFUNCTION RATING SCALE

SPECIFICITY

* * *

TYPE OF INSTRUMENT

Ordinal rating scale
21 items, 6 grades

REFERENCE	**Linn (M.W.), Sculthorpe (W.B.), Evje (M.), Slater (P.H.), Goodman (S.P.).** – A social dysfunction rating scale. *Journal of Psychiatric Research,*, 1969, vol. 6, 299-306.

Language: Original version published in English.
U.S.A.

Location: Enclosed in volume two page 125
See ref. biblio nº 15

For all information concerning the instrument write to the author at the following address:

Margaret Linn,
Social Science Research 151
Veterans Administration Medical Center
1201 N.W. 16th Street
Miami, Florida 33125, U.S.A.

ORIGIN
Rating scale is based on successive modifications added to the experimental instrument, inspired by studies in the literature (ref. 1, 2, 3, 4, 5, 6, 7, 8, 9, 10, 16, 17, 18, 19, 20, 21).

PURPOSE
The purpose of the instrument is to estimate social maladaptation.

POPULATION
Elderly out or inpatients.

ADMINISTRATION
Rater: Social worker.

Time required: 30 minutes.

Training: Is not necessary but is desirable in order to improve reliability.

Scoring: Each item is scored from 1 to 6 according to a scale of increasing severity. The number of points varies from 21 to 126.

VARIABLES
· Low self concept
· Goallessness
· Self-health concern
· Emotional withdrawal
· Hostility
· Manipulation
· Over-dependency
· Anxiety
· Suspiciousness
· Lack of work
· Lack of leisure time activities
· Adaptive rigidity
· Lack of satisfying relationship with significant persons
· Lack of friends, social contacts
· Lack of a satisfying philosophy of meaning of life
· Expressed need for more friends, social contacts
· Expressed need for more leisure, self-enhancing and satisfying activities
· Lack of participation in community activites
· Lack of interest in community affairs and activities which influence others
· Lack of satisfaction from work
· Financial insecurity

VALIDATION
With healthy and mentally diseased persons (ref. 15).
External validity in relation to assessment by 3 social workers.
Factor analysis with psychiatric patients and healthy subjects.
Discriminative sensitivity between healthy and mentally sick persons by discriminative analysis.
Reliability, inter-rater: 2 raters, then 7 raters evaluating schizophrenic patients.

OTHER WORKS
cited by author
Works on out-patient treatment of mentally ill patients following discharge from hospital (ref. 12, 13, 14).

APPLICATION
Clinical: Defining the necessary care for the patient. Screening.
Research: Outcome studies and drug trials
Care planning.

1 Benedek (T.): On the psychic economy of developmental processes. *Archives of General Psychiatry*, 1967, 17, 271-276.

2 Bibring (G.): A study of the psychological processes in pregnancy and of the earliest mother-child relationship: I, II. *Psychoanal. Stud. Child.*, 1961, 16, 9-72.

3 Erikson (E.): Identity and the life cycle. *Psychological Issues*, 1959, 1, n°. 1.

4 Goodman (S.P.), Sculthorpe (W.B.), Evje (M.), Slater (P.), Linn (M.W.): Social dysfunction in psychiatric and medical outpatients. (Abstract). *The Gerontologist*, 1968, 8, 39.

5 Gordon (W.E.): A critique of the working definition. *Soc. Work.*, 1962, 7, 3-13.

6 Grinker (R.), Spiegel (J.): Men under stress. New York: Mc Graw-Hill, 1945.

7 Gurel (L.): Dimensions of psychiatric patient ward behavior. *Journal of Consulting Psychology*, 1967, 31, 328-330.

8 Harman (H.H.): Modern factor analysis. Chicago: Univ. of Chicago Press, 1960.

9 Janis (I.): Psychological stress. New York: John Wiley, 1956.

10 Kaiser (H.F.): The varimax criterion for analytic rotation in factor analysis. *Psychometrika*, 1958, 23, 187-200.

11 Linn (M.W.): Assessing community adjustment in the elderly. In: Raskin (A.), Jarvik (L.F.). Eds: "Psychiatric symptoms and cognitive loss in the elderly: evaluation and assessment techniques". Washington, New York, London: Hemisphere Publishing Corporation, 1979, 187-204.

12 Linn (M.W.), Caffey (E.M.), Klett (C.J.), Hogarty (G.): Hospital vs. community (Foster) care for psychiatric patients. *Archives of General Psychiatry*, jan. 1977, vol. 34, 78-83.

13 Linn (M.W.), Caffey (E.M.), Klett (C.J.), Hogarty (G.), Lamb (R.): Day treatment and psychotropic drugs in the aftercare of schizophrenic patients. *Archives of General Psychiatry*, sept. 1979, vol. 36, 1055-1066.

14 Linn (M.W.), Klett (C.J.), Caffey (E.M.): Foster home characteristics and psychiatric patient outcome. *Archives of General Psychiatry*, feb. 1980, vol. 37, 129-132.

15 Linn (M.W.), Sculthorpe (W.B.), Evje (M.), Slater (P.H.), Goodman (S.P.) A social dysfunction rating scale. *Journal of Psychiatric Research*, 1969, vol. 6, 299-306.

16 Lorr (M.), O'Connor (J.P.): Psychotic symptom patterns in à behavior inventory. *Educ. Psychol. Measur.*, 1962, 22, 139-146.

17 Overall (J.E.), Gorham (D.R.): The brief psychiatric rating scale. *Psychological Reports*, 1962, 10, 799-812.

18 Raskin (A.), Clyde (D.J.): Factors of psycho-pathology in the ward behavior of acute schizophrenics. *Journal of Consulting Psychology*, 1963, 27, 420-425.

19 Sabshin (J.): Psychiatric perspectives on normality. *Archives of General Psychiatry*, 1967, 17, 258-264.

20 Seigel (S.): Non-parametric statistics for the behavioral scientists. New York: Mc Graw-Hill, 1956.

21 Spitzer (R.), Cohen (J.): Common errors in quantitative psychiatric research. *International Journal of Psychiatry*, 1968, 6, 109-118.

INTERVIEW FOR RECENT LIFE EVENTS

SPECIFICITY

*

TYPE OF INSTRUMENT

Interview, semi-structured,
64 questions concerning
64 life events

REFERENCE   Paykel (E.S.), Prusoff (B.A.), Uhlenhuth (E.H.) · – Scaling of life events. *Archives of General Psychiatry,* oct. 1971, 25, 340-347.

Language: Original version published in English.
Great Britain.

Location: Enclosed in volume two page 57
See ref. biblio nº 11

For all information concerning the instrument write to the author at the following address:

Eugene Paykel,
St George's Hospital, Medical School
Dpt of Psychiatry,
Jenner Wing, Cranmer Terrace,
Tooting London SW 17 ORE, Great Britain

ORIGIN   The author was inspired by various life events inventories and particulary by that of **Holmes** and **Rahe** (ref. 3).

PURPOSE   The instrument records the occurence and impact of 64 recent life events, selected according to their affective importance.

POPULATION   All adult populations in addition to the elderly who are able to remember recent life events.

ADMINISTRATION   *Rater:* Physician, psychologist, nurses aide.

Time required: 20 minutes to 1 hour.

Training: with video-cassettes is desirable.

Scoring: 0-20 initially. Nowadays the scoring is much more complex. The author's notes should be consulted.

VARIABLES   Recent life events concerning:

· Work
· Studies
· Health
· Grief

· Material status
· Moving-house
· Family relations
· Social relations.

VALIDATION   Unpublished works on inter-rater reliability by three assessors with 21 patients.

OTHER WORKS cited by author   Evaluation of different populations: depressed patients, schizophrenic patients, attempted suicide, post-partum mothers, in comparison with a control group.

APPLICATION   **Research:** Prospective, retrospective and comparative epidemiological studies.
· Controlled clinical trials.

1 Hinkle (L.E., Jr.), Wolff (H.G.): Ecologic investigations of the relationship between illness, life experiences and the social environment. *Ann. Intern. Med.*, 1958, 49, 1373-1388.

2 Hollingshead (A.B.), Redlich (F.C.): Social class and mental illness. New-York: John Wiley and sons Inc., 1958.

3 Holmes (T.H.), Rahe (R.H.): The social readjustment rating scale. *J. Psychosom. Res.*, 1967, 11, 213-218.

4 Komaroff (A.L.), Masuda (M.), Holmes (T.H.): The social readjustment rating scale: a comparative study of negro, mexican and white americans. *J. Psychosom. Res.*, 1968, 12, 121-128.

5 Masuda (M.), Holmes (T.H.): Magnitude estimations of social readjustment. *J. Psychosom. Res.*, 1967, 11, 219-225.

6 Masuda (M.), Holmes (T.H.): The social readjustment rating scale: a cross-cultural study of japanese and americans. *J. Psychosom. Res.*, 1967, 11, 227-237.

7 National Institute of Mental Health: Handbook of psychiatric rating scales. Public Health Service Publication n°. 1495. U.S. Government Printing Office, 1964.

8 Parloff (M.B.), Kelman (H.C.), Franck (J.D.): Comfort, effectiveness and self-awareness as criteria of improvement in psychotherapy. *Amer. J. Psychiatry*, 1954, 111, 341-351.

9 Paykel (E.S.), Klerman (G.L.), Prusoff (B.): Treatment setting and clinical depression. *Arch. Gen. Psychiat.*, 1970, 22, 11-21.

10 Paykel (E.S.), Myers (J.K.), Dienelt (M.N.), et al.: Life events and depression: a controlled study. *Arch. Gen. Psychiat.*, 1969, 21, 753-760.

11 Paykel (E.S.), Prusoff (B.A.), Uhlenhuth (E.H.): Scaling of life events. *Arch. Gen. Psychiat.*, Oct. 1971, vol. 25, 340-347.

12 Paykel (E.S.), Uhlenhuth (E.H.): Rating the magnitude of life stress. Read before the Research conference on Psychiatric Crossroads, Montreal, 1970.

13 Rahe (R.H.): Life-change measurement as a predictor of illness. *Proc. Roy. Soc. Med.*, 1968, 61, 1124-1128.

14 Stevens (S.S.): A Metric for the social consensus. *Science*, 1966, 151, 530-541.

15 Torgerson (W.S): Theory and methods of scaling. New York: John Wiley and Sons Inc., 1958.

16 Vernon (P.E.): Personality assessment. New-York: John Wiley and Sons Inc, 1964.

PERSONAL HABITS, ENVIRONMENT AND PSYCHO-SOCIAL FACTORS

SPECIFICITY

* *

TYPE OF INSTRUMENT

Ordinal and nominal rating scale 3 grades

REFERENCE	**Kozarević (Dj.), Roberts (A.)** · – Personal habits, environment and psycho-social factors. In: "Respiratory diseases". Beograd: Postgraduate Medical Institute, 1973.
	Language: Original version is in Serbo-Croat, translation in English. **Yugoslavia**
	Location: English version enclosed in volume two page 126 See ref. biblio n⁰ 6
	For all information concerning the instrument and the translation write to the author at the following address:
	Djordje Kozarević, Institute of Chronic Diseases and Gerontology Slobodana Penezica 35 11000 Beograd, Yugoslavia

ORIGIN

The instrument was inspired by a basic questionnaire on cardiovascular and respiratory disease studies (ref. 8).

PURPOSE

The objective of the instrument is to describe the predominant feelings of the interviewees at different moments in their lives, their attitudes in different situations, and the different effects of physical and social environments on their health and frequency of certain diseases, as well as on the incidence of major cardiovascular diseases.

POPULATION

Adults from 45-74 years of age who live in urban and rural settings, as well as out-patients.

ADMINISTRATION

Rater: Psychologist, social worker, nurse

Time required: 10 minutes.

Training: desirable for improvement in reliability

Scoring: different according to the items.

VARIABLES

The principal variables are:
- Pleasantness
- Happiness
- Relaxation
- Peace of mind
- Problems with family
- Problems at work
- Problems with social environment

VALIDATION

Validation studies have examined the relations between different psychosocial factors and arterial hypertension as well as other cardiovascular diseases (ref. 1, 7).

APPLICATION

The instrument has been used in an epidemiological study measuring the effects of the environment on the prevalence and incidence of chronic diseases and functional incapacity.

1 Demirovic (J.), Racic (Z.), Tesanovic (D.), Vojvodic (N.), Milicevic (Lj.): Psychosocial factors and blood pressure levels in urban and rural populations in Yugoslavia. Essential hypertension. Published by Symposia Specialist, Chicago, 1979.

2 Haynes (S.G.) et al.: The relationship of psychosocial factors to coronary heart disease in the Framingham study. *Am. J. Epidemiol.*, 1978, vol. 107, n°. 5.

3 Jenkins (D.C.): Behavioral risk factors in coronary heart disease. *Ann. Rev. Med.*, 1978, 29, 543-562.

4 Kesteloot (H.), Joossens (V.): Epidemiology of arterial blood pressure. The Hague: Martinus Nijhoff Publishers, 1980.

5 Kozarević (Dj.), Pirc (B.), Dawber (Th.) et al.: The Yugoslavia cardiovascular disease study. I. The incidence of coronary heart disease by area. *J. Chron. Dis.*, 1976, 29, 404-414.

6 Kozarević (Dj.), Roberts (A.): Personal habits, environment and psycho-social factors. In: "Respiratory diseases". Beograd: Postgraduate Medical Institute, 1973.

7 Kozarević (Dj.), Roberts (A.), Pirc (B.): Prevalence of chronic obstructive lung diseases in two different areas of Yugoslavia. Symposium on ecology of chronic non-specific lung diseases. Warsaw, sept 1971.

8 Pirc (B.), Kozarević (Dj.), Dawber (Th.), Kahn (H.): The epidemiologic study of cardiovascular diseases in Yugoslavia: Methodology for third examination. Beograd, 1970.

ATTITUDES ET PERCEPTIONS MUTUELLES DES MEDECINS-MALADES-FAMILLES

ATTITUDES AND MUTUAL PERCEPTIONS AMONG PHYSICIANS-PATIENTS-FAMILIES

SPECIFICITY

* * *

TYPE OF INSTRUMENT

Questionnaire
20 questions for each
population

REFERENCE	**Israël (L.), Hugonot (R.)** · − Relations malades-médecins-familles en milieu gériatrique. *Médecine et Hygiène*, 1976, 34, 1196, 846-848.

Language: Original version in French.
                   France

Location: Enclosed in volume two page 58
                   See ref. biblio nº 2

For all information concerning the instrument write to the author at the following address:

     Liliane Israël,
     Pavillon Chissé, C.H.R.U.
     38700 La Tranche,
     Grenoble, France

ORIGIN

The questionnaire was originally developed for INSERM. It is based on the analysis of preliminary non directive interviews and the works of **Pacaud** (ref. 4).

PURPOSE

Evaluation and comparison of data about relationships, reducing as much as possible the observer' subjectivity.

POPULATION

Inpatients, staff and family

ADMINISTRATION

Rater: psychologist or social worker

Time required: 30 minutes

Training: In survey methods for 1 day

DESCRIPTION

The same questions were given to three populations in two different forms (direct and indirect). In the first case the subject is asked for an answer and in the second he is asked to suppose what answers were given by the other groups.
Scoring: Subject is requested to make an order of preference for the 8 possible answers.

VARIABLES

Attitudes:
· Towards frustration and aggressiveness
· Towards existential problems
· Towards a value system

Expectations:
· From institutionalization
· From physician
· From nurse
· From family
· From elderly

Perceptions:
· Image and role of a physician
· Image and role of a nurse
· Image and role of family
· Image and role of patient
· Role of the elderly in family, society, etc.
· Perception of environment
· Perception of life conditions
· Perception of institutions
· Perception of population in institutions.

VALIDATION

The instrument was developed in two phases. The first phase consisted of conducting the non-directive interview on three populations. Analysis of content allowed identification and retention of the principal domains expressed. The second phase was a pre-test on a reduced sample of each population chosen at random, to whom more oriented approaches were administred. A final restructuring preceded a decision on the present definitive form.

OTHER WORKS
cited by author

Summary about organisation of care in hospitals and the relation between physician, patient and family in geriatric care (ref. 1, 2).

APPLICATION

Can be used for training of staff and for making others aware of the specific problems of the elderly. Can also be used for specific surveys.

1 Israel (L.), Gruson (S.), Hugonot (R.): Médecins, malades, familles à l'hôpital gériatrique. Etudes des attitudes, attentes et perceptions mutuelles au moyen d'un questionnaire d'enquête. *Gérontologie*, 1980, n°. 33, 18-30.

2 Israel (L.), Hugonot (R.): Les relations médecins-malades-familles en milieu gériatrique. *Médecine et Hygiène*, 1976, 34, n°. 1196, 846-848.

3 Israel (L.), Prili (C.), Khayat (M.), Hugonot (R.): Le vieillard malade et sa famille dans les structures hospitalières. *Gérontologie*, 1975, n° 19, 7-14.

4 Pacaud (S.): Attitudes, comportements et opinions de personnes âgées dans le cadre de la famille moderne. Paris: C.N.R.S., 1969.

PSYCHODIAGNOSTIC TEST

SPECIFICITY

* *

TYPE OF INSTRUMENT

Projective test
10 cards

REFERENCE	**Rorschach (H.)** · – Psychodiagnostic. Méthode et résultats d'une expérience diagnostique de perception. Interprétation libre de formes fortuites. 5ᵉ éd. française. Paris: Presses Universitaires de France, 1976.

Language: Original version published in German. Translations in French, English and a few other languages.
Germany

Location: See ref. biblio nᵒ 19

For all information concerning the instrument write to the publisher at the following address:

Editions du Centre de Psychologie Appliquée
48, Avenue Victor Hugo
75783 Paris Cedex 16, France

ORIGIN — Original test developed by **Rorschach** in 1921 and based on a person's attitudes in relation to relatively unstructured visual stimuli.

PURPOSE — This projective test, with its non-verbal contents aimed to explore the personality in its structural and dynamic aspects through the interpretation placed by the subject on several ink blots

POPULATION — Children and adults, out and inpatients. Work done by Poitrenaud (ref. 16) concerned persons from 60-84 years of age.

DESCRIPTION — The test consists of ten cards with ink blots on them. Some are black, others black and red, some are in different colours. The interviewee is asked to say all he can see in these blots.
Analysis is done according to three dimensions:
· Way of understanding
· Determinants
· Content analysis

ADMINISTRATION — *Rater:* Psychologist

Time required: about 30 minutes

Training: scoring and interpretation require intensive training.

Scoring: is complex, reference books should be consulted (ref. 18, 19).

VARIABLES — This projective test estimates essentially:
· Perception   · Attitudes
· Adaptation   · Personality

VALIDATION — Numerous works have been done (see Science Citation Index). Numerous studies have been made in order to estimate impact of age on answers to the Rorschach test (ref. 1, 2, 3, 5, 6, 8, 10, 12, 13, 14, 16, 17).

APPLICATION — The instrument is for clinical and research use and allows estimation of personality and its dynamics and adaptational mechanisms.

1 Ames (L.B.): Age changes in the Rorschach responses of a group of elderly individuals. *J. Genet. Psychol.*, 1960, 97, 257-285.

2 Ames (L.B.): Changes in Rorschach response throughout the human life span. *Genet. Psychol. Monogr.*, 1966, 74, 89-125.

3 Ames (L.B.), Learned (J.), Metraux (R.W.), Walker (R.N.): Rorschach responses in old age. New York: Hoeber, 1954.

4 Bendig (A.W.): Age differences in the interscale factor structure of the Guilford-Zimmerman Temperament Survey. *J. Consult. Psychol.*, 1960, 24, 134-138.

5 Caldwell (B. Mc D.): The use of the Rorschach in personality research with the aged. *J. Gerontol.*, 1954, 9, 316-323.

6 Davidson (H.H.), Kruglov (L.): Personality characteristics of the institutionalized aged. *J. Consult. Psychol.*, 1952, 16, 5-12.

7 Dworetzki (G.): Le test de Rorschach et l'évolution de la perception. Genève: Naville, 1939.

8 Eisdorfer (C.): Rorschach performance and intellectual functioning in the aged. *J. Gerontol.*, 1963, 18, 358-363.

9 Friedman (H.): Perceptual regression in schizophrenia: an hypothesis suggested by the use of the Rorschach test. *J. Genet. Psychol.*, 1952, 81, 63-98.

10 Grossman (C.), Warshawsky (F.), Hertz (M.): Rorschach studies of personality characteristics of a group of institutionalized old people. *J. Gerontol.*, 1951, 6 (suppl. n°. 3), 97 (Abstract).

11 Heron (A.), Chown (S.): Age and function. London: Churchill, 1967.

12 Klopfer (W.G.): Personality patterns of old age. *Rorschach Res. Exch.*, 1946, 10, 145-166.

13 Kuhlen (R.G.), Keil (C.): The Rorschach test performance of 100 elderly males. *J. Gerontol.*, 1951, 6 (suppl. n°. 3), 115 (Abstract).

14 Light (B.H.), Amick (J.H.): Rorschach responses of normal aged. *J. Proj. Tech.*, 1956, 20, 185-195.

15 Poitrenaud (J.), Barrère (H.), Moreaux (C.): Influence de l'âge sur quelques-unes des principales dimensions non cognitives de la personnalité. *Gerontologia*, 1973, 19, 31-44.

16 Poitrenaud (J.), Moreaux (C.): Réponses données au test de Rorschach par un groupe de sujets âgés, cliniquement normaux. *Revue de Psychologie Appliquée*, 1975, vol. 25, n°. 4, 267-284.

17 Prados (M.), Fried (E.G.): Personality structure in the older age groups. *J. Clin. Psychol.*, 1947, 3, 113-120.

18 Rausch de Traubenberg (N.): La pratique du Rorschach. Paris: P.U.F., 1970.

19 Rorschach (H.): Psychodiagnostic. Méthode et résultats d'une expérience diagnostique de perception. Interprétation libre de formes fortuites. 5e éd. française. Paris: Presses Universitaires de France, 1976.

20 Siegel (S.): Nonparametric statistics for the behavioral sciences. New York: Mc Graw-Hill, 1956.

LIFE EVENTS INVENTORY

SPECIFICITY

*

TYPE OF INSTRUMENT

Questionnaire 67 items

REFERENCE

Tennant (C.), Andrews (G.) · – A scale to measure the stress of life events. *Australian and New Zealand Journal of Psychiatry*, 1976, 10, 27-32.

Language: Original version published in English.
                Australia

Location: Enclosed in volume two page 60
              See ref. biblio n⁰ 9

For all information concerning the instrument write to the author at the following address:

Christopher Tennant,
Department of Psychiatry
Research Group Hospital
University of New South Wales Teaching Hospitals
Little Bay, New South Wales 2036, Australia

ORIGIN

The author was inspired by the works of **Paykel** (ref. 5, 6) and **Holmes** (ref. 3).

PURPOSE

The aim of the instrument was to adapt to the Australian population the rating scales developed and validated for American populations.
The instrument investigates the hypotheses that the concepts of "change" in life and "stress" are two different entities. Consequently, the importance of change in a person's life caused by an event should be dissociated from emotional impact.

POPULATION

Adults of all ages capable of giving answers.

ADMINISTRATION

Rater: Self administration

Time required: 20 minutes

Training: Not necessary

Scoring: Every event is scored in two respects: changes in an individual's life and their emotional impact (ref. 9).

VARIABLES

Life events concerning:
· Health
· Bereavement
· Family and social relations
· Friends and relatives
· Education
· Work
· Moving house
· Financial and legal aspects

VALIDATION

Validation studies have been conducted with an Australian urban population (ref. 9).

APPLICATION

Research on Australian populations. Surveys on relation of stress to illness.

1 Antonovsky (A.), Kats (R.): The life crisis history as a tool in epidemiological research. *Journal of Health and Social Behaviour*, 1967, 8, 15.

2 Birley (J.L.T.), Brown (G.W.): Crises and life changes preceding the onset or relapse of acute schizophrenia: clinical aspects. *Brit. J. of Psychiat.*, 1970, 116, 327.

3 Holmes (T.H.), Rahe (R.H.): The social readjustment rating scale. *J. of Psychosomatic Research*, 1967, 11, 213.

4 Miller (F.T.), Bentz (W.K.), Aponte (J.F.), Brogan (D.R.): Perception of life crisis events: a comparative study of rural and urban samples. In: Dohrenwend (B.), Dohrenwend (B.P.) Eds.: "Stressful life events: their nature and effects". New York: Wiley and Sons, 1974.

5 Paykel (E.S.), Myers (J.K.), Dienelt (M.N.), Klerman (G.L.), Lindenthal (J.J.), Pepper (M.P.): Life events and depression. *Arch. Gen. Psychiat.*, 1969, 21, 753.

6 Paykel (E.S.), Prusoff (B.A.), Uhlenhuth (E.H.): Scaling of life events. *Arch. Gen. Psychiat*, 1971, 25, 340.

7 Selye (H.): The stress of life. New York: Mc Graw-Hill Book Company, 1956.

8 Stevens (S.S.), Galanter (E.H.): Ratio scales and category scales for a dozen perceptual continua. *J. of Experimental Psychology*, 1957, 54, 377.

9 Tennant (C.), Andrews (G.): A scale to measure the stress of life events. *Australian and New Zealand Journal of Psychiatry*, 1976, 10, 27-32.

10 Theorell (T.), Rahe (R.H.): Psychosocial factors and myocardial infarction. I: an inpatient study in Sweden. *J. of Psychosomatic Research*, 1971, 15, 25.

TEST PROJECTIF
PROJECTIVE TEST

SPECIFICITY

* * *

TYPE OF INSTRUMENT

Projective test
13 items, 21 cards

REFERENCE	**Laforestrie (R.), Missoum (G.)** · – Un test projectif pour personnes âgées. *La Revue de Gériatrie*, nov. 1977, 2, 5, 351-356.

Language: Original version in French
France

Location: See ref. biblio n° 6

For all information concerning the instrument write to the publisher at the following address:

Etablissements d'Applications Psychotechniques
6 bis, rue André Chenier
92130 Issy-Les-Moulineaux, France

ORIGIN
This original test is the result of the author's clinical practice. It differs by its specific content and presentation from the thematic traditional tests dealing with the main characteristics of personality, especially from **Bellak's** works (ref. 1).

PURPOSE
The purpose of this projective test is to allow an understanding of an old person's adaptation to old age.

POPULATION
Out or inpatients from 60 to 95 years.

ADMINISTRATION
Rater: Psychologist only

Time required: 30 to 45 minutes.

Training: Theoretical and practical training of one year or 300 hours.

DESCRIPTION
The interviewee is shown 15 cards, each representing old people in undefined situations. These situations cover different themes: death, loneliness, sexuality, communication, loss of job, groups, couples, the body. The person is asked to say freely everything suggested by the cards.

Scoring: Classification given by the authors allows quick interpretation of answers on each card. A person's adaptability is assessed in relation to each situation given in the test, and then classified into one of seven groups devised by the authors (positive, situational, adaptive, control, negative, psychologically fragile, pathological).

VARIABLES
Thirteen variables have been evaluated:

1. Death in hospital
2. Death in family context
3. Grief
4. Sexuality
5. Sexuality between young and old
6. Contacts with social environment
7. Contacts with family
8. Retirement
9. Desire for preserving activity
10. Isolation in town
11. Loneliness at home
12. Physical decline
13. Social life

This test measures the importance of emotional projection in 13 situations. It enables classification of an old person in relation to each of these factors.

VALIDATION
Has established norms and factor analysis of the elderly living at home, in institutions for the aged and hospitals (ref. 6, 7, 8, 9, 10, 11).

OTHER WORKS
cited by author
Individual results and surveys.

APPLICATION
Diagnosis, prognosis, therapy.

1 Bellak (L.), Bellak (S.S.): Manual for the Senior Apperception Technique. Larchmont, N.Y.: CPS, 1973.

2 Evans (R.B.), Marmorston (J.): Rorschach signs of brain damage in cerebral thrombosis. *Percep. Motor Skills*, 1964, 181, 977-988.

3 Fischer (J.), Gonda (T.A.), Little (H.): The Rorschach and central nervous system pathology. A cross validation study. *Am. J. Psychiat.*, 1955, 111, 487-492.

4 Hugues (R.M.): Rorschach signs for the diagnosis of organic pathology. *Rorschach Res.*, 1948, 12, 165-167.

5 Hugues (R.M.): A factor of Rorschach diagnostic signs. *J. Genet. Psychol.*, 1950, 43, 85-103.

6 Laforestrie (R.), Missoum (G.): Un test projectif pour personnes âgées. *La Revue de Gériatrie*, novembre 1977, tome 2, n° 5, 351-356.

7 Laforestrie (R.), Missoum (G.): Une tentative de compréhension de la démence à travers un test projectif pour personnes âgées. *La Revue de Gériatrie*, avril 1978, tome 3, n° 2, 65-75.

8 Laforestrie (R.), Missoum (G.): La mère et la mort. A propos de l'histoire d'une démente. *Psychanalyse à l'Université*, mars 1979, 4, 14, 325-340.

9 Laforestrie (R.), Missoum (G.), Berthaux (P.): Psychological diagnosis and clinical evaluation. Elaboration and validation of a new projective test suitable for old people. XII International Congress of Gerontology, Hamburg, Germany, July 12-17, 1981.

10 Laforestrie (R.), Missoum (G.), Piette (F.), Moulias (R.): Evaluation psychologique du sujet âgé en institution gériatrique. *Médecine et Hygiène*, juin 1981, n° 1427, 2133-2138.

11 Missoum (G.), Laforestrie (R.), Beruard (F.), Lenoir (H.), Moulias (R.), Berthaux (P.): L'influence psychologique de la pratique des activités physiques chez les personnes âgées. *La Revue de Gériatrie*, décembre 1981, tome 6, n° 10, 493-500.

12 Poitrenaud (J.): L'appréciation psychométrique de l'affaiblissement intellectuel chez le sujet âgé. In: Bourlière (F.) Ed.: "Progrès en gérontologie". Paris: Flammarion, 1969.

13 Piotrowski (Z.): The Rorschach inkblot in organic disturbances of the central nervous system. *J. Nerv. Ment. Dis.*, 1937, 86, 525-537.

14 Ross (D.), Ross (S.): Some Rorschach ratings of clinical values. *Rorschach Res. Exch.*, 1944, 8, 1-9.

15 Walton (D.): On the validity of the Rorschach test in the diagnosis of intracranial damage and pathology. *J. Ment. Sci*, 1955, 101, 370-382.

ASPECTS PSYCHOLOGIQUES ET SOCIAUX DU VIEILLISSEMENT
PSYCHOLOGICAL AND SOCIAL ASPECTS OF AGING

SPECIFICITY

* * *

TYPE OF INSTRUMENT

Questionnaire
85 questions

REFERENCE	Unpublished manuscript (1978).

Language: Original version French.
France.

Location: Enclosed in volume two page 61

For all information concerning the instrument write to the author at the following address, or directly to Gamma Group:

Liliane **Israël**,
Pavillon Chissé, C.H.R.U.
38700 La Tronche,
Grenoble, France

Groupe Gamma
M.G. Vandenborre
Secrétaire Général Adjoint
Centre Public d'Aide Sociale
Rue Haute 298 a
1000 Bruxelles, Belgium

ORIGIN
This original questionnaire has been developed by the Gamma Group (European Group for Gerontological Actions). Its origin has two sources, analyses of content of non directive interviews previously conducted in Aosta (Italy), and works by **Paillat** (ref. 5, 6, 7).

PURPOSE
To study living conditions of the elderly, their fundamental needs and ways of satisfying them in rural and urban settings.

POPULATION
Ambulant population over 65 years living at home.

ADMINISTRATION
Rater: Social worker or non-specialised interviewer
Time Required: 45 minutes
Training: In survey methods for 1 day.
Scoring: Open questions are coded according to classifying criteria.

DESCRIPTION
The questionnaire is divided into two parts: The first part concerned with living conditions includes 65 questions. The second part of 20 questions concerns psychological and social aspects, assessing the following topics:
· Subjective psychological needs
· Anxiety
· Scale of values
· Perception and meaning of ageing
· Hopes and wishes
· Integration, relationships, communication,
· Autonomy, dependency and need for help

VARIABLES
The entire questionnaire estimates the following aspects:
· Needs
· Resources
· Assistance and help
· Dependency
· Integration
· Housing
· Professional activities and leisure
· Environment and health.

VALIDATION
This questionnaire has been pre-tested and administered to a small population sample from Aosta with the purpose of defining categories for scoring open answers. It has been administered to 80 people chosen at random in different communities of Valley of Aosta. Final restructuring has been made according to information selected from analysis of content.

OTHER WORKS
cited by author
A survey of elderly citizens from Valley of Aosta.

APPLICATION
All kinds of psychosocial surveys concerning needs and attitudes of the elderly and their families towards environment and ageing.

1 Clément (F.): Conditions de vie, désirs et besoins des retraités agricoles de la Sarthe. Paris: Fondation Nationale de Gérontologie, 1971,154 p.

2 Guillemard (A.M.): La retraite: une mort sociale. Paris: Mouton, 1972, 303 p.

3 Guillemard (A.M.), Orlic (F.): Conditions de vie et comportements des retraités de l'agriculture. 2 tomes. Paris: Laboratoire de Sociologie Industrielle, 1969, 214 et 149 p.

4 Maslowski (J.), Paillat (P.): Conditions de vie et besoins des personnes âgées en France. Tome 3: Les ruraux âgés non agricoles. Paris: P.U.F., Cahiers de l'INED, 1973, 246 p.

5 Paillat (P.): Conditions de vie des ruraux âgés en France. Situation en 1974. *Aktuelle Gerontologie*, 1974, n° 4. 189-195.

6 Paillat (P.), Parant (A.), Delbes (C.): Le vieillissement de la campagne française. Paris: P.U.F., Travaux et documents, 1980, n° 88, 294 p.

7 Paillat (P.), Wibaux (C.): Les citadins âgés, conditions de vie et besoins des personnes âgées en France. Paris: INED, Cahier n° 52, 281 p.

8 Zarca (B.): La retraite, révélatrice du mode de vie et de la nature des relations familiales en milieu paysan. Paris: Université René-Descartes, thèse de 3e cycle, 1974, 394 p.

RELATIVES' STRESS SCALE

SPECIFICITY

* * *
to family

TYPE OF INSTRUMENT

Ordinal rating scale
15 items, 5 degrees

REFERENCE	**Greene (J.G.), Smith (R.), Gardiner (M.), Timbury (G.C.)** · – Measuring behavioural disturbance of elderly demented patients in the community and its effects on relatives: a factor analytic study. *Age and Ageing*, 1982, 11, 121-126.

Language: Original version published in English.
Great Britain

Location: Enclosed in volume two page 127
See ref. biblio n⁰ 4

For all information concerning the instrument write to the author at the following address:

John Greene,
Department of Psychology
Gartnavel Royal Hospital
1055 Great Western Road
Glasgow G12 OXH, Great Britain

ORIGIN
: The existing literature (ref. 1, 2, 6, 7, 8, 9, 10).

PURPOSE
: To enable relatives to make a standard assessment of the stress they are experiencing as a result of having to care for an elderly demented person living at home. It can also be used in research projects.

POPULATION
: Relatives of demented elderly persons living at home.

ADMINISTRATION
: *Rater:* Relatives living with or caring for the elderly person in the community.

Time required: 10 to 15 minutes.

Training: Not required

Scoring: Each item rated 0 to 4 according to severity.

VARIABLES
: · Personal distress
· Domestic upset
· Negative feelings

VALIDATION
: Scale developed by means of a factor analysis and a test-retest reliability study carried out on relatives' self-ratings of degree of stress being experienced (ref. 4).

OTHER WORKS
cited by author
: Longitudinal study of therapeutic programme being carried out in a day hospital for elderly demented patients.

APPLICATION
: · Assessment of strain on relatives and the home.
· Assessment of attitudes to elderly demented persons.
· Assessment of therapy and intervention
· Any research projects being carried out on elderly demented persons living in the community with relatives.

1 Bergmann (K.): How to keep the family supportive. *Geriat. Med.*, 1979, 23, 53-57.

2 Bergmann (K.), Foster (E.M.), Justice (A.W.), Matthews (V.): Management of the elderly demented patient in the community. *Brit. J. Psychiat.*, 1978, 132, 441-449.

3 Greene (J.G.), Smith (R.), Gardiner (M.): Evaluating reality orientation with psychogeriatric day hospital patients. In: Taylor (R.), Gilmore (A.) Eds: "Recent trends in social gerontology". Gower Publishing Co., 1982.

4 Greene (J.G.), Smith (R.), Gardiner (M.) Timbury (G.C.): Measuring behavioural disturbance of elderly demented patients in the community and its effects on relatives: a factor analytic study. *Age and Ageing*, 1982, 11, 121-126.

5 Greene (J.G.), Timbury (G.C.): A geriatric psychiatry day hospital service: a five-year review. *Age and Ageing*, 1979, 8, 49-53.

6 Gurel (L.), Linn (M.W.), Linn (B.S.): Physical and mental impairment of function evaluation in the aged: The PAMIE scale. *J. Geront.*, 1972, 1, 83-90.

7 Lawton (M.P.), Brody (E.M.): Assessment of older people: self-maintaining and instrumental activities of daily living. *Gerontologist*, 1969, 179-186.

8 Meer (B.), Baker (J.): The Stockton geriatric rating scale. *J. Gerontol.*, 1966, 21, 372-403.

9 Pattie (A.H.), Gilleard (C.): Manual of the Clifton assessment procedures for the elderly. Sevenoaks, Kent: Hodder and Stoughton, 1979.

10 Wilkinson (I.A.), Graham-White (J.): Psychogeriatric dependency rating scales (P.G.D.R.S.). A method of assessment for use by nurses. *Brit. J. Psychiat.*, 1980, 137, 558-565.

PHYSICAL MENTAL

III.1	Nursing Load Score (*)	HULTEN	1969
III.2	Instrumental Activities of Daily Living Scale (*)	LAWTON - BRODY	1969
III.3	Index of A.D.L. (*)	KATZ	1970
III.4	Physical and Mental Health Questionnaire	MILNE	1972
III.5	Disability Rating Scale (*)	AKHTAR	1973
III.6	Geriatric Profile	MISSOURI INSTITUTE	1973
III.7	Performance Test of Activities of Daily Living (*)	KURIANSKY	1976
III.8	Ward Function Inventory (*)	NORTON	1977
III.9	Echelle Clinique de Gérontologie	CROCQ	1980
III.10	Evaluation de l'Autonomie (*)	DELOMIER	1980
III.11	Fischer Symptom Check-list	FISCHER	1981
III.12	Geriatric Rating Scale	GÖTESTAM	1981
III.13	Bilan-Test d'Appréciation de la Perte d'Autonomie (*)	GRAUX	1981
III.14	G.B.S. Scale (*)	GOTTFRIES	1982
III.15	Drug Dependency and Overdose Assessment	IDÄNPÄÄN-HEIKKILÄ	1982
III.16	Evaluation de la Dépendance en Institution (*)	KUNTZMANN	1982
III.17	Rapid Disability Rating Scale-2 (*)	LINN	1982
III.18	Echelle de Dépendance C.E.N.T.S. (*)	HUGONOT	1982

(*) Instruments evaluating primarily dependency.

NURSING LOAD SCORE

SPECIFICITY

| * * |

TYPE OF INSTRUMENT

Ordinal rating scale
9 items from 2 to 5
grades

REFERENCE   **Hulten (A.), Kerstell (J.), Olsson (R.), Svanborg (A.)** · – A method to calculate nursing load. *Scandinavian Journal of Rehabilitation Medicine*, 1969, 1, 117-125

Language: Original version published in Swedish. Translation in English. **Sweden**

Location: Enclosed in volume two page 129

For all information concerning the instrument and the translation write to the authors at the following addresses:

A. Hulten,
Geriatric Clinic II
Vasa Hospital
University of Göteborg
Göteborg, Sweden

Alvar Svanborg
Vasa Sjukhus
Aschebergsgatan 46
S 41133 Göteborg
Sweden

ORIGIN
The original instrument is based on the experience of different hospital nursing teams concerning the parameters considered to increase nursing load.

PURPOSE
To evaluate arithmetically the quantity of work a nurse devotes to each patient, based on the judgement of the patient's state of physical dependence and the condition resulting in this state of dependence.

POPULATION
Elderly persons in need of nursing care.

ADMINISTRATION
Rater: Nurse and physician.

Time required: A few minutes.

Training: No training is necessary

Scoring: Each of the nine aspects covered by situations numbered from 2 to 5. Each situation has its score indicated. The total "Nursing Load Score" varies from 0 (independent patients) to 41 (very dependent patients).

VARIABLES
· Disturbing behavior
· Faecal incontinence
· Urinary incontinence
· Dressing and undressing
· Bedsores

· Personal hygiene
· Toilet visits
· Walking ability
· Feeding

VALIDATION
The instrument was applied to a hospitalised geriatric population, and the following was established:
External validity was based on the quantity of time spent on each patient by the nursing team. An equation permits the calculation of "nursing time" as a function of the total score of the "nursing load".

Observation of the inpatient population during 45 days. The nursing load score was calculated according to the type of care considered most adequate (home-care, residential home, hospital, specialised institution or none) after the necessary staff and type of care were determined.

APPLICATION
For hospital administration.
For planning types of care in hospital.
To evaluate the effects of treatment aimed to increase the degree of autonomy of the elderly.

INSTRUMENTAL ACTIVITIES OF DAILY LIVING SCALE (I.A.D.L.)

SPECIFICITY

TYPE OF INSTRUMENT

* * *

Ordinal rating scale
14 items

REFERENCE	**Lawton (M.P.), Brody (E.M.)** · – Assessment of older people: self-maintaining and instrumental activities of daily living. *Gerontologist*, 1969, 9, 179-186.

Language: Original version published in English. Translated into French by L. Israël. **U.S.A.**

Location: Enclosed in volume two page 130
See ref. biblio nº 8

For all information concerning the instrument write to the author at the following address:

M. Powell Lawton,
Philadelphia Geriatric Center
5301 Old York Road
Philadelphia, Pennsylvania 19141, U.S.A.

ORIGIN

The I.A.D.L. scale is original: it was inspired by works on instrumental activities by **Barrabee** et al. (ref. 1) and by **Phillips** (ref. 11). The authors use it together with the "Physical Self Maintenance Scale" (P.S.M.S.), originating from an instrument designed by **Lowenthal** et al. (ref. 10).
A modified scoring system has been developed by the authors.

PURPOSE

To evaluate the functional abilities of elderly persons on different levels of competence, in particular physical and instrumental autonomy in activities of daily living.

POPULATION

Elderly out-patients and elderly inpatients.

ADMINISTRATION

Rater: Mental health workers, social workers, nurses.

Time required: 5 minutes

Training: Takes about half a day and consists of evaluating 3 aspects: presentation, enquiries or observation, discussion before and after assessment.

Scoring: Is based on information obtained from the subject himself if his cognitive functions are preserved, from persons surrounding him or from staff. For each item the score can be only 0 or 1. The score for the P.S.M.S. scale varies from 0 to 6 and the score for the I.A.D.L. scale from 0 to 5 for men, and 0 to 8 for women.

VARIABLES

I.A.D.L.: Current activities such as:
ability to telephone, shopping, food preparation, housekeeping, laundry, mode of transportation, responsibility for own medication, ability to handle finances.
P.S.M.S.: Toilet, feeding, dressing, grooming, physical ambulation, bathing.

VALIDATION

The instrument was applied on a population of persons aged 60 or more years, both inpatients and out-patients.
Validity was tested by comparing results with another 3 instruments: "Physical Classification", a medical rating scale (ref. 12), "Mental Status Questionnaire", an orientation and memory test (ref. 4), and "Behavior and Adjustment Rating Scale", a rating scale testing intellectual adaptation, personal behavioral and social adaptation (ref. 12).
Compliance with Guttman's criteria for P.S.M.S. (ref. 2).
Inter-rater reliability tested with two evaluaters (ref. 8).

APPLICATION

Clinical: This instrument can be used as an indicator for determining the type and level of care necessary, and for determining the necessity of placing a person under institutional care. Decisions can be made according to periodic assessment and its results.
Research: Training and educating staff, care planning.

1 Barrabee (P.), Barrabee (E.), Finesinger (J.): A Normative social adjustment scale. *American Journal of Psychiatry*, 1955, 112, 252-259.

2 Guttman (L.): On Festinger's evaluation of scale analysis. *Psychological Bulletin*, 1947, 44, 451-465.

3 Howell (S.C.): Assessing the function of the aging adult. *Gerontologist*, 1958, 8, 60-62.

4 Kahn (R.L.), Goldfarb (A.I.), Pollock (M.), Gerber (I.E.): The relationship of mental and physical status in institutionalized aged persons. *American Journal of Psychiatry*, 1960, 117, 120-124.

5 Lawton (M.P.): Problems in the functional assessment of older people. Paper presented at the 21st annual meeting of Gerontological Society, Denver, 1968.

6 Lawton (M.P.): The functional assessment of elderly people. *Journal of the American Geriatrics Society*, 1971, vol. 19, n° 6, 465-481.

7 Lawton (M.P.): Assessing the competence of older people. In: Kent (D.P.), Kastenbaum (R.), Sherwood (S.) Eds.: "Research, planning and action for the elderly: the power and potential of social science". New York: Behavioral Publications, 1972, 122-143.

8 Lawton (M.P.), Brody (E.M.): Assessment of older people: self-maintaining and instrumental activities of daily living. *Gerontologist*, 1969, 9, 179-186.

9 Liebowitz (B.), Brody (E.): Proposal for the establishment of a geriatric day care center for mentally impaired and mentally retarded. Philadelphia Geriatric Center, 1968 (mimeo).

10 Lowenthal (M.F.): Lives in distress. New York: Basic Books, 1964.

11 Phillips (L.G.): Human adaptation and its failures. New York: Academic Press, 1968.

12 Waldman (A.), Fryman (E.): Classification in homes for the aged. In: Shore (H.), Leeds (M.) Eds: "Geriatric institutional management". New York: Putnam's, 1964.

INDEX OF A.D.L.

SPECIFICITY

* * *

TYPE OF INSTRUMENT

Ordinal rating scale
6 items 7 grades

REFERENCE	**Katz (S.), Downs (T.D.), Cash (H.R.), Grotz (R.C.)** · – Progress in development of the index of ADL. *Gerontologist*, Spring 1970, Part 1, 20-30.

Language: Original version published in English
              U.S.A.

Location: Enclosed in volume two page 132
              See ref. biblio nº 6

For all information concerning the instrument write to the author at the following address:

Sidney Katz,
Office of Health Services Education and Research
College of Human Medicine
Michigan State University
A110 East Fee Hall
East Lansing, Michigan 48824, U.S.A.

ORIGIN

The instrument is original and is based on earlier works done by the author himself (ref. 7, 8, 9, 10) and other publications by **Dyar** (ref. 1), **Ford** (ref. 2), **Steinberg** (ref. 15); it was produced by the team at the Benjamin Rose Hospital of the University of Cleveland. It has been used several times as a basic reference to more recent developments in the field of instruments concerning activities of daily living (ref. 5).

PURPOSE

It is designed to serve as a measure for objective evaluation of activities of daily living.

POPULATION

Concerns all elderly persons living in institutions.

ADMINISTRATION

Rater: Physician, nurse, social worker.

Time required: 20 minutes

Training: Necessary

Scoring: Six items, 7 grades each expressing a level of dependence.

VARIABLES

Variables that are assessed deal with the six following activities:
· Bathing   · Transfer
· Dressing   · Continence
· Toileting   · Feeding

APPLICATION

Clinical:
For prognostic purposes and prevention.
For evaluating effectivness of treatment.

Research:
For epidemiological enquiries – as a survey instrument.
As a teaching aid.
For training in types of care and rehabilitation.

1 Dyar (R.): Problems in the measurement of the progression of chronic disease. *Milbank Memorial Fund Quarterly*, 1953, 31, 239-241.

2 Ford (A.B.), Katz (S.), Adams (M.): Research design and strategy in a controlled study of nursing care. *American Journal of Public Health*, 1965, 55, 1295.

3 Havighurst (R.J.): A social-psychological perspective in aging. *Gerontologist*, 1968, 8, 67-71.

4 Hollingshead (A.B.): Two-factor index of social position. New Haven, Conn.: A.B. Hollingshead, 1957.

5 Katz (S.), Akpom (C.A.): A measure of primary sociobiological functions. *International Journal of Health Services*, 1976, vol. 6, n° 3, 493-508.

6 Katz (S.), Downs (T.D.), Cash (H.R.), Grotz, (R.C.): Progress in development of the index of ADL. *Gerontologist*, Spring 1970, Part I, 20-30.

7 Katz (S.), Ford (A.B.), Chinn (A.B.), Newill (V.A.): Prognosis after strokes. Part II: Long-term course of 159 patients. *Medicine*, 1966, 45, 236-246.

8 Katz (S.), Ford (A.B.), Moskowitz (R.W.), Jackson (B.A.), Jaffe (M.W.): Studies of illness in the aged: the index of ADL, a standardized measure of biological and psychosocial function. *Journal of the American Medical Association*, 1963, 185, 914-919.

9 Katz (S.), Heiple (K.G.), Downs (T.D.), Ford (A.B.), Scott (C.P.): Long-term course of 147 patients with fracture of the hip. *Surgery, Gynecology and Obstetrics*, 1967, 124, 1219-1230.

10 Katz (S.), Vignos (P.J.Jr.), Moskowitz (R.W.), Thompson (H.M.), Svec (K.H.): Comprehensive outpatient care in rheumatoid arthritis, a controlled study. *Journal of the American Medical Association*, 1968, 206, 1249-1254.

11 Krech (D.), Crutchfield (R.S.): Elements of psychology. New York: Alfred A. Knopf, 1958.

12 Kuhlen (R.G.): Aging and life-adjustment. In: Birren (J.E.) Ed.: "Handbook of aging and the individual". Chicago: University of Chicago Press, 1959.

13 Mac Mahon (B.), Pugh (T.F.), Ipsen (J.): Epidemiologic methods. Boston: Little, Brown and Co., 1960.

14 Raven (J.C.): Coloured progressive matrices (sets A, Ab1, B of revised order 1956). London: H.K. Lewis and Co., 1962.

15 Steinberg (F.U.), Frost (M.): Rehabilitation of geriatric patients in a general hospital: a follow-up study of 43 cases. *Geriatrics*, 1963, 18, 158-164.

16 Stevens (S.): Measurement, statistics, and the schemapiric view. *Science*, 1968, 161, 849-856.

17 Wallis (W.A.), Roberts (H.V.): Statistics, a new approach. New York: Free Press, 1956.

18 Wechsler (D.): A standardized memory scale for clinical use. *Journal of Psychology*, 1945, 19, 87-95.

PHYSICAL AND MENTAL HEALTH QUESTIONNAIRE (P.M.H.Q.)

SPECIFICITY

```
* * *
```

TYPE OF INSTRUMENT

Questionnaire and examination
Physical health: 10 sections
Mental health: 25 questions

REFERENCE	**Milne (J.S.), Maule (M.M.), Cormack (S.), Williamson (J.)** · – The design and testing of a questionnaire and examination to assess physical and mental health in older people using a staff nurse as the observer. *Journal of Chronic Diseases*, 1972, 25, 385-405.

Language: Original version published in English
Great Britain

Location: Enclosed in volume two page 62
See ref. biblio nº 14

For all information concerning the instrument write to the author at the following address:

J.S. Milne,
Department of Geriatric Medicine
City Hospital
Greenbank Drive,
Edinburgh EH10 5SB, Great Britain

ORIGIN

This is an instrument derived from 2 sources: longitudinal study of ageing persons begun by the authors in 1968-69 and published work mainly about questionnaire enquiries:
· The questionnaire about ischaemic heart disease and intermittent claudication by **Rose** (ref. 18) and the reading of ECG by the **Minnesota Code** (ref. 20). The questionnaires of the **Medical Research Council** on chronic bronchitis (ref. 12) and of **Epstein** on the diagnosis of duodenal ulcer (ref. 6).
· The papers of **Dyer** and **Pride** (ref. 5) on hiatus hernia. The studies of **Cobb** et al. (ref. 3) regarding arthropathy.

The Mental Status Questionnaire of **Kahn** et al. (ref. 9). The Mental Impairment Measurement of **Isaacs** et al. (ref. 8). The Intellectual Rating Scale of **Robinson** (ref. 17). The Psychological Test Proforma of **Blessed, Roth** et al. (ref. 2). The Signs Symptoms Inventory of **Foulds** (ref. 7). The Beck Depression Inventory of **Beck** et al. (ref. 1).

PURPOSE

To develop for research purposes, a questionnaire to measure physical and mental health in older people which will be brief and accurate and which will not upset persons examined with it.

POPULATION

Old people, except those who are grossly demented.

ADMINISTRATION

Rater: Nurse (male or female).

Time required: 30 minutes.

Training: Necessary and important. Training explains the purpose of the questions and specifies how to ask them. This is done using audio-visual methods (ref. 14).

Scoring: This varies with the section of the instrument which is in use. In the section on mental health, the observer is asked to record the exact words of the subjects. Interpretation of these is left to the psychiatrist.

VARIABLES

Physical health: Questionnaire records ischaemic heart disease, obliterative arterial disease of lower limbs, chronic bronchitis, smoking, duodenal ulcer, hiatus hernia, urinary tract infection, arthropathy, cerebrovascular accident and previous hospital admission.
Examination records: blood pressure, height, weight, triceps skinfold thickness, handgrip and examination of joints.
Mental health: Dementia. Emotional and depressive illness.

VALIDATION

Questions regarding physical health had already been validated elsewhere. As regards mental health, the four rating scales, listed under the heading "Origin", were examined with respect to specificity and sensitivity (ref. 14). The Mental Impairment Measurement was regarded as the most suitable of the four. As regards emotional and depressive illness, the validity of each item of the S.S.I. (ref. 7) and of the Beck Inventory (ref. 1) was studied by comparison with full psychiatric clinical assessment. Subjects examined in this work were those in the longitudinal study of ageing persons mentioned above.
· Mental health questionnaire was validated by comparison with the results of psychiatric examination.
· An inter-observer study of doctors and nurses carried out with the observers each performing the tests on the same subjects on the same day. Tests done in studies of reproducibility of any one observer were repeated after two weeks (ref. 14).

APPLICATION

Fundamental and applied research:
· Epidemiological studies either of disability in a sample or in prospective longitudinal studies.
· Detection and prevention of disability; care programmes.

BIBLIOGRAPHY

1 Beck (A.J.), Ward (C.H.), Mendelson (M.) et al: An inventory for measuring depression. *Arch. Gen. Psychiat.*, 1961, 41, 561-571.

2 Blessed (G.), Tomlinson (B.E.), Roth (M.): The association between quantitative measures of dementia and of senile change in cerebral grey matter of elderly subjects. *Brit. J. Psychiat.*, 1968, 144, 797-811.

3 Cobb (S.), Warren (J.E.), Merchant (W.R.) et al.: An estimate of the prevalence of rheumatoid arthritis. *J. Chron. Dis.*, 1957, 5, 636-643.

4 Dunn (J.P.), Etter (L.E.): Inadequacy of the medical history in the diagnosis of duodenal ulcer. *New. Eng. J. Med.*, 1962, 266, 68-72.

5 Dyer (N.H.), Pridie (R.B.): Incidence of hiatus hernia in asymptomatic subjects. *Gut*, 1968, 9, 696-699.

6 Epstein (L.M.): Validity of a questionnaire for diagnosis of peptic ulcer in an ethnically heterogeneous population. *J. Chron. Dis.*, 1969, 22, 49-55.

7 Foulds (G.A.): Personality and personal illness. London: Tavistock, 1965.

8 Isaacs (B.), Walkey (F.): The assessment of the mental state of elderly hospital patients using a simple questionnaire. *Amer. J. Psychiat.*, 1963. 120, 173-174.

9 Kahn (R.L.), Goldfarb (A.I.), Pollock (M.) et al.: Brief objective measures for the determination of mental status in the aged. *Amer. J. Psychiat.*, 1960, 117, 326-328.

10 Kay (D.W.), Beamish (P.), Roth (M.): Old age mental disorders in Newcastle-upon-Tyne. *Brit. J. Psychiat.*, 1964, 110, 146-158.

11 Kellgren (J.H.): Epidemiology of chronic rheumatism. Oxford: Blackwell, 1963, 293.

12 Medical Research Council Committee on Actiology of Bronchitis: Definition and classification of chronic bronchitis for clinical and epidemiological purposes. A report to the Medical Research Council by their committee on the actiology of chronic bronchitis. Lancet, vol. 1, n° 3, 775-779.

13 Milne (J.S.), Hope (K.), Williamson (J.): Variability in replies to a questionnaire on symptoms of physical illness. *J. Chron. Dis.*, 1970, 22, 805-810

14 Milne (J.S.), Maule (M.M.), Cormack (S.), Williamson (J.): The design and testing of a questionnaire and examination to assess physical and mental health in older people using a staff nurse as the observer. *J. Chron. Dis.*, 1972, vol. 25, 385-405.

15 Milne (J.S.), Maule (M.M.), Williamson (J.): Method of sampling in a study of older people with a comparison of respondents and nonrespondents. *Brit. J. Prev. Soc. Med.*, 1966, 25, 37-41.

16 Pridie (R.B.): Incidence and coincidence of hiatus hernia. *Gut*, 1966, 7, 188-189.

17 Robinson (R.A.): Problems of drug trials in elderly people. *Geront. Clin.*1961, 3, 247-257.

18 Rose (G.A.): The diagnosis of ischaemic heart pain and intermittent claudication in field surveys. *Bull. WHO*, 1962, 27, 645-658.

19 Rose (G.A.): Standardization of observers in blood-pressure measurement. *Lancet*, 1965, 1, 673-674.

20 Rose (G.A.), Blackburn (H.): Cardiovascular survey methods. Geneva: WHO, 1968.

21 Seltzer (C.C.), Mayer (J.): Greater reliability of the triceps over the subscapular skinfold as an index of obesity. *Amer. J. Clin. Nutr.*, 1967, 20, 950-953.

22 Walbaum (P.R.), McCormack (R.J.M.): Hiatus hernia. *Scot. Med. J.*, 1968, 13, 103-109.

23 Williamson (J.), Stokoe (I.H.), Gray (S.) et al.: Old people at home, their unreported needs. *Lancet*, 1964, 1, 1117-1120.

24 Witts (L.J.): Medical surveys and clinical trials. 2nd ed. London: Oxford University Press, 1964.

25 Wright (B.M.), Dore (C.F.): A random - zero sphygmomanometer. *Lancet*, 1970, 1, 337-338.

DISABILITY RATING SCALE

SPECIFICITY

* * *

TYPE OF INSTRUMENT

Ordinal rating scale
11 items 3, 5, 6,
grades

REFERENCE	**Akhtar (A.J.), Broe (G.A.), Crombie (A.), Mc Lean (W.M.R.), Andrews (G.R.), Caird (F.I.)** · – Disability and dependence in the elderly at home. *Age and Ageing,* 1973, vol. 2, 102-111.

Language: Published in English.
Great Britain

Location: Enclosed in volume two page 134
See ref. biblio nº 2

For all information concerning the instrument write to the author at the following address:

Anthony Broe,
Lidcombe Hospital,
Joseph Street
Lidcombe, New South Wales 2141, Australia

ORIGIN   The author was inspired by the works of **Harris** (ref. 6), **Bennet** and **Garrad** (ref. 4).

PURPOSE   The instrument was developed for epidemiological investigations to assess the prevalence of functional incapacity and the dependency of elderly out-patients.

POPULATION   Elderly persons living at home

ADMINISTRATION *Rater:* Physician, nurse or social worker.
Time required: 5-10 minutes.
Training: Not necessary if the staff are experienced.
Scoring: Varies according to the item in question.

VARIABLES   The following activities are assessed:
· Mobility
· Continence
· Domestic care
· Self care
· Psychiatric disability

VALIDATION   **Concurrent validity** was established according to comparisons with other studies (ref. 4, 6).
Inter-rater reliability between physicians and social workers (ref. 2).

OTHER WORKS   Study on a group of 808 elderly people over 65 years of age, living at home in a village in Scotland
cited by author (ref. 2).

APPLICATION   Epidemiological studies.
Training of staff.

1 Akhtar (A.J.): Refusal to participate in a survey of the elderly. *Gerontol. clin.*, 1972, 14, 205.

2 Akhtar (A.J.), Broe (A.), Crombie (A.), McLean (W.M.R.), Andrews (G.R.), Caird (F.I.): Disability and dependence in the elderly at home. *Age and Ageing*, 1973, vol. 2, 102-111.

3 Andrews (G.R.), Cowan (N.R.), Anderson (W.F.): The practice of geriatric medicine in the community: an evaluation of the place of health centres. In: "Problems and progress in medical care". Essays on current research, 5th series. Ed. McLachlan, G. Oxford University Press, 1971, p. 58.

4 Bennett (A.E.), Garrad (J.), Halil (T.): Chronic disease and disability: a prevalence study. *British Medical Journal*, 1970, 3, 762

5 Carstairs (V.), Morrison (M.): The elderly in residential care. Scottish Health Service Studies n° 19. Scottish Home and Health Department, 1971.

6 Harris (A.I.): Handicapped and impaired in Great Britain. London: Her Majesty's Stationery Office, 1971.

7 Hobson (W.), Pemberton (J.): The health of the elderly at home. London: Butterworth, 1955.

8 Isaacs (B.): Studies of illness and death in the elderly in Glasgow. Scottish Health Service Studies n° 17. Scottish Home and Health Department, 1971.

9 Milne (J.S.), Maule (M.M.), Williamson (J.): Method of sampling in a study of older people with a comparison of respondents and non-respondents. *Br. J. Prev. Soc. Med.*, 1971, 25, 37.

10 Sheldon (J.H.): The social medicine of old age. London: Oxford University Press, 1948.

11 Slater (E.), Roth (M.): Clinical psychiatry. London: Bailliere, Tindall and Cassell, 1969.

12 Stout (C.), Wight (M.A.), Bruhn (J.G.): The Cornell Medical Index in the disability evaluation. *Br. J. Prev. Soc. Med*, 1969, 23, 251.

13 Taylor (P.J.), Fairrie (A.J.): Chronic disability in men of middle age. A study of 165 men in a general practice and a refinery. *Br. J. Prev. Soc. Med.*, 1968, 22, 183.

14 Williamson (J.), Stokoe (I.H.), Gray (S.), Fisher (M.), Smith (A.), McGhee (A.), Stephenson (E.): Old people at home: their unreported needs. *Lancet*, 1964, 1, 1117.

GERIATRIC PROFILE (G.P.)

SPECIFICITY

* * *

TYPE OF INSTRUMENT

Rating scale of
84 items, 4 grades

REFERENCE	Unpublished manual.
	Language: Original in English.
	Location: Enclosed in volume two page 135 See ref. biblio nᵒ 8

For all information concerning the instrument write to the author at the following address:

Richard **Evenson,**
Missouri Institute of Psychiatry
5400 Arsenal Street
Saint Louis, Missouri 63139, U.S.A.

ORIGIN

The instrument consists of items adapted from other scales: "Missouri Inpatient Behaviour Scale" (ref. 9), "Stockton Geriatric Rating Scale" (ref. 7), "Geriatric Rating Scale" (ref. 10), "Self Care Inventory" (ref. 4) and additional items suggested by personnel of the Department of Mental Health, Missouri. The provisional form of the scale has been subjected to statistical analysis that resulted in the "Geriatric Profile".

PURPOSE

To quantify the conduct and behavior of hospitalized psychogeriatric patients; to appraise changes with regard to symptomatology and day to day activities.

POPULATION

Aged patients hospitalized on psychiatric or psychogeriatric wards.

ADMINISTRATION

Rater: Administered by nurses, attendants or other members of treatment team.

Time required: 10 minutes

Training: Desirable, though brief. See directions in the instruction manual.

Scoring: Based on observation of patients conduct and behavior in preceeding 48 to 72 hours. Every item is rated from 0 (never) to 3 (almost always). Items 1 to 38 assess undesirable (symptomatic) behavior, items 39 to 64 assess adjustment level and adaptive behavior of every day life. Eighteen items of physical symptomatology are rated 0-3 and include typical medication side effects. The global ratings are rated 1-4 for level of general functioning.

VARIABLES

Factor analysis of data resulted in the identification of 10 scales:
- Depression
- Paranoid thinking
- General competence
- Confusion
- Physical disability
- Hostile irritability
- Agitation
- Sociability
- Sleep disturbance
- Total maladjustment

VALIDATION

Observations obtained from a population of psychogeriatric patients hospitalized in 5 state hospitals were subjected to **factor analysis** of a preliminary form of the scale which yielded 10 factors. The preliminary form has been presented elsewhere (ref. 11).
Normative data are presented in the manual, based on a sample of 520 patients from state hospitals in Missouri. Items are simply added together for each scale, based on the key in the manual. The scales are added for the total maladjustment score.
Inter-rater reliability: Independent ratings by two observers, and for the measure of total maladjustment.

APPLICATION

Clinical follow-up initial symptoms, main symptoms as indications for treatment, progress, outlook for discharge, prognosis.
The Geriatric Profile has been used in the Missouri Department of Mental Health to provide routine assessment, and later follow-up, of geriatric admissions to public psychiatric hospitals (ref. 6). It has also been used to measure the effects of drug holidays in psychiatric patients (ref. 14) and the presence of iatrogenic symptoms in hospitalized patients. The author recommends a reduced version of 50 items for research or for use in non-automated clinical settings.

1 Altman (H.), Mehta (D.), Evenson (R.C.), Sletten (I.W.): Behavioral effects of drug therapy on psychogeriatric inpatients. I: Chlorpromazine and thioridazine. *Journal of the American Geriatrics Society*, 1973, vol. 21, n° 6, 241-248.

2 Altman (H.), Mehta (D.), Evenson (R.C.), Sletten (I.W.): Behavioral effects of drug therapy on psychogeriatric inpatients. II: Multivitamin supplement. *Journal of the American Geriatrics Society*, 1973, vol. 21, n° 6, 249-252.

3 Data processing in the Missouri Division of Mental Health. IBM, August 1973.

4 Gurel (L.), Davis (J.E.), Stumpf (J.C.): Survey of the self-care dependent in selected VA hospitals. Psychiatric evaluation project. Washington, 1963, 18-19.

5 Gurel (L.), Linn (M.W.), Linn (B.S.): Physical and mental impairment of function evaluation of the aged: the PAMIE scale. *Journal of Gerontology*, 1972, vol. 27, n° 1, 83-90.

6 Hedlund (J.), Sletten (I.), Evenson (R.), Altman (H.), Cho (D.W.): Automated psychiatric information systems: a critical review of Missouri's standard system of psychiatry (SSOP). *Journal of Operational Psychiatry*, 1977, vol. 8, n° 1, 5-26.

7 Meer (B.), Baker (J.A.): The Stockton Geriatric rating scale. *Journal of Gerontology*, 1966, vol. 21, n° 3, 392-403.

8 Missouri Institute of Psychiatry: Geriatric Profile. Unpublished manuscript, 1973.

9 Missouri Institute of Psychiatry: Missouri Inpatient Behavior Scale Manual. Unpublished manuscript, revised 1973.

10 Plutchik (R.), Conte (H.), Lieberman (M.) et al.: Reliability and validity of a scale for assessing the functioning of geriatric patients. *Journal of the American Geriatrics Society*, 1970, vol. 18, n° 6, 491-500.

11 Salzman (C.), Kochansky (G.E.), Shader (R.I.): Rating scales for geriatric psychopharmacology: a review. *Psychopharmacology Bulletin*, 1972, vol. 8, n° 3, 3-50.

12 Sletten (I.W.), Evenson (R.C.): The Missouri automated Standard System of Psychiatry (SSOP): an overview. *Computer Medicine*, july 1972.

13 Ulett (G.A.), Sletten (I.W.): A statewide electronic data – processing system. *Hospital and Community Psychiatry*, march 1969, 26-29.

PERFORMANCE TEST OF ACTIVITIES OF DAILY LIVING

SPECIFICITY

* * *

TYPE OF INSTRUMENT

Ordinal rating scale
3 grades 16 items

REFERENCE	**Kuriansky (J.), Gurland (B.)** · – The performance test of activities of daily living. *International Journal of Aging and Human Development*, 1976, 7, 4, 343-352.
	Language: Original version published in English. **U.S.A.**
	Location: Enclosed in volume two page 136 See ref. biblio nº 10
	For all information concerning the instrument write to the author at the following address:
	Judith Kuriansky, Columbia University Center for Geriatrics and Gerontology 100 Haven Avenue Tower 3-29F New York, New York 10032, U.S.A.

ORIGIN

The instrument was directly inspired by the works of **Goldfarb** (A.I.) (ref. 9), and to an even greater extent by a collection of investigations whose aim was to assess, on the basis of interviews, the ability of subjects to manage independently their daily needs (ref. 7, 8, 14, 16, 21, 23, 24).

PURPOSE

The instrument was developed to enable objective assessment of the degree of autonomy of elderly psychiatric subjects in activities of daily living.

POPULATION

Elderly inpatients suffering from organic brain syndrome.

ADMINISTRATION

Rater: Psychologist, physician, nurse, nurse's aide.

Time required: Approximately 20 minutes.

Training: Two half days of training.

Scoring: Each item is coded as 0,1 or 9 depending on the degree of autonomy of the subject for simple activities (0 = dependency, 1 = autonomy, 9 = cannot be scored), general score can be assigned concerning the percent of answers for each of these categories.

DESCRIPTION

The instrument is presented as a praxia test containing 16 sub-tests. The subject is asked to choose from certain objects, such as a fork, a glass and a comb, those which he would use in the course of simple activities of daily living as: eating with a spoon, drinking from a glass, combing his hair etc. Each action is divided into simple actions (items) which the rater assesses. Time is not taken into account. The instrument includes the performance of 16 activities of everyday living.

1. Drink from a cup
2. Use a tissue to wipe nose
3. Comb hair
4. File nails
5. Shave
6. Lift food into spoon and to mouth
7. Turn faucet (tap) on and off
8. Turn light switch on and off
9. Put on and remove a jacket with buttons
10. Put on and remove a slipper
11. Brush teeth, including removing false teeth
12. Make a phone call
13. Sign name
14. Turn key in lock
15. Tell time
16. Stand up and walk a few steps and sit back down.

VARIABLES

Degree of autonomy or dependency.

VALIDATION

Face validity of the instrument has been assessed. Studies concerning **inter-rater reliability** and a study of **concurrent** and **content validity** have been carried out (ref. 5, 10, 11).

APPLICATION

The instrument was conceived for clinical and research purposes to assess the degree of autonomy on the physical and mental level of elderly patients in different activities of daily living. It can be used by itself or included in a battery of tests for diagnostic, therapeutic, planning or management purposes, for care and treatment in and out of hospital.

1 Alberts (D.), Howard (G.), Pasewar (R.): The Geriatric Profile Index: a system for identifying, managing and planning for geriatric patients in state hospitals. *Journal of the American Geriatrics Society*, 1969, 17, 1108-1112.

2 Anderson (D.): Hospital discharge of the geriatric patient: a team process. *Journal of the American Geriatrics Society*, 1963, 11, 266-277.

3 Brody (E.), Kleban (M.), Lawton (M.P.), Moss (M.): A longitudinal look at excess disabilities in the mentally impaired aged. *Journal of Gerontology*, 1974, 29, 79-84.

4 Busse (E.): Psychoneurotic reactions and defense mechanisms in the aged. In: Hoch (P.), Zubin (J.) Eds.: "Psychopathology of aging". New York: Grune and Stratton, 1964.

5 Copeland (J.R.M.), Kelleher (M.J.), Kellett (J.M.), Fountain-Gourlay (A.J.), Cowan (D.W.), Barron (G.), De Gruchy (J.), Gurland (B.J.), Sharpe (L.), Simon (R.J.), Kuriansky (J.B.), Stiller (P.): Diagnostic differences in psychogeriatric patients in New York and London. *Canadian Psychiatric Association Journal*, 1974, 19, 267-271.

6 Copeland (J.R.M.), Kelleher (M.J.), Kellett (J.M.), Gourlay (A.J.), Gurland (B.J.), Fleiss (J.L.), Sharpe (L.): A semi-structured clinical interview for the assessment of diagnosis and mental state in the elderly: the geriatric mental state schedule. I: Development and reliability. *Psychological Medicine*, 1976, 6, 451-459.

7 Council of Jewish Federations and Welfare Funds: Mental impairment in homes for the aged: a pilot study. Unpublished manuscript.

8 Epstein (L.J.), Robinson (S.C.), Simon (A.): Predictors of survival in geriatric mental illness during the eleven years after initial hospital admission. *Journal of the American Geriatrics Society*, 1971, 19, 913-922.

9 Goldfarb (A.I.): The evaluation of geriatric patients following treatment. In: Hoch (P.), Zubin (J.) Eds.: "The Evaluation of psychiatric treatment". New York: Grune and Stratton, 1964.

10 Kuriansky (J.B.), Gurland (B.J.): The performance test of activities of daily living. *International Journal of Aging and Human Development*, 1976, vol. 7, n° 4, 343-352.

11 Kuriansky (J.B.), Gurland (B.J.), Fleiss (J.L.), Cowan (D.W.): The assessment of self-care capacity in geriatric psychiatric patients. *Journal of Clinical Psychology*, 1976, 32, 95-102.

12 Lawton (E.B.): Activities of daily living for physical rehabilitation. New York: Mc Graw-Hill, 1963.

13 Lawton (M.P.), Brody (E.M.): Assessment of older people: self-maintaining and instrumental activities of daily living. *Gerontologist*, 1969, 9, 179-186.

14 Lowenthal (M.F.): Indices of social and physical self-maintenance. Personal communication, 1975.

15 Markson (E.), Grevert (P.): Circe's terrible island of change: self-perceptions of incapacity. *International Journal of Aging and Human Development*, 1972, 3, 261-271.

16 Meer (B.), Krag (G.): Correlates of disability in a population of hospitalized geriatric patients. *Journal of Gerontology*, 1964, 19, 440-446.

17 Plutchik (R.), Conte (H.), Lieberman (M.), Bakur (M.), Grossman (J.), Lehrman (N.): Reliability and validity of a scale for assessing the functioning of geriatric patients. *Journal of the American Geriatrics Society*, 1970, 18, 491-500.

18 Roth (M.), Kay (D.W.K.): Affective disorders arising in the senium. II: Physical disability as an aetiological factor. *Journal of Mental Science*, 1952, 102, 141-150.

19 Staff of Benjamin Rose Hospital: Multidisciplinary study of illness in aged persons. I: Methods and preliminary results. *Journal of chronic diseases*, 1958, 7, 322-345.

20 Stotsky (B.): A controlled study of factors in the successful adjustment of mental patients to nursing homes. *American Journal of Psychiatry*, 1967, 123, 1243-1251.

21 Townsend (P.): The last refuge. London: Routledge and Kegan Paul, 1962.

22 Trier (T.): A study of change among elderly psychiatric inpatients during their first year of hospitalization. *Journal of Gerontology*, 1968, 23, 354-362.

23 Wilson (L.A.), Grant (K.), Whitney (P.M.), Kerridge (D.F.): Mental status of elderly hospital patients related to occupational therapist's assessment of activities of daily living. *Gerontologia Clinica*, 1973, 17, 197-202.

24 Zeman (F.D.): The functional capacity of the aged: its estimation and practical importance. *Journal of Mount Sinaï*, 1947, 14, 721.

WARD FUNCTION INVENTORY (W.F.I.)

SPECIFICITY	TYPE OF INSTRUMENT
* * *	Ordinal rating scale 12 items, 5 grades

REFERENCE **Norton (J.C.), Romano (P.O.), Sandifer (M.G.)** · – The Ward Function Inventory (W.F.I.): A scale for use with geriatric and demented inpatients. *Diseases of the Nervous System*, 1977, 38, 1, 20-23.

Language: Original version published in English.
U.S.A.

Location: Enclosed in volume two page 137
See ref. biblio nº 6

For all information concerning the instrument write to the author at the following address:

James Norton,
Veterans Administration Medical Center (116A - CDD)
Lexington, Kentucky 40511, U.S.A.

ORIGIN

This is an original instrument constructed through the method of successive revisions based on studies on interjudge reliability. It results in a consensus among different members of the health care team concerning the specific problems posed by patients with organic brain syndrome.

PURPOSE

This clinical tool contributes to facilitating communication among the health care team.

POPULATION

The population appropriate for this instrument are aged hospitalized patients with organic brain syndrome or dementia.

ADMINISTRATION

Rater: All hospital personnel, but preferably nurses.

Time required: 5 minutes.

Training: Not necessary but training increases the accuracy of the ratings.

Scoring: Each item is rated on a scale of 1 to 5, based on increasing severity. The total score varies from 12 to 60.

VARIABLES

The scale covers a group of cognitive deficiencies and general behaviors observed in this group of illnesses.

· Orientation   · Attention
· Continence   · Memory
· Following commands   · Management of money
· Personal hygiene   · Future planning
· Socialization   · Feeding
· Inappropriate behavior   · Verbal skills

VALIDATION

The instrument is effective with psychiatric, neurologic and institutionalized population (ref. 6):
Face validity: built into the instrument.
External validity: discriminates among psychiatric, neurologic and institutionalized patients; correlates with a preexisting classification of patients with regard to level of deficiency.
Inter-rater reliability: for each of the items and for the total score, the numbers of observers varies from 6 to 15.

APPLICATION

Research: Can be used in the evaluation of the effect of treatment on the functional autonomy of patients.
Clinical application: Can be used in making determinations regarding the needs of patients for nursing care and in estimating their degree of functional autonomy.

III.8

1 Honigfeld (G.), Klett (C.J.): The Nurses'observation scale for inpatient observation, a new scale for measuring improvement in chronic schizophrenia. *Journal of Clinical Psychology*, 1965, 21, 65-71.

2 Lawton (M.P.), Brody (E.M.): Assessment of older people: self maintaining and instrumental activities of daily living. *Gerontologist*, 1969, 9, 179-186.

3 Lorr (M.), Klett (C.J.): Inpatient multidimensional psychiatric scale: manual. Revised ed. Palo Alto, California: Consulting Psychologists Press, 1966.

4 Lowenthal (M.F.): Lives in distress. New York: Basic Books, 1964.

5 Meer (B.), Baker (J.A.): Stockton geriatric rating scale. *Journal of Gerontology*, 1966, 21, 392-403.

6 Norton (J.C.), Romano (P.O.), Sandifer (M.G.): The Ward Function Inventory (WFI): a scale for use with geriatric and demented inpatients. *Diseases of the Nervous System*, jan. 1977, vol. 38, n° 1, 20-23.

7 Plutchik (R.), Conte (H.), Lieberman (M.), Bakur (M.), Grossman (J.), Lehrman (N.): Reliability and validity of a scale for assessing the functioning of geriatric patients. *Journal of the American Geriatrics Society*, 1970, 18, 491-500.

8 Robinson (R.A.): Some problems of clinical trials in elderly people. *Gerontologia Clinica*, 1961, 3, 247-257.

9 Wittenborn (J.R.): Reliability, validity, and objectivity of symptom rating scales. *Journal of Nervous and Mental Disease*, 1972, 154, 79-87.

ECHELLE CLINIQUE DE GERONTOLOGIE
CLINICAL SCALE IN GERONTOLOGY

SPECIFICITY

** *

TYPE OF INSTRUMENT

Ordinal rating scale
87 items

REFERENCE	**Crocq (L.), Bugard (P.), Fondarai (J.), Boscredon (J.), Bruneaux (J.), Charazac (P.) Clerc (G.), Darondel (A.), Drevet (M.), Fraud (J.P.), Gallet (G.), Louppe (A.), Martin (A.), Meisart (P.), Oules (J.), Patay (M.), Piel (E.), Reverzy (J.P.), Treisser (C.), Werquin (G.)** · – Traitement des états asthéno-dépressifs: Etude multicentrique de 248 cas évalués par l'échelle clinique G.E.F.4. *Psychologie Médicale*, 1980, 12, 12, 2643-61.

Language: Original version published in French.
France

Location: Enclosed in volume two page 138
See ref. biblio n° 3

For all information concerning the instrument write to the author at the following address:

Louis Crocq,
Ministère de la Défense
Direction des Recherches, Etudes et Techniques (D.R.E.T.)
26, Bd Victor
75996 Paris Armées, France

ORIGIN
The instrument is original and is derived from clinical experience. The form consisting of 20 items is derived from earlier versions written by the author (ref. 1).

PURPOSE
The instrument has a dual purpose: to standardise clinical observations and to quantify symptoms

POPULATION
All fatigue, somatic, psychological, reactive and psycho-social syndromes in young and elderly adults.

ADMINISTRATION
Rater: Physician.

Time required: 30 minutes.

Training: Not necessary.

Scoring: Out of the total number of 97 items, 67 are descriptive, 20 involve a 5 point assessment (1 corresponds to a global evaluation and 1 is an index of fatigue).

VARIABLES
The following variables are assessed:
· Fatigue
· Will
· Mood
· Cognitive functions
· Somatic functions
· Appearance-contact-speech
· Existential inventory (10 items)

VALIDATION
External validity according to clinical diagnosis (ref. 2).

OTHER WORKS
cited by author
A number of therapeutic trials.

APPLICATION
Clinical: To differentiate effects among diagnostic groups.
Research: Drug trials
Epidemiological studies.

1 Crocq (L.): Méthode objective d'appréciation des médications psychotoniques de la fatigue. *Sem. Hôp. Paris Thér.*, 1976, 10, 52, 557-564.

2 Crocq (L.), Bugard (P.): Fiche clinique standard pour l'appréciation des syndromes asthéniques et de leur évolution. *Psychol. Méd.*, 1977, 9, 9, 1757-1775.

3 Crocq (L.), Bugard (P.), Fondarai (J.), Boscredon (J.), Bruneaux (J.), et al.: Traitement des états asthéno-dépressifs par la minaprine. Etude multicentrique de 248 cas évalués par l'échelle clinique G.E.F.4. *Psychologie Médicale*, 1980, 12, 12, 2643-2661.

4 Crocq (L.), Bugard (P.), Fondarai (J.), Fraud (J.Ph.), Patay (M.), et al.: Essais cliniques de la minaprine (Cantor) dans les états asthéno-dépressifs ambulatoires (étude multicentrique quantifiée par l'échelle d'évaluation clinique "G.E.F.4". Congr. Psychiatr. Neurol. Langue Fr., Reims, 22-28 juin 1980.

5 Crocq (L.), Bugard (P.), Viaud (P.): Enquête du groupe d'études de la fatigue sur l'asthénie en pratique généraliste. *Psychol. Méd.*, 1978, 10, 10, 1943-1953.

6 Crocq (L.), Fondarai (J.): Exploitation par ordinateur des échelles d'appréciation psychiatrique. Congr. Psychiat. Neur. Langue Fr., LXXIe session, Monaco, 2-7 juillet 1973. Paris: Masson, 1974, 403-415.

7 Israel (L.): A novel method for drug trials using a rating scale for measuring the memory activity of elderly outpatients. XIth Int. Congr. Gerontol., Tokyo, 24 Aug. 1978.

8 Laborit (H.): Anxiété, dépression et Ag. 1240. *Agressologie*, 1972, 13, 275-283.

EVALUATION DE L'AUTONOMIE
EVALUATION OF AUTONOMY

SPECIFICITY

* * *

TYPE OF INSTRUMENT

Ordinal rating scale
10 items, 4 grades

REFERENCE — **Delomier (Y.), Gagne (A.), Girtanner (C.)** · – Evaluation de l'autonomie au Centre de Jour de Saint Etienne. *La Revue de Gériatrie*, 1980, tome 5, n° 8, 389-392.

Language: Published in French.
France

Location: Enclosed in volume two page 141
See ref. biblio n° 1

For all information concerning the instrument write to the author at the following address:

Yves Delomier,
Service de Gériatrie, C.H.R.U.
Hôpital de la Charité
40, rue Pointe Cadet
42022 Saint-Etienne Cedex, France

ORIGIN — Was inspired by the **Exton-Smith** rating scale (ref. 2), but was adapted according to the specific needs of the Day Center in question.

PURPOSE — To study the development of autonomy of elderly persons frequenting a day center by using an instrument adapted to services for long term patients.

POPULATION — Elderly inpatients in long-term care.

ADMINISTRATION — *Rater:* Nurse.

Time required: 5 minutes.

Training: Not necessary.

Scoring: Rating scale with 4 grades of severity, questions being coded from 1 (absence of autonomy) to 4 (autonomy). The score can vary from 10 to 40.
To the extent that a coded score is reliable, the following was established: the mean score for those returning to their homes is 35 points, 32 points for those going to homes for the aged and 25 points for those using services for long-term patients.

VARIABLES — The following aspects are assessed:
· General state
· Sleep
· Feeding
· Walking
· Dressing
· Continence
· Memory
· Language
· Activity
· Autonomy

VALIDATION — The instrument is in an experimental phase.

APPLICATION — Assessment of the development of the state of autonomy of a patient. Evaluation of changes.

1   Delomier (Y.), Gagne (A.), Girtanner (C.): Evaluation de l'autonomie au Centre de jour de Saint-Etienne. *La Revue de Gériatrie*, 1980, tome 5, n° 8, 389-392.

2   Exton-Smith (A.N.), Norton (D.), McLaren (R.): An investigation of geriatric nursing problems in hospital. London: National Corporation for the Care of Old People, 1962.

FISCHER SYMPTOM CHECK-LIST (F.S.C.L.)

SPECIFICITY

| * * |

TYPE OF INSTRUMENT

A 4 grade rating scale containing 41 items (plus 1 supplementary and provision for 6 "discretionary" items)

REFERENCE   **Fischer-Cornelssen (K.A.)** · – F.S.C.L.: Fischer symptom check-list. In: Collegium Internationale Psychiatriae Scalarum (C.I.P.S.) Hrsg.: "Internationale Skalen für Psychiatrie". 2nd ed. Weinheim, Germany: Beltz-Test, 1981.
And in: "Manual NCDEU assessment battery". 3rd ed. Chevy Chase, Maryland: NIMH, in print.

Language: Original version published in German. Translations in English, French, Spanish and Chinese with description and instructions. Glossary of Symptoms. **Switzerland**

Location: Enclosed in volume two page 143
See ref. biblio nº 4

For all information concerning the instrument or translations write to the author at the following address:

Kurt A. Fischer Cornelssen,
Sandoz Ltd, Medical Research Department
Kohlenstrasse, 386,
4002 Basel, Suisse

ORIGIN   An original instrument based on the published literature as well as on own sample populations, dealing with symptom frequency and severity in the main psychiatric disorders, especially depressions, anxiety and geriatric disturbances.

PURPOSE   To provide an instrument of quantitative evaluation for the symptoms, syndromes and severity of psychiatric disturbances (endogenous/non-endogenous depressions, anxiety neuroses or reactions, geriatric disturbances/depressions). The FSCL is a detailed and sensitive tool for clinical research purposes and for use in drug trials.

POPULATION   "Psychiatric" patients (in and out-patients). The FSCL must be supplemented by a somatic rating scale e.g. the FSUCL (Fischer Somatic Symptoms and Untoward Effects) (ref. 10). For use in geriatric patients appropriate cognitive tests and scale for rating daily-living activities should be included.

ADMINISTRATION   *Rater:* Physician, not necessarily a psychiatrist, or other medically qualified person; possibly by a psychologist (up to date no experience available).

Time required: During or immediately after the interview with the patient; completion of FSCL itself takes 2-5 minutes.

Training: Before using the FSCL for the first time the rater should familiarize himself with the check-list and its scoring system and with the necessary interview technique by means of a "trial run" with a few patients.

Scoring: Based on a non-suggestive, semi-structured interview with the subject, possibly supplemented by information obtained from nursing staff and relatives. The rating relates to the patient's state on the day of the interview or over the preceding week (or the interval to the last control). Each item is scored from 0 (none, not present) to 3 (severe). The totals for each of the 7 groups of symptoms into which the checklist is divided are then obtained by addition of the individual item scores, and the grand total for the whole FSCL is obtained by adding up all 41 item scores. This grand total represents the overall severity of the patient's conditions, but does not – as experience proved – differentiate diagnoses. Scores for "discretionary" items are not included in the overall total and have to be evaluated separately.

VARIABLES   Forty one symptoms or items (see vol. 2); "external stress" as an additional item for assessing the effect of his/her environment on the patient's condition (separate evaluation); up to 6 "discretionary" items determined by the rater (separate evaluation).
Symptoms arranged in 7 groups underlined by cluster analysis: mood / affect; time dependent variability; sleep; psychomotor status; thought processes; thought content; social behaviour.

VALIDATION
· **Construct validity** in patients (ref. 9, 11); six factors obtained by factor analysis – principal component analysis and Varimax rotation (50% of total variance); in a population of 344 geriatrics (mean age 72 years), which led to the detection of the factors:

anxiety / excitation (14%)
retardation / depression (13%)
impaired social behavior (7%)

abnormal thought processes and contents (7%)
agitation / aggression (5%)
auto-aggressiveness (4%)

Results in more than 700 geriatric patients demonstrate that common geriatric scales do not cover sufficiently important symptoms.

· In 188 **endogenous depressions,** with the following 6 factors (52%) of total variance, same method as above; mean age 46 years; (ref. 7):

retardation / depression (16%)
(including social behaviour
anxiety / excitation (9%)

somatic depression (8%)
auto-aggressiveness (7%) phobias / obsessions (6%)
hypochondriasis (7%)

Content validity: guaranteed by the fact that the check-list is based on the frequency distribution data for psychiatric and geriatric signs and symptoms given in the literature and in own sample populations, and on observations of its sensitivity in detecting changes in disease status.

Concurrent and **external validity**: correlated well with Zung's SDS or SAS, correlated well in clinical use with the global scores of a 4-point overall clinical rating scale.

Inter-rater and intra-rater (test-retest) reliability: using SAPE (Standardized Audiovisual Psychiatric Evaluation) with 34 trained and untrained raters (ref. 7), good agreement was found for both, symptom groups and individual symptoms.

· Calibration: specimen values or samples are available for the following, based on data from various countries: depressions, anxiety neuroses and reactions, geriatric disturbances.

OTHER WORKS
cited by author
· On going evaluations in large populations multicentre double-blind studies in psychiatric patients (ref. 2, 5, 6, 7, 8, 9, 10). Video-recordings in psychiatry and psychopharmacology (ref. 6, 7).

· Multicentre trials and studies: specimen values or samples for basic data, individual symptoms, symptom groups, total scores (frequency, intensity) before and during treatments, comparative data for placebo and standard treatments.

APPLICATION
Clinical: Symptom/syndrome profiles and assessment of severity of disease; prevention.
Research: Clinical drug trials (profiles of action, improvement and comparative effect). Differentiation between normal and pathological

BIBLIOGRAPHY

III.11

1 Bech (P.), Gram (L.F.), Dein (E.), Jacobsen (O.), Vitger (J.), Bolwig (T.G.): Quantitative rating of depressive states. *Acta Psychiat. Scand.*, 1975, 51, 161-170.

2 Berchier (P.), Fischer-Cornelssen (K.A.): Factor and cluster analysis of the german version of the FSCL in geriatric patients. Internal report. Basle: Sandoz Ltd, 1980.

3 Fischer-Cornelssen (K.A.): Einige Gesichtspunkte zur Gerontopsychiatrie: Hypothesen und Methodologie Klinischer Prüfüngen. *Arzneimittel-Forsch. (Drug Research)*, 1980, vol. 30, n° 8, 1215-1216.

4 Fischer-Cornelssen (K.A.): F.S.C.L.: Fischer Symptom Check-List. In: Collegium Internationale Psychiatriae Scalarum (C.I.P.S.) Hrsg: "Internationale Skalen für Psychiatrie". 2nd ed. Weinheim, Germany: Beltz-Test, 1981.

5 Fischer-Cornelssen (K.A.): Methods of multicenter trials in psychiatry. Part I: Review. *Prog. Neuro-Psychopharmacol.*, 1981, vol. 4, 545-560.

6 Fischer-Cornelssen (K.A.): Multicenter trials and complementary studies of Cloxazolam, a new anxiolytic drug. *Arzneimittel-Forsch. (Drug Research)*, 1981, vol. 31, n° 10, 1757-1765.

7 Fischer-Cornelssen (K.A.), Abt (K.): Television in psychiatry and psychopharmacology, presentation of a new method: SAPE. *Drug exp. clin. Res.*, 1977, 1, 173-182.

8 Fischer-Cornelssen (K.A.), Abt (K.): Videotape recording in psychiatry and psychopharmacology: review and presentation of a new method. *Acta Psychiat. Scand.*, 1980, 61, 228-238.

9 Fischer-Cornelssen (K.A.), Berchier (P.): Geriatrische Patienten mit depressiven Störungen: Doppelblinde Multizenterstudie und Langzeitstudie mit Vergleich Pizotifen, Plazebo, Doxepin und Cinnarizin. *Arzneimittel-Forsch. (Drug Research)*, 1980, vol. 30, n° 8, 1216-1217.

10 Fischer-Cornelssen (K.A.), Berchier (P.): Validität und Reliabilität einer Symptom-Checkliste (FSCL): Anwendung in der Psychogeriatrie. *Zeitschrift für Gerontologie*, 1982, 15, 31-37.

11 Fischer-Cornelssen (K.A.), Ferner (U.), Steiner (H.): Multifokale Psychopharmakaprüfung: Multihospital trial. *Arzneimittel-Forsch. (Drug Research)*, 1974, 24, 1706-1724.

12 Fischer-Cornelssen (K.A.), Hole (G.), Abt (K.): New audiovisual method: testing reliability of rating scales. Paper read at the 5th World Congress of Psychiatry in Mexico. Prens. med. mex. Congress volume, 291-292.

GERIATRIC RATING SCALE (G.R.S.)

SPECIFICITY

* * *

TYPE OF INSTRUMENT

Ordinal rating scale 20 items

REFERENCE

Götestam (K.G.) · – A geriatric rating scale empirically derived from three rating scales for geriatric behaviour. *Acta Psychiatrica Scandinavica, Supplementa,*, 1981, 294, 54-63

Language: Published in English.
Norway.

Location: Enclosed in volume two page 144
See ref. biblio nº 2

For all information concerning the instrument write to the author at the following address:

K. Gunnar Götestam,
Department of Psychiatry
Östmarka Hospital
P.O. Box 3008
N.–7001 Trondheim, Norway

ORIGIN

The instrument comprises items from the following scales: "Crichton Geriatric Rating Scale" (ref. 9), "Gottfries Cronholm Psychogeriatric Rating Scale" (ref. 5), and "Plutchik Geriatric Rating Scale" (ref. 8): Selection of items was done on the basis of their validity, sensitivity to changes, reliability and/or their correlation with a general clinical assessment index of the severity of disorders.

PURPOSE

The instrument was developed to assess, on the physical, mental and social levels, behavioral pathology in elderly subjects, and to test the effectiveness of certain therapeutic programmes.

POPULATION

Geriatric inpatients.

ADMINISTRATION

Rater: All members of hospital staff.

Time required: Brief.

Training: Not necessary.

Scoring: The grades for scoring vary according to the items.

VARIABLES

The instrument assesses 7 factors:
· Confusion
· Memory/orientation
· Activity and communication
· Sleep
· Mood
· Eating
· Psychotic symptoms and disturbing behavior

VALIDATION

Was composed on a population of elderly people (ref. 2):
Concurrent validity of the rating scale
Inter-rater reliability

APPLICATION

Clinical: Indications for placement or kinds of treatment, effectiveness of drug treatments. Diagnosis. Differentiation between chronic psychoses and senile dementia.
Describing clinical groups (Leon-principle, "heaviness of care" economic questions with regards to care cost-benefit).
Research: Epidemiological studies. Treatment evaluation: clinical drug trials, psychotherapy, etc.

1 Asberg (M.), Montgomery (S.A.), Perris (C.), Schalling (D.), Sedvall (G.): A comprehensive psychopathological rating scale. *Acta Psychiat. Scand.*, 1978, Suppl. 271, 5-27.

2 Götestam (K.G.): A geriatric rating scale empirically derived from three rating scales for geriatric behaviour. *Acta Psychiat. Scand.*, 1981, Suppl. 294, 54-63.

3 Götestam (K.G.), Forslund (B.A.), Käll (L.G.): Reliabilitet og validitet hos ett geriatriskt skattningsschema applicerat pa kroniska psyko-geriatriska patienter. *Nord. Geron.*, 1975, 2, 29-31.

4 Götestam (K.G.), Ljunghall (S.), Olsson (B.): A double-blind comparison of the effects of haloperidol and cis(Z)-clopenthixol in senile dementia. *Acta Psychiat. Scand.*, 1981, Suppl. 294.

5 Gottfries (C.G.), Cronholm (B.): Skattningsschema för geriatriska patienter. 1974. Manuscript unpublished.

6 Middelfart (E.), Götestam (K.G.): A rating scale for geriatric behaviour. (Abstract). Submitted to VII World Congress of Psychiatry, 1983.

7 Montgomery (S.A.), Asberg (M.): A new depression scale designed to be sensitive to change. *Brit. J. Psychiat.*, 1979, 134, 382-389.

8 Plutchik (R.), Conte (H.), Lieberman (M.), Bakur (M.), Grossman (J.), Lehrman (N.): Reliability and validity of a scale for the assessing of functioning of geriatric patients. *J. Amer. Geriat. Soc.*, 1970, 18, 491-500.

9 Robinson (R.A.): Some problems of clinical trials in elderly people. *Geront. Clin,*, 1961, 3, 247-251.

BILAN-TEST D'APPRECIATION DE LA PERTE D'AUTONOMIE

TEST – ASSESSMENT OF LOSS OF AUTONOMY

SPECIFICITY

* * *

TYPE OF INSTRUMENT

Questionnaire
20 questions

REFERENCE	**Graux (P.), Frigard (B.)** · – Bilan-test permettant d'apprécier la perte d'autonomie. In: "Accidents vasculaires cérébraux. Recherche épidémiologique". Premier congrès francophone de gérontologie, Paris, 17-18 septembre 1979. Paris: Masson, 1981, 548-552.

Language: Published in French.
France.

Location: Enclosed in volume two page 64
See ref. biblio n° 2

For all information concerning the instrument write to the author at the following address:

Pierre Graux
254 rue Solférino
59000 Lille, France

ORIGIN | The original instrument was constructed for use in geriatrics by Professor **Graux**, Lille (France).

PURPOSE | To establish an instrument which evaluates physical and mental status of the elderly as indicators of the level of their dependence.

POPULATION | Both geriatric inpatients and geriatric out-patients.

ADMINISTRATION | *Rater:* Physician, psychologist.
Time required: 10 minutes.
Training: Takes about 1 hour.
Scoring: Indicators of 4 degrees separately determine each variable, except psychiatric status where the indicator depends on the number of positive answers.

VARIABLES | The variables assessed are:
· Physical mobility
· Psychic functions
· Continence
· Eyesight
· Hearing

VALIDATION | On a population of elderly persons with an average age of 80 years, or patients in a geriatric ward.

APPLICATION | Can be applied in all cases concerning research and evaluation of physical status and level of loss of autonomy.

1 Graux (P.), Frigard (B.): Etude de l'autonomie des personnes âgées. *Revue de Gériatrie*, 1980, tome 5, n° 9, 419-421.

2 Graux (P.), Frigard (B.): Bilan-test permettant d'apprécier la perte d'autonomie. In: "Accidents vasculaires cérébraux – Recherche épidémiologique". Premier Congrès Francophone de Gérontologie, Paris, 17 – 18 septembre 1979. Paris: Masson, 1981, 548-552.

G.B.S. SCALE

SPECIFICITY

* * *

TYPE OF INSTRUMENT

Ordinal rating scale
26 items, 7 grades

REFERENCE   **Gottfries (C.G.), Brane (G.), Steen (G.)** · – A new rating scale for dementia syndromes. *Gerontology*, 1982, 28, Suppl. 2, 20-31.

Language: Original version published in Swedish.
Sweden.

Location: English version enclosed in volume two page 147
See ref. biblio nº 5 and 6
Write to author

For all information concerning the instrument write to the author at the following address:

C.G. Gottfries,
Department of Psychiatry and Neurochemistry
St. Jörgen's Hospital
S-422 03 Hisings Backa, Sweden

ORIGIN   The scale derives from the following literature (ref. 1, 2, 3, 7, 9, 10, 11, 12).

PURPOSE   To rate the degree of physical inactivity, impairment of intellectual and emotional capacities and mental symptoms common in dementia.

POPULATION   Hospitalized or non-hospitalized patients with dementia syndromes.

ADMINISTRATION   *Rater:* Physician, psychologist, registered nurse.

Time required: 30 minutes

Training: One session of training is necessary, especially concerning the emotional functions.

Scoring: Every item has 7 scale steps (0-6). 0, 2, 4 and 6 are clearly defined. 0 is equivalent to normal function or absence of symptoms, while 6 means maximal disturbance or presence of symptoms. The total score varies from 0 - 156.

VARIABLES   Four subscales:

· Motor functions: Motor insufficiency in undressing and dressing; Motor insufficency in taking food; Impaired physical activity; Deficiency of spontaneous activity; Motor insufficiency in managing personal hygiene; Inability to control bladder and bowel.

· Intellectual functions: Impaired orientation in space; Impaired orientation in time; Impaired personal orientation; Impaired recent memory; Impaired distant memory; Impaired wakefulness; Impaired concentration; Inability to increase tempo; Absentmindedness; Long-windedness; Distractability.

· Emotional functions; Emotional blunting; Emotional lability; Reduced motivation.

· Different symptoms common in dementia: Confusion; Irritability; Anxiety; Agony; Reduced mood; Restlessness.

VALIDATION   Reliability and the validity patients in a somatic and in a psychogeriatric hospital were rated.
Inter-rater reliability: Four independent nurses, one physician and one psychologist rated the patient at different occasions.

APPLICATION   **Clinical:** To get a quantitative measure of dementia and a dementia profile.
Research: Evaluation of psycho-pharmacological and other treatment.

1 Adolfsson (R.), Gottfries (C.G.), Nyström (L.), Winblad (B.): Prevalence of dementia disorders in institutionalized swedish old people. The work imposed by caring for these patients. *Acta Psychiat. Scand.*, 1981, 63, 225-244.

2 Asberg (M.), Montgomery (S.A.), Perris (C.), Schalling (D.), Sedvall (G.): A comprehensive psychopathological rating scale. *Acta Psychiat. Scand.*, Suppl. 271, 5,-27.

3 Berg (S.), Svensson (T.): An orientation scale for geriatric patients. *Age and Ageing*, 1980, 9, 215-219.

4 Gottfries (C.G.), Brane (G.), Steen (B.), Steen (G.): A new rating scale for assessment of the degree of dementia. Paper presented at 12th International Congress of Gerontology, Hamburg, 12-17 July 1981.

5 Gottfries (C.G.), Brane (G.), Steen (G.): A new rating scale for dementia syndromes. *Gerontology*, 1982, 28, Suppl. 2, 20-31.

6 Gottfries (C.G.), Brane (G.), Steen (G.): G.B.S. scale. *Archives of Gerontology and Geriatrics*, 1982, 1, 4, 311-330.

7 Gottfries (C.G.), Gottfries (I.): Geriatriskt skattningsschema. Manuscript unpublished, 1968.

8 Hamilton (M.): Use of rating scale in geriatric patients. *Gerontology*, 1982, 28, Suppl. 2, 42-48.

9 Kahn (R.L.), Goldfarb (A.I.), Pollak (M.), Peck (A.): Brief objective measures for the determination of mental status in the aged. *Am. J. Psychiat.*, 1960, 117, 326.

10 Plutchik (R.), Conte (H.), Lieberman (M.), Bakur (M.), Grossman (J.), Lehrman (N.): Plutchik geriatric rating scale. In: Guy (W.) Ed.: «ECDEU Assessment manual for psychopharmacology». Revised ed. Kensington, Maryland: George Washington University, 1976.

11 Robinson (R.A.): Some problems of clinical trials in elderly people. *Gerontologia Clinica*, 1961, 3, 247-251.

12 Shader (R.I.), Harmatz (J.), Salzman (C.): A new scale for clinical assessment in geriatric populations: Sandoz clinical assessment – geriatric (SCAG). *Journal of the American Geriatrics Society*, 1974, 22, 3, 107-113.

DRUG DEPENDENCY AND OVERDOSE ASSESSMENT

SPECIFICITY

* *

TYPE OF INSTRUMENT

Questionnaire
22 questions

REFERENCE   **Idänpään-Heikkilä (J.), Khan (I.)** · − Psychotropic substances and public health problems. Report of a seminar convened by the World Health Organization with the collaboration of the Government of Finland and the United Nations Fund for Drug Abuse Controll. Helsinki: Government of Finland, 1982.

Language: Finnish, English
Finland

Location: Enclosed in volume two page 66
See ref. biblio nº 12

For all information concerning the instrument or translation, write to:

Juhana Idänpään – Heikkilä   Inayat Khan,
National Board of Health   World Health Organization
Helsinki   1211 Geneva 27
Finland   Switzerland.

ORIGIN   This questionnaire was derived from an earlier version which was used in the course of specific studies investigating the misuse of psychotropic drugs and drug abuse control (ref. 7, 9, 13).

PURPOSE   The instrument was conceived for the assessment of the role of psychotropic substances in the cases of severe overdosing and the causes of this (suicide attempts or accidents). It enables the regrouping of information and the coordination of research of drug dependency and overdose throughout the world.

POPULATION   Patients of all ages suffering from deliberate or accidental overdosing and drug dependents who are requesting drugs or who are hospitalised because of complications arising from their drug dependency.

ADMINISTRATION   *Rater:* Physician from the casualty department.

Time required: 30-45 minutes

Training: Necessary

Scoring: Varies according to the sections being assessed.

VARIABLES   The following variables are assessed:
· State of consciousness   · Drug dependency
· Suicidal intention   · Alcohol dependency
· Aggression in casualty

These variables were assessed bearing in mind the type of drug, the source of overdosing, the manner of administration, and the source of supply.

VALIDATION   The instrument was used on different populations and various studies were published (ref. 14, 16, 21).

APPLICATION   Epidemiological studies concerning, above all, morbidity and mortality caused by psychotropic substances.

1 Bewley (B.R.), Bewley (T.H.): Dependence as a public health problem (alcohol, tobacco, and other drugs). In: Hobson (W.) Ed.: "The theory and practice of public health". 5th. ed. Oxford University Press, 1979, 480-500.

2 Connell (P.H.): Amphetamine psychosis. London: Chapman and Hall, 1958.

3 Cooper (J.R.): Sedative hypnotic drugs: risks and benefits. Washington, DC: US Department of Health Education, and Welfare (NIDA), 1977.

4 De Alarcon (R.), Rathod (N.H.): Prevalence and early detection of heroin abuse. *British Medical Journal*, 1968, 2, 549-553.

5 Drug abuse warning network. Phase VI report. Washington, DC: US Department of Health, Education and Welfare (NIDA), May 1977-April 1978.

6 Eddy (N.B.) et al.: Drug dependence: its significance and characteristics. *Bulletin of the World Health Organization*, 1965, 32, 721-733.

7 Edwards (G.), Gattoni (F.), Hensman (C.): Correlates of alcohol dependence scores in a prison population. *Quarterly Journal on study of alcohol*, 1972, 33, 417-429.

8 Ellinwood (E.), Cohen (S.) Eds.: Current concepts on amphetamine use. Washington, DC: US Government Printing Office, 1972.

9 Ghodse (A.H.): Drug problems dealt with by 62 London casualty departments. A preliminary report. *British Journal of Preventive and Social Medicine*, 1976, 30, 251-256.

10 Ghodse (A.H.): Casualty departments and the monitoring of drug dependence. *British Medical Journal*, 1977, 1, 1381-1382.

11 Ghodse (A.H.): Morbidity and mortality of drug dependent individuals. In: Edwards (G.), Busch (C.) Eds.: "The british drug problem and the responses 1969-1976". London: Academic Press, 1981.

12 Idänpään-Heikkilä (J.), Khan (I.): Psychotropic substances and public health problems: report of a seminar convened by the World Health Organization with the collaboration of the Government of Finland and the United Nations Fund for Drug Abuse Control. Helsinki: Government of Finland, 1982.

13 Lader (M.): Benzodiazepine dependence. In: Murray (R.) et al. Eds.: "The misuse of psychotropic drugs". Gaskell: The Royal College of Psychiatrists, Service Publication, 1981.

14 Mohan (D.): Pattern and prevalence of drug overdosage in casualty emergency services: a collaborative study of Delhi hospitals. New Delhi: Indian Council of Medical Research, 1981.

15 Murray (R.M.): The use and abuse of analgesics. *Scottish Medical Journal*, 1972, 17, 393-396.

16 National Institute on Drug Abuse: Drug dependence in pregnancy: clinical management of mother and child. Washington, DC: US Department of Health, Education and Welfare, 1979.

17 Oswald (I.) et al.: Drugs of dependence though not of abuse. In: Singh (J.M.) et al. Eds.: "Drug addiction: clinical and socio-legal aspects". Vol. 2. New York: Futura, 1972, 75-82.

18 Perlin (M.J.), Simon (K.J.): The epidemiology of drug use during pregnancy. *International Journal of Addictions*, 1979, 14, 3, 355-364.

19 Schuster (C.R.), Bergman (I.), Hartel (C.R.): Assessing the impact on public health, individual deficit, and organ system damage associated with psychoactive substance use. Washington, DC: US Department of Health, Education and Welfare (NIDA), 1980.

20 Sellers (E.M.), Marshman (J.A.), Kaplan (H.L.), Giles (H.G.), Kapur (B.M.), Busto (U.), Mac Leod (S.M.), Stapleton (C.), Sealey (F.): Acute and chronic drug abuse emergencies in Metropolitan Toronto. *International Journal of Addictions*, 1981, 16, 2, 283-303.

21 World Health Organization: Technical report series, n° 656, 1981.

EVALUATION DE LA DEPENDANCE EN INSTITUTION
ASSESSMENT OF NEEDS OF GERIATRIC UNITS PATIENTS

SPECIFICITY

* * *

TYPE OF INSTRUMENT

Ordinal rating scale
5 indicators

REFERENCE **Kuntzmann (F.), Rudloff (H.), Etheve (M.), Berthel (M.), Gitz (A.M.), Strubel (D.), Artzner (M.)** · − Evaluation des besoins des pensionnaires des établissements gériatriques. *La Revue de Gériatrie*, 1982, tome 7, n̊ 6, 263-271.

Language: Original version published in French.
France.

Location: Enclosed in volume two page 152
See ref. biblio n̊ 7

For all information concerning the instrument write to the author at the following address:

Francis Kuntzmann,
Service de Gériatrie
Pavillon Ch. Schutzenberger
Centre Hospitalier Régional
Hôpital de la Robertsau
67015 Strasbourg Cedex, France

ORIGIN   This is based on the deliberations of different members of the French Gerontological Society in May 1980, the Gerontological Societies of the Rhone-Alpes region and the East in October 1980 and March 1981 (ref. 6). The instrument was also inspired by the works of **Svanborg** (ref. 4).

PURPOSE   To assess the physical and psychological dependency of pensioners living in geriatric institutions with the aim of determining the means which would enable that institution to fulfill the subject's needs. This instrument, which was developed for pragmatic purposes, identifies the necessary equipment and staff required to meet the various needs of different institutions which vary from year to year.

POPULATION   Elderly population living in a geriatric institution.

ADMINISTRATION   *Rater:* Combined efforts of a team are necessary.
A minimum of 3 raters is required: physician, nurse, nurse's aide.

Time required: 2 minutes per rater.

Training: Special training is not necessary. After 10-20 observations, assessment becomes easier.

Scoring: The scale is scored from 0 to 2, or A, B, C.

VARIABLES   Five principal indicators:
· Needs concerning self care: · Bladder and bowel control
   Feeding   · Transfer and mobility
   Grooming   · Psychological dependency
   Dressing   · Need for medical care and indications for rehabilitation

VALIDATION   A multicentre study conducted in France on a population of elderly people in long-term units, residential and nursing homes (ref. 9).

OTHER WORKS
cited by author   Longitudinal studies have been made, identifying the number of pensioners living in residential homes requiring nursing home accommodation.
Study of the population of all the units for long-term care in Alsace.

APPLICATION   The instrument is to be used exclusively for the following puposes:
· Adapting the various institutions according to the needs of the populations living in them.
· Comparison of various population groups living in different institutions.
· Comparison of population groups living in the same institutions at different times.

1 Delcros (M.), Lanoe (R.): Une nouvelle échelle d'évaluation de la dépendance des patients dans les établissements de Long Séjour. *Revue de Gériatrie*, 1980, tome 5, n° 8, 395-400.

2 Dubos (G.), Hugonot (R.): Evaluation de la dépendance des personnes âgées. Analyse des échelles actuellement utilisées dans les services de gériatrie. *Revue de Gériatrie*, 1980, tome 5, n° 8, 367-370.

3 Henrard (J.C.), Cassou (B.), Colvez (A.), Lazar (P.): Perte d'autonomie en handicap, problèmes conceptuels. *Revue de Gériatrie*, 1980, tome 5, n° 8, 375-378.

4 Hulten (A.), Kerstell (J.), Olsson (R.), Svanborg (A.): A Method to calculate nursing load. *Scand J. Rehab. Med.*, 1969, 1, 117-125.

5 Gitz (A.M.), Etheve (M.), Kissel (C.), Bucher (M.E.), Niederberger (M.P.), Charras (D.), Kuntzmann (F.): L'évaluation de l'autonomie des vieillards en unité de Long Séjour, facteur de communication et d'information de l'équipe soignante. A propos d'une technique d'évaluation. *Revue de Gériatrie*, 1980, tome 5, n° 9, 423-424.

6 Kuntzmann (F.): Objectifs de l'évaluation de la perte d'autonomie des personnes âgées. *Revue de Gériatrie*, 1980, tome 5, n° 8, 363-365.

7 Kuntzmann (F.), Rudloff (H.), Etheve (M.), Berthel (M.), Gitz (A.M.), Strubel (D.), Artzner (M.): Evaluation des besoins des pensionnaires des établissements gériatriques. *Revue de Gériatrie*, 1982, tome 7, n° 6, 263-271.

8 Leroux (R.), Viau (G.), Fournier (M.), Bergeot (R.), Attalli (G.): Visualisation d'une échelle simple d'autonomie: Géronte. *Revue de Gériatrie*, 1981, tome 6, n° 9, 433-436.

9 Rudloff (H.), Etheve (M.), Gitz (A.M.), Kuntzmann (F.): Evaluation de la dépendance des personnes âgées vivant en institution en vue de l'appréciation de leurs besoins d'assistance. Présentation d'une grille expérimentale dans plusieurs établissements. *Revue de Gériatrie*, 1982, tome 7, n° 2, 88.

10 Stähelin (H.B.), Seiler (W.), Kelterborn (P.), Peter (S.): Aussagekraft von Beurteilungs-Kriterien der Pflegebedürftigkeit. *Akt. Gerontol.*, 1980, 10, 419-422.

RAPID DISABILITY RATING SCALE 2

SPECIFICITY

* *

TYPE OF INSTRUMENT

Ordinal rating scale
I: 16 items, 3 grades
II: 18 items, 4 grades

REFERENCE

Linn (M.W.) · – A rapid disability rating scale. *Journal of the American Geriatrics Society*, 1967, 15, 2, 211-214.
Linn (M.W.), Linn (B.S.) · – The rapid disability rating scale – 2. *Journal of the American Geriatrics Society*, 1982 30, 6, 378-382

Language: Original version published in English
U.S.A.

Location: Enclosed in volume two page 154
See ref. biblio nº 15, 19

For all information concerning the instrument write to the author at the following address:

Margaret Linn,
Social Science Research 151
Veterans Administration Medical Center
1201 N.W. 16th Street
Miami, Florida 33125, U.S.A.

ORIGIN — The original instrument is based on a number of published works (ref. 1, 2, 3, 4, 5, 6, 7, 8, 9, 10, 11, 13, 22, 23, 24, 25).

PURPOSE — To measure disability in relation to activities of daily living and dependence, with the aid of a brief and simple instrument, constructed on the basis of a number of observations which are found in different research works.

POPULATION — Geriatric inpatients and out-patients.

ADMINISTRATION — *Rater:* Nurse. Any person who is familiar with the subject.
Time required: 5 minutes.
Training: Getting familiar with the items.
Scoring: Each item is coded from 1 to 3 according to increasing severity. The global score varies from 16-48 for scale 1, and from 18 to 72 for scale 2.

VARIABLES — Twelve variables common for 2 scales:

· Eating	· Hearing	· Incontinence
· Diet	· Sight	· Mental confusion
· Medication	· Bathing	· Uncooperativeness
· Walking	· Dressing	· Depression

Four variables specific for scale I:
Verbal expression; Shaving; Confined to bed; Safety supervision

Six variables specific for scale II:

· Toileting	· Adaptive tasks	· In bed during day
· Grooming	· Communication	· Mobility

VALIDATION — Was tested on a population of elderly out-patients and inpatients (ref. 15, 19):
Factor analyses
Content validity of items was tested in studies on their distribution and intrapersonal sensitivity.
External validity, concurrent and predictive, based on judgements made by physicians made on each patient on the number of previous hospitalisations, the length of current hospitalisation and the number of deaths within a six-month period.
Inter-rater reliability (60 independent raters), inter-rater reliability and test retest (scoring done by 2 different teams in a 4 day interval).

OTHER WORKS cited by author — Research on institutional care (ref. 12, 14, 16, 21), on late-stage cancer patients (ref. 20). Cultural studies in the elderly (ref. 17).

APPLICATION — **Research:** Treatment assessment, Organization of care, Screening of needs.

1 Bergner (M.), Bobbit (R.A.), Kressel (S.) et al.: The sickness impact profile: a conceptual formulation and methodology for development of a health status measure. *Int. J. Health Serv.*, 1976, 6, 393.

2 Brook (R.H.), Ware (J.E.), Davies-Avery (A.) et al.: Overview of adult health status measures fielded in Rand's health insurance study. *Med. Care*, 1979, 17, Suppl.: whole issue.

3 Burack (B.): Interdisciplinary classification for the aged. *J. Chronic Dis.*, 1965, 18, 1059.

4 Committee on Medical Rating of Physical Impairment: a guide to the evaluation of permanent impairment of the extremities and back. *J.A.M.A.*, 1958, (special edition), 166, 1.

5 Gauger (A.B.), Brownwell (W.M.), Russell (W.W.) et al.: Evaluation of levels of substance. *Arch. Phys. Med. Rehabil.*, 1964, 45, 286.

6 Gurel (L.), Linn (M.W.), Linn (B.S.): Physical and mental impairment-of-function evaluation in the aged: the Pamie scale. *J. Gerontol.*, 1972, 27, 1, 83.

7 Kaiser (H.F.): The varimax criterion for analytic rotation in factor analysis. *Psychometrika*, 1958, 23, 187.

8 Katz (S.), Ford (A.B.), Moskowitz (R.W.) et al.: Studies of illness in the aged: the index of ADL, a standardized measure of biological and psychosocial function. *J.A.M.A.*, 1963, 185, 914.

9 Kleh (J.): A classification for the aged and other patients with chronic disease or disability. *J. Am. Geriatrics Soc.*, 1963, 11, 638.

10 Krauss (T.C.): Use of a comprehensive rating scale system in the institutional care of geriatric patients. *J. Am. Geriatrics Soc.*, 1962, 10, 95.

11 Lawton (M.P.), Brody (E.): Assessment of older people: self-maintaining and instrumental activities of daily living. *Gerontologist*, 1969, 9, 179.

12 Linn (B.S.), Linn (M.W.), Greenwald (S.R.), Gurel (L.): Validity of impairment ratings made from medical records and from personal knowledge. *Med. Care*, 1974, 12, 4, 363-368.

13 Linn (B.S.), Linn (M.W.), Gurel (L.): Cumulative illness rating scale. *J. Am. Geriat. Soc.*, 1968, 16, 622.

14 Linn (B.S.), Linn (M.W.), Gurel (L.): Correlates of prognosis: a study of the physician's clinical judgment. *Med. Care*, 1973, 11, 5, 430-435.

15 Linn (M.W.): A rapid disability rating scale. *Journal of the American Geriatrics Society*, 1967, vol. 15, n° 2, 211-214.

16 Linn (M.W.), Gurel (L.), Linn (B.S.): Patient outcome as a measure of quality of nursing home care. *A.J.P.H.*, 1977, 67, 4, 337-344.

17 Linn (M.W.), Hunter (K.I.), Linn (B.S.): Self-assessed health, impairment and disability in Anglo, Black and Cuban elderly. *Med. Care*, 1980, 18, 3, 282-288.

18 Linn (M.W.), Linn (B.S.): Problems in assessing response to treatment in the elderly by physical and social function. *Psychopharmacology Bulletin*, 1981, 17, 4, 74-81.

19 Linn (M.W.), Linn (B.S.): The rapid disability rating scale-2. *Journal of the American Geriatrics Society*, 1982, 30, 6, 378-382.

20 Linn (M.W.), Linn (B.S.), Harris (R.): Effects of counseling for late stage cancer patients. *Cancer*, 1982, 49, 5, 1048-1055.

21 Linn (M.W.), Linn (B.S.), Stein (S.): Ratings of impairment and functional status in prediction of mortality. *Psychological Reports*, 1975, 37, 998.

22 Mahoney (R.I.), Barthel (D.W.): Functional evaluation: the Barthel index. *Md State Med. J.*, 1965, 14, 61.

23 Meer (B.), Baker (J.A.): The Stockton geriatric rating scale. *J. Gerontol.*, 1966, 21, 392.

24 OARS community survey questionnaire. Mimeographed. Durham, North Carolina: Duke University, Center for the Study of Aging and Human Development, 1972.

25 Overall (J.E.), Gorham (D.R.): The brief psychiatric rating scale. *Psychol. Rep.*, 1962, 10, 799.

ECHELLE DE DEPENDANCE C.E.N.T.S.

RATING SCALE FOR DEPENDENCY

SPECIFICITY

* * *

TYPE OF INSTRUMENT

Ordinal rating scale 5 items, 6 grades

REFERENCE	The instrument was not published
	Language: Written in French. **France.**
	Location: Enclosed in volume two page 155
	For all information concerning the instrument write to the author at the following address:
	Robert Hugonot, Pavillon Elisée Chatin C.H.R.U. 38700 La Tronche, France

ORIGIN

This was derived through joint efforts of different members of the French Society of Gerontology to produce scales for the assessment of dependency.

PURPOSE

The instrument was conceived to assess global dependency and the burden of care which results inside an institution.

POPULATION

Elderly inpatients.

ADMINISTRATION

Rater: Nurse's aide. The instrument is completed by the whole team.

Time required: Less than 5 minutes.

Training: Not necessary.

Scoring: Each item is scored from 0-5.
If one or more items have a score over 3, the patient belongs to the category requiring long-term hospitalisation. If no items exceed 3, the patient belongs to the category of residential homes.

VARIABLES

Dependency: From neurological and psychiatric causes.
Motor activity

Degree of care: Nursing
Medical treatment
Special care

VALIDATION

The instrument was tested on 400 subjects living in medical geriatric establishments in the Rhone-Alpes region, long-term hospitals, hospices or nursing homes.

OTHER WORKS
cited by author

Daily use to assess the burden of caring for an individual in a sector of care.

APPLICATION

Indications for placement in a given institution.

PHYSICAL MENTAL SOCIAL

IV.1	Stockton Geriatric Rating Scale (*)	MEER	1966
IV.2	Parkside Behaviour Rating Scale	FINE	1970
IV.3	Geriatric Rating Scale (*)	PLUTCHIK	1970
IV.4	P.A.M.I.E. Scale (*)	GUREL	1972
IV.5	Functional Life Scale (*)	SARNO	1973
IV.6	Parachek Geriatric Behavior Rating Scale	PARACHEK-MILLER	1974
IV.7	Sandoz Clinical Assessment Geriatric	SHADER	1974
IV.8	Psychogeriatric Assessment Program	DOUGLAS HOSPITAL	1975
IV.9	Geriatric Functional Rating Scale (*)	GRAUER	1975
IV.10	Echelle d'Appréciation Clinique en Gériatrie	GEORGES-LALLEMAND	1977
IV.11	Comprehensive Assessment and Referral Evaluation	GURLAND	1977
IV.12	Multidimensional Functional Assessment Questionnaire (*)	CENTER FOR AGING	1978
IV.13	Geriatric Resident Goals Scale (*)	CORNBLETH	1978
IV.14	London Psychogeriatric Rating Scale	HERSCH	1978
IV.15	Origine de la Dépendance (*)	ISRAEL	1978
IV.16	Geriatric Rapid Diagnostic Battery (*)	MURKOFSKY	1978
IV.17	Batterie de Fiches d'Evaluation (*)	ZAY	1978
IV.18	Disability Assessment Schedule (*)	W.H.O.	1979
IV.19	Echelle de Dépendance - Autonomie (*)	DELCROS-LANOË	1980
IV.20	Comprehensive Health Questionnaire	KOZAREVIĆ	1980
IV.21	Evaluation Globale de l'Autonomie (*)	PATRON	1980
IV.22	Edinburgh Psychogeriatric Dependency Rating Scale (*)	WILKINSON	1980
IV.23	Système d'Information C.T.M.S.P. (*)	E.R.O.S.	1981
IV.24	Echelle d'Expression de l'Autonomie: Géronte (*)	LEROUX-ATTALLI	1981
IV.25	Clifton Assessment Procedures for Elderly (*)	PATTIE	1981
IV.26	Questionnaire d'Enquête pour Etude Epidémiologique	VIGNAT-ISRAEL	1981
IV.27	Self Assessment Scale - Geriatric	YESAVAGE	1981
IV.28	Multilevel Assessment Instrument (*)	LAWTON	1982
IV.29	Nürnberger-Alters-Inventar	OSWALD	1982
IV.30	Functional Activities Questionnaire (*)	PFEFFER	1982
IV.31	Grille pour l'Evaluation du Degré de Dépendance (*)	C.I.C.P.A.	
IV.32	Grille de Dépendance (*)	CENTRE DE GERIATRIE	
IV.33	Bilans de Bel Air 1960-1982	ECOLE DE BEL AIR	

(*) Instruments evaluating primarily dependency.

STOCKTON GERIATRIC RATING SCALE (S.G.R.S.)

SPECIFICITY

* * *

TYPE OF INSTRUMENT

Ordinal rating scale
3 grades
Form I: 30 items
Form II: 33 items

REFERENCE	**Meer (B.), Baker (J.A.)** · − The Stockton Geriatric Rating Scale. *Journal of Gerontology*, 1966, 21, 392-403.

Language: Original version published in English. French translation by: P. Pichot, B. Girard, J.C. Dreyfus (ref. 22).
Dutch translation by P. Van der Kam (ref. 27).
U.S.A.

Location: Enclosed in volume two page 156
See ref. biblio n⁰ 20

For all information concerning the instrument write to the following addresses:

Cletus Krag   California Dpt of Mental Hygiene
1215 W. Swain Rd   Sacramento, U.S.A.
Stockton, CA 95207 U.S.A.

ORIGIN
Form I of the instrument consisted of 30 items, 14 of which were used in a previous study to measure physical disability (ref. 21). The 16 new items were generated first from clinical experience, and then from a review of current behavioral rating scales (ref. 2, 6, 19, 23). After factor analysis was completed, 5 items were excluded and another 8 added to constitute form II of the scale consisting of 33 items.

PURPOSE
To construct a scale measuring the patient's daily behavior in geriatric hospitals in order to determine the patients needs concerning type of care. Assessment is done in the course of evaluating the intensity of disturbed behavior

POPULATION
Geriatric inpatients aged 65 and over.

ADMINISTRATION
Rater: Nurse. For clinical use or research it is necessary to have 2 independent evaluations for each patient.
Time required: 10 minutes.
Training: Not necessary.
Scoring: Each item is coded 0,1 or 2. The scale measures severity; 2 indicates the severest state concerning each item, 0 the absence of any anomaly. The higher the total score, the more severe the deterioration. Rating of the patient's behavior should be based on the one-week period preceding the rating.

VARIABLES
Factor analysis determined 4 factors:
1. Physical disability (10 items)   3. Communication failure (4 items)
2. Apathy (10 items)   4. Socially irritating behavior (9 items)

VALIDATION
Was done on 3 random samples of geriatric inpatients (ref. 20). Patients not suffering from organic brain syndrome or functional psychosis were excluded. These studies included:
Factor analyses (4 above listed factors)
External validity and sensitivity based on the results of E.C.T. on depressed patients.
Predictive validity: based on length of hospitalisation.
Inter-rater validity for each factor and for global score.
Studies on internal consistency of the factors.

OTHER WORKS
cited by author
Concerns the application of a shortened version of this scale in psychiatric surroundings (ref. 8), completed in Great Britain by C.J. Gilleard (ref. 9).

APPLICATION
Clinical: Programming treatment, predicting outcome, measuring changes in the patient's behavior.
Research: Changes in behavior of patients in the course of drug trials. Epidemiological studies and enquiries.

1 Berger (L.), Bernstein (A.), Klein (E.), Cohen (J.), Lucas (G.): Effects of aging and pathology on the factorial structure of intelligence. *Journal of Consulting Psychology*, 1964, 28, 199-207.

2 Burdock (E.I.), Elliott (H.E.), Hardesty (A.S.), O'Neill (F.J.), Sklar (J.): Biometric evaluation of an intensive treatment program in a state mental hospital. *Journal of Nervous and Mental Diseases*, 1960, 130, 271-277.

3 Burdock (E.I.), Hardesty (A.S.), Hakerem (G.), Zubin (J.): A ward behavior rating scale for mental patients. *Journal of Clinical Psychology*, 1960, 16, 246-247.

4 Burt (C.): The factorial study of temperamental traits. *British Journal of Psychology, Statist. Sec.*, 1948, 1, 178-203.

5 Dixon (J.C.): Cognitive structure in senile conditions with some suggestions for developing a brief screening test of mental status. *Journal of Gerontology*, 1965, 20, 41-49.

6 Ellsworth (R.B.): The MACC behavioral adjustment scale (Manual). Beverly Hills, Calif.: Western Psychological Services, 1962, 14 p.

7 Ellsworth (R.B.), Clayton (W.H.): Measurement of improvement in mental illness. *Journal of Consulting Psychology*, 1959, 23, 15-20.

8 Freyens (R.): Application d'une échelle d'appréciation gériatrique aux patients d'un hôpital psychiatrique fermé. *Acta Psychiat. Belg.*, 1976, 76, 586-598.

9 Gilleard (C.J.), Pattie (A.H.): The Stockton geriatric rating scale: a shortened version with british normative data *Brit. J. Psychiat.*, 1977, 131, 90-94.

10 Guilford (J.P.): Fundamental statistics in psychology and education. 3rd ed. New York: Mc Graw-Hill, 1956, 565 p.

11 Guttman (L.): "Best possible" systematic estimate of communalities. *Psychometrika*, 1956, 21, 273-285.

12 Kaiser (H.F.): The varimax criterion for analytic rotation in factor analysis. *Psychometrika*, 1958, 23, 187-200.

13 Kral (V.A.), Cahn (C.), Mueller (H.): Senescent memory impairment and its relation to the general health of the aging individual. *Journal of the American Geriatrics Society*, 1964, 12, 101-113.

14 Lewandowski (T.): Evaluation of patients in a geriatric rehabilitation unit of a state mental hospital: use of a rating scale system. *Journal of the American Geriatrics Society*, 1962, 10, 526-531.

15 Lorr (M.): The Psychotic Reaction Profile (PRP): Manual. Beverly Hills, Calif.: Western Psychological Services, 1961, 10 p.

16 Lorr (M.), O'Connor (J.P.), Stafford (J.): The psychotic reaction profile. *Journal of clinical Psychology*, 1960, 16, 241-245.

17 Lowenthal (M.F.): Lives in distress. New York: Basic Books, 1964, 266 p.

18 Lucero (R.J.), Meyer (B.T.): A Behavioral rating scale suitable for use in mental hospitals. *Journal of clinical Psychology*, 1951, 7, 250-254.

19 Mc Reynolds (P.), Ferguson (J.T.): Clinical manual for the hospital adjustment scale. Stanford, Calif.: Stanford Univ. Press, 1953, 12 p.

20 Meer (B.), Baker (J.A.): The Stockton Geriatric Rating Scale. *Journal of Gerontology*, 1966, 21, 392-403.

21 Meer (B.), Krag (C.L.): Correlates of disability in a population of hospitalized geriatric patients. *Journal of Gerontology*, 1964, 19, 440-446.

22 Pichot (P.), Girard (B.), Dreyfus (J.C.): L'échelle d'appréciation gériatrique de Stockton (S.G.R.S.): Etude de sa version française. *Revue de Psychologie Appliquée*, 4e trim. 1970, vol. 20, n° 4, 245-254.

23 Scott (T.), Devereaux (C.P.), Janes (E.): Potential social habilitation of elderly patients. Res. Div., Dept. of Mental Hyg., State of Calif., Sacramento, 1962, Res. Monogr. n° 2, 90 p. (Mimeogr.).

24 Shatin (L.), Freed (E.X.): A behavioral rating scale for mental patients. *J. ment. Sci.*, 1955, 101, 644-653.

25 Trites (D.K.), Sells (S.B.): A note on alternative methods for estimating factor scores. *J. appl. Psychol.*, 1955, 39, 454-456.

26 Tryon (R.C.): Reliability and behavior domain validity: reformulation and historical critique. *Psychol. Bull.*, 1957, 54, 229-249.

27 Van Der Kam (P.), Mol (F.) Wimmers (M.): Beoordelingsschaal voor Oudere Patiënten. Deventer, Holland: Van Loghum Staterus, 1971.

PARKSIDE BEHAVIOUR RATING SCALE

SPECIFICITY

| * * * |

TYPE OF INSTRUMENT

Nominal rating scale
5 grades

REFERENCE   **Fine (E.W.), Lewis (D.), Villa-Landa (I.), Blakemore (C.B.)** · − The effect of cyclandelate on mental function in patients with arteriosclerotic brain disease. *British Journal of Psychiatry*, 1970, 117, 157-161.

Language: Original version published in English.
Great Britain

Location: See ref. biblio n° 2

For all information concerning the instrument write to the publisher at the following address:

Brocades & Co Ltd
Trend House
Pyrford Road
West Byfleet,
Surrey, Great Britain

PURPOSE   This instrument is designed to measure changes in the subject's behaviour in relation to his environment.

POPULATION   Elderly persons living in a residential home.

ADMINISTRATION   *Rater:* Nursing staff.

Time required: 15 minutes.

Training: None.

Scoring: Parameters graded in severity up to 5.
Several sub-headings are included. Against each sub-heading, is indicated a description of that parameter graded in severity from 1 (severest) to 5 (least severe).
For example: Under the main heading of Self Care as sub-headings the following descriptions appear:
1. Requiring every form of nursing care.
2. Requiring regular nursing supervision.
3. Usually attends to own personal habits.
4. Verbal nursing care only.
5. Border.

VARIABLES: Six main headings:
· Self Care
· Orientation
· Communication and socialisation
· Psychotic behavior
· Cooperation and occupation
· Mood and reaction to environment

OTHER WORKS
cited by author   The instrument was used together with the tests of Bender (ref. 1) and Wechsler digits (ref. 3) in a study on the effect of a cerebral vasodilator in 40 elderly subjects with arteriosclerotic brain disease.

APPLICATION   Drug trials.
Monitoring of changes.

1 Bender (L.): A visual motor gestalt test and its clinical use. New Yok: American Orthopsychiatric Association, 1938.

2 Fine (E.W.), Lewis (D.), Villa-Landa (I.), Blakemore (C.B.): The effect of Cyclandelate on mental function in patients with arteriosclerotic brain disease. *Brit. J. Psychiat.*, 1970, 117, 157-161.

3 Wechsler (D.): Manual for the Wechsler Adult Intelligence Scale. New York: The Psychological Corporation, 1955.

GERIATRIC RATING SCALE (G.R.S.)

SPECIFICITY

* * *

TYPE OF INSTRUMENT

Ordinal rating scale
31 items, 3 grades

REFERENCE	**Plutchik (R.), Conte (H.), Lieberman (M.), Bakur (M.), Grossman (J.), Lehrman (N.)** · – Reliability and validity of a scale for assessing the functioning of geriatric patients. *Journal of the American Geriatrics Society*, 1970, 18, 6, 491-500.

Language: Original version published in English.
                  U.S.A.

Location: Enclosed in volume two page 160
                  See ref. biblio nº 9

For all information concerning the instrument write to the author at the following address:

Robert Plutchik,
Department of Psychiatry
Albert Einstein College of Medicine of Yeshiva University
1300 Morris Park Avenue
Bronx, New York 10461, U.S.A.

ORIGIN

A modified version of the "Stockton Geriatric Rating Scale" represented the first model of this instrument (ref. 2). Reflections on the general validity of the scale resulted in the definitive form. Compared with this model the scale includes 3 items which are identical, 19 where the formulation is modified and 9 new items.

PURPOSE

To evaluate the geriatric patient's level of mental, physical and social functioning with the aid of brief, objective and simply formulated items, intended to verify the efficacy of certain therapeutic programmes.

POPULATION

Geriatric inpatients.

ADMINISTRATION

Rater: Any member of the hospital medical staff.

Time required: Short time.

Training Not necessary.

Scoring: Each item is coded 0,1 or 2. A score of 0 means the symptom is absent, 2 means it is accentuated. The global score varies from 0 to 62. It is proportional to the degree of physical, mental and social disability. The patient's cooperation or presence is not necessary for scoring.

VARIABLES

Concern physical, mental and social status of the patient (eating, walking, communication, cooperativeness, activity)

VALIDATION

Was tested on a representative sample of geriatric inpatients:
Factor analysis accounts for 87.5% of the variance of items and includes 3 factors (ref. 11).
     · Apathy
     · Social behavior
     · Activities of daily living
External validity based on psychological and psychiatric clinical evaluation.
Specificity of the instrument based on comparisons between scores of geriatric patients and non geriatric patients.
Predictive validity by comparison with the phase of disease (death, discharge from hospital) (ref. 5).
Sensitivity: patients in a state of severe disability and those whose state is satisfactory (ref. 9).
Inter-rater reliability with 2 raters. Studies on stability and sensitivity, test-retest over one year period (ref. 5).

APPLICATION

Clinical: As indicators for placement of patients and selecting patient groups.
              Evaluation of medical or other treatment.
Research: Epidemiological studies.

IV.3

1   Characteristics of residents in institutions for the aged and chronically ill. U.S. Dept. of Health, Education and Welfare, Public Health Service-Publication n° 1000, Series 12, n° 2, April-June 1963.

2   Meer (B.), Baker (J.A.): The Stockton geriatric rating scale. *J. Gerontol.*, 1966, 21, 392-403.

3   Meer (B.), Krag (C.L.): Correlates of disability in a population of hospitalized geriatric patients. *J. Gerontol.*, 1964, 19, 440-446.

4   Plutchik (R.), Bakur-Weiner (M.), Conte (H.): Studies of body image. I: Body worries and body discomforts. *Journal of Gerontology*, 1971, vol. 26, n° 3, 344-350.

5   Plutchik (R.), Conte (H.): Change in social and physical functioning of geriatric patients over a one-year period. *The Gerontologist*, Summer 1972, part I, vol. 12, n° 2, 181-184.

6   Plutchik (R.), Conte (H.), Bakur-Weiner (M.): Studies of body image. II: Dollar values of body parts. *Journal of Gerontology*, 1973, vol. 28, n° 1, 89-91.

7   Plutchik (R.), Conte (H.), Bakur-Weiner (M.): Studies of body image. III: Body feelings as measured by the semantic differential. *Int'l. Aging and Human Development*, 1973, vol. 4, n° 4, 375-380.

8   Plutchik (R.), Conte (H.), Bakur – Weiner (M.), Teresi (J.): Studies of body image. IV: Figure drawings in normal and abnormal geriatric and nongeriatric groups. *Journal of Gerontology*, 1978, vol. 33, n° 1, 68-75.

9   Plutchik (R.), Conte (H.), Lieberman (M.), Bakur (M.), Grossman (J.), Lehrman (N.): Reliability and validity of a scale for assessing the functioning of geriatric patients. *Journal of the American Geriatrics Society*, 1970, vol. 18, n° 6, 491-500.

10 Plutchik (R.), Mc Carthy (M.), Hall (B.M.): Changes in elderly welfare hotel residents during a one-year period. *Journal of the American Geriatrics Society*, 1975, vol. 23, n° 6, 265-270.

11 Smith (J.M.), Bright (B.), Mc Closkey (J.): Factor analytic composition of the geriatric rating scale (GRS). *Journal of Gerontology*, 1977, vol. 32, n° 1, 58-62.

P.A.M.I.E. SCALE

SPECIFICITY

$* \quad * \quad *$

TYPE OF INSTRUMENT

Check-list of
77 items

| REFERENCE | **Gurel (L.), Linn (M.W.), Linn (B.S.)** · – Physical and mental impairment-of-function evaluation in the aged: The P.A.M.I.E. Scale. *Journal of Gerontology*, 1972, 27, 1, 83-90.

Language: Original version published in English. **U.S.A.**

Location: Enclosed in volume two page 89. See ref. biblio n° 7

For all information concerning the instrument write to the author at the following address:

Lee Gurel,
3123 South 14th Street
Arlington, Virginia 22204, U.S.A. |

ORIGIN

This instrument is inspired by the **Stockton** and **Plutchik** scales; it is derived from the "Patient Evaluation scale", based on the results of the functional analysis (ref. 4, 5, 25). The "Patient Evaluation Scale" consisting of 43 items is based on the "Self Care Inventory" (ref. 2, 6, 12, 24).

PURPOSE

This instrument assesses a variety of behavioral characteristics in patients suffering from chronic diseases, especially geriatric patients; evaluation is multifunctional, reflecting comprehensive behavioral disabilities based on physical, mental and social functioning. Assessment is completed with the aid of simply formulated items and does not require the rater's interpretation (ref. 7).

The author's intentions were to improve assessment using the 7 previously used items, to acquire supplementary information and include additional items facilitating decisions for placement of elderly patients (ref. 7).

POPULATION

Geriatric inpatients and elderly people living in residential homes.

ADMINISTRATION

Rater: Nurse familiar with the patient.
Training: Not necessary.
Time required: 45 minutes.
Scoring: Most items have a yes-no answer, some (3) are graded from 3 to 6.

VARIABLES

Ten factors:
· Self care (10 items)
· Irritability (13 items)
· Confusion (12 items)
· Anxiety-depression (7 items)
· Bedridden-moribund (6 items)
· Behavioral deterioration (5 items)
· Paranoid ideas (6 items)
· Psychomotor disability (4 items)
· Withdrawal-apathy (5 items)
· Mobility (3 items)

These 10 factors are correlated and can be regrouped into 3 general aspects:
Physical disability; Psychological deterioration; Agitation.

VALIDATION

Was done on the whole population of male V.A. patients being placed in a nursing home during the course of 6 months, from 9 psychiatric hospitals and 9 general hospitals:
Factor analysis was done on the whole population, with separate analyses of patients suffering from general medical and surgical disturbances, and separate analyses of psychiatric patients. Analyses results were almost identical in all cases pointing out the 10 factors mentioned above.
External validity based on information obtained by subjective assessment done by the nursing team (type of care required, favourable or unfavourable prognosis, adequate or inadequate placement).
Concurrent validity based on the medical rating scale "C.I.R.S." (Cumulative Illness Rating Scale) by Linn (ref. 16).
Predictive validity correlated with mortality during the interval of 6 months to 1 year upon evaluation with the P.A.M.I.E. Scale (ref. 7).
Studies on **internal consistency** and intercorrelation of factors.

APPLICATION

In all cases concerning multidimensional assessment of comprehensive behavioral disabilities of the elderly and chronically ill patients who are disabled; Therapeutic programmes; Epidemiological surveys.

1 Cohen (J.), Gurel (L.), Stumpf (J.C.): Dimensions of psychiatric symptom ratings determined at thirteen timepoints from hospital admission. *Journal of Consulting Psychology*, 1966, 30, 39-44.

2 Dobson (W.R.), Patterson (T.): A Behavioral evaluation of patients living in a nursing home as compared to a hospitalized group. *Gerontologist*, 1961, 1, 135-139.

3 Gurel (L.): Dimensions of psychiatric patient ward beha-vior. *Journal of Consulting Psychology*, 1967, 31, 328-331.

4 Gurel (L.): Community resources and VA outplacement. In: Proceedings of 13th Annual Conference, VA Cooperative studies in psychiatry, Denver, April 1968. Washington, DC: Veterans Administration, 1968, 85-89.

5 Gurel (L.): Dorothea Dix revisited: extended care in the community as an alternative to hospitalization. Paper read at Gerontological Society meetings, Denver, october 1968.

6 Gurel (L.), Davis (J.E.): A survey of self-care dependency in psychiatric patients. *Hospital and Community Psychiatry*, 1967, 18, 135-138.

7 Gurel (L.), Linn (M.W.), Linn (B.S.): Physical and mental impairment-of-function evaluation in the aged: the PAMIE scale. *Journal of Gerontology*, 1972, vol. 27, n° 1, 83-90.

8 Gurel (L.), Linn (M.W.), Linn (B.S.), Davis (J.E.), Maroney (R.J.): Patients in nursing homes: multidisciplinary characteristics and outcomes. *Journal of the American Medical Association*, 1970, 213, 73-77.

9 Harman (H.H.): Modern factor analysis. Chicago: University of Chicago Press, 1960.

10 Kahn (R.L.), Goldfarb (A.I.), Pollack (M.), Gerber (I.E.): The relationship of mental and physical status in institutionalized aged persons. *American Journal of Psychiatry*, 1960, 117, 120-124.

11 Kaiser (H.F.): The varimax criterion for analytic rotation in factor analysis. *Psychometrika*, 1958, 23, 187-200.

12 Katz (S.), Downs (T.D.), Cash (M.R.), Grotz (R.C.): Progress in development of the index of ADL. *Gerontologist*, 1970, 10, 20-30.

13 Katz (S.), Ford (A.B.), Moskowitz (R.W.), Jackson (B.A.), Jaffe (M.W.): Studies of illness in the aged: the index of ADL, a standardized measure of biological and psychosocial function. *Journal of the American Medical Association*, 1963, 185, 914-919.

14 Kelman (H.R.): An experiment in the rehabilitation of nursing home patients. *Public Health Reports*, 1962, 77, 356-366.

15 Kelman (H.R.), Muller (J.N.): Rehabilitation of nursing home residents. *Geriatrics*, 1962, 17, 402-411.

16 Linn (B.S.), Linn (M.W.), Gurel (L.): Cumulative illness rating scale. *Journal of the American Geriatrics Society*, 1968, 16, 622-626.

17 Lyerly (S.B.), Abbott (P.S.): Handbook of psychiatric rating scales (1950-1964). Washington, DC: PHS Publication n° 1495, 1966.

18 Meer (B.), Baker (J.A.): The Stockton geriatric rating scale. *Journal of Gerontology*, 1966, 21, 392-403.

19 Miller (M.B.): Physical, emotional and social rehabilitation in a nursing-home population. *Journal of the American Geriatrics Society*, 1965, 13, 176-185.

20 Muller (J.N.): Rehabilitation evaluation: some social and clinical problems. *American Journal of Public Health*, 1961, 51, 403-410.

21 Nunnally (J.C.): Psychometric theory. New York: Mc Graw-Hill, 1967.

22 Plutchik (R.), Conte (H.), Lieberman (M.), Bakur (M.), Grossman (J.), Lehrman (N.): Reliability and validity of a scale for assessing the functioning of geriatric patients. *Journal of the American Geriatrics Society*, 1970, 18, 491-500.

23 Walker (R.), Dempsey (M.): Ward behavior in schizophrenic patients ready for release and in those requiring further hospitalization. *Nursing Research*, 1967, 16, 174-178.

24 Watson (C.G.), Fulton (J.R.): Treatment potential of the psychiatric-medically infirm. I: self- care independence. *Journal of Gerontology*, 1967, 22, 449-455.

25 Watson (C.G.), Fulton (J.R.): Treatment potential of the psychiatric-medically infirm. II: Psychiatric symptomatology. *Journal of Gerontology*, 1968, 23, 226-230.

FUNCTIONAL LIFE SCALE (F.L.S.)

SPECIFICITY

> *

TYPE OF INSTRUMENT

> Ordinal rating scale
> 44 items, 5 grades

REFERENCE	**Sarno (J.E.), Sarno (M.T.), Levita (E.)** · – The functional life scale. *Archives of Physical Medicine and Rehabilitation*, 1973, 54, 214-220.
	Language: Original version published in English. **U.S.A.**
	Location: Enclosed in volume two page 161 See ref. biblio nº 6

ORIGIN

The instrument is inspired by published works (ref. 1, 3, 4, 5) and works from the author (ref. 7).

PURPOSE

The instrument is designed to provide a quantitative measure of an individual ability to participate in basic daily activities; the scale attempts to describe what a patient actually does and not what he may have the capacity to do; for clinical purposes, teaching and research purposes.

POPULATION

Out-patients either before, during or after the rehabilitation process.

ADMINISTRATION

Rater: Physician, physiotherapist, psychologist, nurse, speech therapist, occupational therapist.

Time required: 45 minutes.

Training: Necessary to improve scoring.

Scoring: From 0 to 4 for qualities assessed for each item: overall efficiency, speed, frequency, self-initiative. For each of these scoring is on a 5 point scale from 0 (unable to perform this activity) to 4 (normal). There are 6 global scores, one for each of the 5 groups of variables and 1 total score.

VARIABLES

Five groups of variables are assessed:
· Cognitive functions (orientation, the appropriate use of words yes or no, arithmetical ability, verbal communication and gestural communication, reading. writing, social behavior, fluent speech, self criticism and memory).
· Activities of daily living (mobility, transferring, feeding, use of toilet, dressing, bathing).
· Home activities (preparing food, housekeeping, odd jobs around or in the house, hobbies, use of telephone, use of television set, use of record player).
· Outside activities (leisure activities, shopping, spectator events, use of transportation, trips).
· Social interaction (games, meetings, going out, work).

VALIDATION

Was done on 2 populations of subjects going through the rehabilitation process, mean age 46 and 58.5 years (ref. 6):
Concurrent validity based on a 9 point graphic rating scale made by a psychiatrist.
Reliability: · **Inter-rater** with 11 raters of various professions.
      · **Test-retest:** during a 2-3 week interval with the same rater.
      · **Internal consistency:** between scores for each group for total score and for scores of each quality assessed.

APPLICATION

Clinical: Estimating the global functional status of each disabled subject.
      Evaluating rehabilitation efficacy.
Research: For estimation of the impact of specific physical, mental and social factors on the success or failure of treatment.
      Medical training.

1 Anderson (T.P.), Bourestom (N.), Greenberg (F.R.): Rehabilitation predictors in completed stroke. Final report to the Social and Rehabilitation Service and Welfare. Washington, DC, March 1970, 247-264.

2 Cronbach (L.J.): Essentials of psychological testing. New York: Harper, 1960, 96-153.

3 Doll (E.A.): Vineland social maturity scale. Minneapolis: Educational Test Bureau, 1947.

4 Gersten (J.W.), Miller (B.), Cenkovich (F.), Dinken (H.): Comparison of home and clinic rehabilitation for chronically ill and physically disabled persons. *Arch. Phys. Med. Rehabil.*, nov 1968, 49, 615-642.

5 Lawton (E.B.): Activities of daily living for physical rehabilitation. New York: Mc Graw-Hill Book Co, 1963.

6 Sarno (J.E.), Sarno (M.T.), Levita (E.): The functional life scale. *Arch. Phys. Med. Rehabil.*, 1973, 54, 214-220.

7 Sarno (M.T.): Functional communication profile manual of directions. Rehab. Monograph 42. New York University Medical Center, 1969.

8 Selltiz (C.), Jahoda (M.), Deutsch (M.), Cook (S.W.): Research methods in social relations. New York: Holt, Rinehart and Winston, 1959, 186-198.

PARACHEK GERIATRIC BEHAVIOR RATING SCALE (P.G.B.R.S.)

SPECIFICITY

* * *

TYPE OF INSTRUMENT

Ordinal rating scale 10 items, 5 grades

REFERENCE	**Miller (E.R.), Parachek (J.F.)** · – Validation and standardization of a goal oriented, quick-screening geriatric scale. *Journal of the American Geriatrics Society* 1974, 22, 6, 278-283.
	Language: Original version published in English. **U.S.A.**
	Location: Enclosed in volume two page 163 See ref. biblio nº 2

ORIGIN

The instrument presents a shortened version of the "Geriatric Rating Scale" from **Plutchik** (ref. 4), and is considered to be one of the briefest known scales in current use.

PURPOSE

To determine efficiently individual patient capacities, also to detect behavioral changes occuring as a result of the effect of therapeutic programmes.

POPULATION

Elderly inpatients.

ADMINISTRATION

Rater: Nurse's aide.

Time required: 3 to 5 minutes.

Training: Not necessary.

Scoring: The meaning of each of the 5 grades is explained for each item, the scoring varying from 1 to 5. The global score can range from 10 (state of severe disability) to 50 (absence of anomalies). Grading is presented graphically.
The patient's presence is not necessary for scoring.

VARIABLES

· Physical status: ambulation, eyesight, hearing.
· General self-care: continence, feeding, hygiene, grooming.
· Social behavior: attitudes towards others, sociability, group activities.

VALIDATION

The authors chose a representative sample from a population of geriatric inpatients. Patients suffering from degenerative neurological diseases (Pick's disease, Alzheimer's disease, Parkinson's disease) as well as patients who were in a critical state were excluded. Validation works (ref. 2) included:
Concurrent validity with the Plutchik Geriatric Rating Scale, for pre and post-therapeutic scores.
External validity:
· by comparing initial scores obtained by applying diagnostic classification established in the "Geriatric Psychology Diagnostic Profile of Behavior" (G.P.D.P.B.).
· by comparing opinions of clinicians who classified patients into several different treatment groups depending on type of pathology.
Predictive validity of tables constructed in regard to clinicians' classification of different groups and the obtained scores and for success or failure of treatment.

APPLICATION

Clinical: For studies concerning treatment programmes, and care programming.
Research: Longitudinal statistical studies of geriatric patients.
           Epidemiological studies.

1 Helmstadter (G.C.): Principles of psychological measurement. New York: Appleton-Century-Crofts, 1964.

2 Miller (E.R.), Parachek (J.F.): Validation and standardization of a goal-oriented, quick-screening geriatric scale. *J. of the Amer. Geriat. Soc.*, 1974, 22, 6, 278-283.

3 Oberleder (M.): Adapting current psychological techniques for use in testing the aging. *Gerontologist*, 1967, 7, 188.

4 Plutchik (R.), Conte (H.), Lieberman (M.) et al: Reliability and validity of a scale for assessing the functioning of geriatric patients. *J. of the Amer. Geriatr. Soc.*, 1970, 18, 491.

5 Salzman (C.), Kochansky (G.E.), Shader (R.I.): Rating scales for geriatric pharmacology. A review. *Psychopharmacol. Bull.*, 1972, 8, 3, 3.

6 Sandler (J.): A test of the significance of the difference between the means of correlated measures based on a simplification of student's t. *Brit. J. Psychol.*, 1955, 46, 225.

7 Trier (T.R.): A study of change among elderly psychiatric inpatients during their first year of hospitalization. *J. Gerontol.*, 1968, 23, 354.

SANDOZ CLINICAL ASSESSMENT GERIATRIC (S.C.A.G.)

SPECIFICITY

```
* * *
```

TYPE OF INSTRUMENT

Ordinal rating scale
19 items, 7 grades

REFERENCE	**Shader (R.l.), Harmatz (J.S.), Salzman (C.)** · – A new scale for clinical assessment in geriatric populations: Sandoz clinical assessment – geriatric (SCAG). *Journal of the American Geriatrics Society*, 1974, 22, 3, 107-113.

Language: Original version published in English.
Translations in French (ref. 4, 5), German (ref. 15) and Swedish (ref. 1).
U.S.A.

Location: Enclosed in volume two page 164
See ref. biblio n⁰ 11

For all information concerning the instrument and the translations, write to the author at the following address:

Richard Shader,
New England Medical Center
171 Harrison Avenue, Box 1007
Boston, Massachusets 02111, U.S.A.

ORIGIN   This original instrument was developed at Sandoz Laboratories.

PURPOSE   For clinical assessment related to psychopharmacological research. Enables rapid evaluation of psychopathological states in elderly patients, especially where it is necessary to discriminate early senile deterioration and depressive disorders.

POPULATION   Elderly persons, especially out-patients.

ADMINISTRATION   *Rater:* Physician, psychologist, nurse, social worker.

Time required: 20 minutes

Training: Scoring on 5 patients together with rater-experimenter.

Scoring: Each item is coded from 1 to 7. Seven indicates severe symptom, 1 that it is absent.

VARIABLES   The first 18 items are related to symptoms, the 19th represents the rater's overall impression of the patient:

- Confusion
- Mental alertness
- Impairment of recent memory
- Disorientation
- Mood depression
- Emotional lability
- Self-care
- Anxiety
- Motivation & initiative
- Irritability
- Hostility
- Bothersome
- Indifference to surroundings
- Sociability
- Uncooperativeness
- Fatigue
- Appetite
- Dizziness
- Overall impression of patient

VALIDATION   A study was done with 2 groups of patients. The first was with voluntary elderly persons, who were divided into those in good health and those with mild senile deterioration, compatible with leading an independant life in the community. The second group consisted of inpatients divided into those with depressive disorders and those with senile dementia. Validation included (ref. 11):
Concurrent validity based on "Mental Status Examination Record" (M.S.E.R.).
External validity based on clinical classification, by "comparing pairs" (volunteer-inpatient, volunteer in good health, deteriorated volunteer, inpatient with depressive disorders, inpatient with dementia).
Inter-rater reliability based on the scoring of 4 psychiatrists done on the same patients.

OTHER WORKS
cited by author
- Drug trials with hydergine (ref. 6).
- Retrospective study on drug trials after a decade of research and on the factor structure of S.C.A.G.: Interpersonal relations – Cognitive disorders – Affectivity – Apathy – Physical status – Self-care (ref. 13).

APPLICATION   · Psychopharmacological research; Drug trials.

1 Berg (S.), Landahl (S.), Steen (B.), Steen (G.): SCAG-S. Rating scale of activity for geriatric and psychogeriatric patients. Jönköping: Institute of Gerontology, 1980.

2 Dunn (O.J.): Multiple comparisons among means. *J. Am. Stat. Assoc.*, 1961, 56, 52.

3 Ebel (R.L.): Estimation of the reliability of ratings. *Psychometrika*, 1951, 16, 407.

4 Georges (D.), Lallemand (A.), Coustenoble (J.), Loria (Y.): Validation par l'analyse factorielle d'une échelle d'évaluation clinique des troubles de la sénescence cérébrale: application à l'essai thérapeutique. *Thérapie*, 1977, 32, 173-180.

5 Henry (J.F.), Loria (Y.), Lallemand (A.), Georges (D.), Berthaux (P.): Etude de la fiabilité inter-juges d'une échelle d'évaluation clinique des troubles de la sénescence cérébrale. *La Revue de Gériatrie*, février 1978, tome 3, n° 1, 20-22.

6 Loew (D.M.), Weil (C.): Hydergine in senile mental impairment. *Gerontology*, 1982, 28, 54-74.

7 Maurer (W.), Ferner (U.), Patin (J.), Hamot (H.B.): Sandoz clinical assessment geriatric scale (SCAG): eine transkulturelle faktorenanalytische Studie: *Zeitschrift für Gerontologie*, 1982, 15, 26-30.

8 Mental Health Facilities Report: Patients in state and county mental hospitals 1967, NIMH-Mental Health Statistics Series A n° 2, PHS Publication n° 1921. Washington, DC: U.S. Government Printing Office, 1969, 1-89.

9 Salzman (C.), Kochansky (G.E.), Shader (R.I.): Rating scales for geriatric psychopharmacology. *Psychopharmacology Bulletin*, 1972, 8, 3.

10 Shader (R.I.), Ebert (M.H.), Harmatz (J.S.): Langner's psychiatric impairment scale: a short screening device. *Am. J. Psychiat.*, 1971, 128, 596.

11 Shader (R.I.), Harmatz (J.S.), Salzman (C.): A new scale for clinical assessment in geriatric populations: Sandoz clinical assessment geriatric (SCAG). *Journal of the American Geriatrics Society*, 1974, vol. 22, n° 3, 107-113.

12 Shader (R.I.), Harmatz (J.S.), Tammerk (H.A.): Towards an observational structure for rating dysfunction and pathology in ambulatory geriatrics. *Interdiscipl. Topics Gerontol.*, 1979, vol. 15, 153-168.

13 Singer (J.), Hamot (H.): Problems and opportunities in geriatric clinical trial methodology after a decade of research. In: «Drugs and methods in C.V.D.»: Procceedings of the International Symposium on experimental and clinical methodologies for study of acute and chronic cerebrovascular diseases, Paris, 24-26 march 1980. New York, Oxford, Toronto: Pergamon Press, 1981, 337-343.

14 Spitzer (R.L.), Endicott (J.): An Integrated group of forms for automated psychiatric case records. *Arch. Gen. Psychiat.*, 1971, 24, 540-547.

15 Warschawski (P.): Die geriatrische Test-Batterie (G.T.B.). Diss. Universität Zürich, 1978.

PSYCHOGERIATRIC ASSESSMENT PROGRAM

SPECIFICITY

| * * * |

TYPE OF INSTRUMENT

Compound Instrument:
Rating Scales
Clinical examination EEG
Laboratory findings

REFERENCE   **Dastoor (D.P.), Norton (S.), Boillat (J.), Minty (J.), Papadopoulou (F.), Muller (H.F.)** · – A psychogeriatric assessment program. I, II, III, IV., V. *Journal of the American Geriatrics Society*, 1975, vol 23, nº 10, 11; 1976, vol 24, nº 1, 2; 1979, vol. 27, nº 4.

Language: Original version published in English.
Canada

Location: Enclosed in volume two page 196
See ref. biblio nº 3, 4, 11, 12, 16

For all information concerning the instrument write to the author at the following address:

Dolly Dastoor,
Geriatric and Medical Services
Douglas Hospital Centre
6875 Boul. La Salle
Verdun, Québec H4H 1R3, Canada

ORIGIN   Scales from different sources were used for evaluating the patients: "Minimal Social Behavior Scale", modified by **Farina** (ref. 8), "Integrative Social Functioning Scale" (ref. 5), "Plutchik Nurses Observation Scale for Geriatric Patients" (ref. 22), "Hamilton Depression Scale" (ref. 10), "Brief Psychiatric Rating Scale" (ref 20).

PURPOSE   A multidisciplinary approach for determining the differential diagnosis of elderly geriatric patients in a hospital population.

POPULATION   Geriatric patients with psychiatric problems, hospitalized and ambulatory.

ADMINISTRATION   *Rater:* A multidisciplinary team comprising psychiatrist, physician, psychologist, social worker and nurse.

Time required: A 2-day out-patient evaluation followed by a team meeting and discussion with the family.

Training: Professional training of the various team members.

VARIABLES
· General physical health and laboratory test results including neurological assessment
· Psychological and psychiatric status including electro-encephalographic findings
· Social functioning and relationships

VALIDATION   **Factor analysis** (ref. 12, 16).
Predictive validity of the scales for diagnosis, treatment planning and theory in 80 newly admitted psychogeriatric patients (ref. 1, 6, 7, 17, 19) – reevaluation of 35 of the 40 survivors, three years later, using the same scales.

Correlation between results of examination done by psychiatrist, general practioner, psychologist, social worker and nurse together with the results of the 5 above mentioned scales.

APPLICATION
· Diagnostic, prognostic.
· Prevention of hospitalization.
· Development of appropriate treatment and placement plans for the patient.
· Training of personnel.
· Consultation to community agencies for the management of psychogeriatric problems.
· Interaction with social and community agencies and personnel.

1 Bartko (J.J.), Patterson (R.D.): Survival among healthy old men: a multi-variate analysis. In: Granick (S.), Patterson (R.D.) Eds: "Human Aging. II: An Eleven-year follow-up biomedical and behavioral study". NIMH, DHEW Publ. n° (HSM) 71-9037. Washington, DC: U.S. Govt. Printing Office, 1971.

2 Dastoor (D.P.): Psychogeriatric assessment program. Presented at the 9th annual meeting of the Canadian Association on Gerontology, Saskatchewan, October 16-19, 1980.

3 Dastoor (D.P.), Klingner (A.), Müller (H.F.), Kachanoff (R.): A Psychogeriatric assessment program. V: Three-year follow-up. *Journal of the American Geriatrics Society*, 1979, vol. 27, n° 4, 162-169.

4 Dastoor (D.P.), Norton (S.). Boillat (J.) et al.: A Psychogeriatric assessment program. I: Social functioning and ward behavior. *Journal of the American Geriatrics Society*, 1975, vol. 23, n° 10, 465-571.

5 Doll (E.A.): Vineland social maturity scale:manual of directions. (rev.ed.). Minneapolis: Educational Test Bureau (now American Guidance Service), 1965.

6 Epstein (L.J.), Robinson (B.C.), Simon (A.): Predictors of survival in geriatric mental illness during eleven years after initial hospital admission. *Journal of the American Geriatrics Society*, 1971, 19, 913.

7 Epstein (L.J.), Simon (A.): Prediction of outcome of geriatric mental illness. *Interdiscipl. Topics Gerontol.*, 1969, 3, 51.

8 Farina (A.), Arenberg (D.), Guskin (S.): A Scale for measuring minimal social behavior. *J. Consulting Psychol.*, 1957, 21, 265.

9 Granick (S.): Psychological test functioning. In: Granick (S.), Patterson (R.D.) Eds: «Human Aging. II: An Eleven-year follow-up biomedical and behavioral study». NIMH, DHEM Publ. n° (HSM) 71-9037. Washington, DC: U.S. Govt. Printing Office, 1971.

10 Hamilton (M.): A Rating scale for depression. *J. Neurol. Neurosurg. Psychiat.*, 1960, 23, 56.

11 Hontela (S.), Müller (H.F.), Grad (B.) et al.: A Psychogeriatric assessment program. II: Clinical and laboratory findings. *Journal of the American Geriatrics Society*, 1975, vol. 23, n° 11, 519-524.

12 Klingner (A.), Kachanoff (R.), Dastoor (D.P.) et al.: A Psychogeriatric assessment program. III: Clinical and experimental psychologic aspects. *Journal of the American Geriatrics Society*, 1976, vol. 24, n° 1, 17-24.

13 Lehmann (H.E.), Ban (T.A.): Psychometric tests in the evaluation of brain pathology, response to drugs. *Geriatrics*, 1970, 25-142.

14 Libow (L.S.): Pseudo-senility: acute and reversible organic brain syndromes. *Journal of the American Geriatrics Society*, 1973, 21, 112.

15 Müller (H.F.): The electroencephalogram in senile dementia. In: Nandy (K.) Ed.: "Senile dementia: a biomedical approach." New York, Amsterdam: Elsevier, 1978.

16 Müller (H.F.), Dastoor (D.P.), Hontela (S.) et al.: A psychogeriatric assessment program. IV: Interdisciplinary aspects. *Journal of the American Geriatrics Society*, 1976, vol. 24, n° 2, 54-57.

17 Müller (H.F.), Grad (B.), Engelsmann (F.): Biological and psychological predictors of survival in a psychogeriatric population. *Journal of Gerontology*, 1975, vol. 30, n° 1, 47-52.

18 Müller (H.F.), Schwartz (G.): Electroencephalograms and autopsy findings in gerontopsychiatry. *Journal of Gerontology*, 1978, vol. 33, n° 4, 504-513.

19 Neiditch (J.), White (L.): Prediction of short-term outcome in newly admitted psychogeriatric patients. *Journal of the American Geriatrics Society*, 1976, vol. 24, 72.

20 Overall (J.E.), Gorham (D.R.): The brief psychiatric rating scale. *Psychol. Rep.*, 1962, vol. 10, 799.

21 Patterson (R.D.), Freeman (L.C.), Butler (R.N.): Psychiatric aspects of adaptation, survival, and death. In: Granick (S.), Patterson (R.D.) Eds.: "Human aging. II: An eleven-year follow-up biomedical and behavioral study". NIMH, DHEM Publ. n° (HSM) 71.9037. Washington, DC: U.S. Govt. Printing Office, 1971.

22 Plutchik (R.), Conte (H.), Lieberman (M.) et al.: Reliability and validity of a scale for assessing the functioning of geriatric patients. *Journal of the American Geriatrics Society*, 1970, vol. 18, 491.

GERIATRIC FUNCTIONAL RATING SCALE

SPECIFICITY

* * *

TYPE OF INSTRUMENT

Nominal rating scale
30 items

REFERENCE **Grauer (H.), Birnbom (F.)** · – A geriatric functional rating scale to determine the need for institutional care. *Journal of the American Geriatrics Society*, 1975, 23, 10, 472-476.

Language: Original version published in English.
Canada

Location: Enclosed in volume two page 166
See ref. biblio n° 3

For all information concerning the instrument write to the author at the following address:

H. Grauer,
Institute of Community and Family Psychiatry
The Sir Mortimer B. Davis - Jewish General Hospital
4333 Chemin de la Côte Ste-Catherine
Montréal, Québec H3T 1E2, Canada

ORIGIN Original instrument. In its conception, the author was influenced by the work of **Katz et al** (ref. 4), **Lowenthal** (ref. 6), **Lawton** (ref. 5), who have studied activities of daily living, but also by his experience in evaluating patients with the help of a multidisciplinary team.

PURPOSE To evaluate the aged, in terms of their needs for institutionalization or their need for community resources in terms of domiciliary care, group or foster homes, day hospitals, etc.

POPULATION Urban aged.

ADMINISTRATION *Rater:* Social worker, nurse, members of a home care team, family practitioner.

Training: Not required. A guide for the utilization of the scale is available.

Time required: 15 to 20 minutes.

Scoring: The scale is composed of two parts; the first part measures physical and mental capabilities, the second part activities of daily living, social and community supports. The scores in the first section are given minus values. There are three degrees of severity assigned to each item. In the absence of debility the score remains 0. As debility increases, scores increase from minus 3 to minus 20. The items in the second part are given plus values. They range from plus 1 to plus 10. After the total score is determined, the patients can be grouped into 3 categories. Those under 20 are unable to function in the community and require institutionalization. Those between 20-40 can manage in the community with the support of domiciliary care, day hospital or home care help. A score over 40 indicates that no outside help is required and the person can usually function independently.

VARIABLES
· Physical state
· Mental state
· Functional ability
· Social support

· Living quarters
· Community resources
· Relatives and friends
· Financial situation

VALIDATION The predictive aspect of the rating scale was validated in an 18 month follow-up study. Predictions held for those who died, were institutionalized or continued independently in the community (ref. 3).

APPLICATION Mainly clinical: to help determine the need for institutionalization, to determine the appropriate type of institutional setting and where appropriate, the type of community resources required.

IV.9

1 Blenkner (M.): Proceedings V: I. Abstracts of Symposium and lectures, p. 417. (Fed. Am. Soc. Exper. Biol. Bethesda, MD): 8th International Congress of Gerontology. Washington, D.C., 1969.

2 Goldfarb (A.I.): Predicting mortality in the institutionalized aged. *Arch. Gen. Psychiat*, 1969, 21, 172.

3 Grauer (H.), Birnbom (F.): A geriatric functional rating scale to determine the need for institutional care. *J. of the American Geriatrics Society*, 1975, 23, 10, 472-476.

4 Katz (S.), Downs (T.D.), Cash (H.R.), et al.: Progress in development of the index of A.D.L. *Gerontologist*, 1970, part 1, 20-30.

5 Lawton (M.P.), Brody (E.): Assessment of older people: self-maintaining instrumental activities of daily living. *Gerontologist*, 1969, 9, 179.

6 Lowenthal (M.F.): Lives in distress. New York: Basic Books, 1964.

7 Maddox (G.): Self-assessment of health status. *J. Chron. Dis.*, 1964, 17, 449.

8 Wyler (A.R.), Masuda (M.), Holmes (T.H.): Seriousness of illness rating scale. *J. Psychosom. Res.*, 1968, 11, 363.

ECHELLE D'APPRECIATION CLINIQUE EN GERIATRIE (E.A.C.G.)
SCALE FOR CLINICAL ASSESSMENT IN GERIATRIC POPULATIONS

SPECIFICITY

* * *

TYPE OF INSTRUMENT

Ordinal rating scale
17 items, 7 grades

REFERENCE   **Georges (D.), Lallemand (A.), Coustenoble (J.), Loria (Y.)** · – Validation par l'analyse facto-rielle d'une échelle d'évaluation clinique des troubles de la sénescence cérébrale. Application à l'essai thérapeutique. *Thérapie*, 1977, 32, 173-180.

Language: Original version published in French.
France

Location: Enclosed in volume two page 168
See ref. biblio nº 3

For all information concerning the instrument (copyright) write to the following address:

Laboratoire Sandoz,
Service Expérimentations Cliniques
14, Boulevard Richelieu
92506 Rueil Malmaison, France

ORIGIN   The instrument is derived from the "S.C.A.G.", Sandoz Clinical Assessment Geriatric (ref. 8), modified in the following way: two items from S.C.A.G. are joined into one (item 3 in E.A.C.G., Orientation-Confusion), 4 are excluded (irritability, hostility, indifference, bothersome), 4 are new and present physical symptoms (mobility, headache, sleeping troubles, tinnitus).

PURPOSE   To measure the effects of therapy in regard to cerebral impairments. Includes homogeneous groups of patients undergoing drug trials.

POPULATION   Elderly persons above 65 years, both out-patients and inpatients suffering from psychosocial disorders due to cerebral insufficiency.

ADMINISTRATION   *Rater:* Physician.

Time required: 20 minutes.

Training: Necessary. Consists of getting acquainted with this method of quantified assessment.

Scoring: Each of the items is coded up to 7 points, with increasing severity: "normal" (1), "severely impaired" (7). Scoring should vary from 3-5 if a patient is to be included in the trial.
It can diverge from this on a maximum of six items

VARIABLES   The following 17 items assessed are:
· Mental alertness
· Impairment of recent memory
· Orientation-confusion
· Anxiety
· Depression
· Emotional Stability
· Motivation-initiative
· Cooperation
· Sociability

· Self care
· Mobility
· Appetite
· Dizziness
· Fatigue
· Headache
· Sleep
· Tinnitus

VALIDATION   **Factor analysis** was done on an elderly population, selected according to inclusion criteria at the be-ginning, (ref. 3), and revealed 4 factors responsible for 56.3% of the total variance.
· Mental deterioration (23% of the variance)
· Affective disorders (13.5% of the variance)
· Decrease in dynamism (10.5% of the variance)
Concurrent validity. Correlation measured with psychometric tests (ref. 5).
Inter-rater reliability done with 9 physicians – raters exploring the 13 items of the scale occurring most often and having the highest score values in an elderly population (ref. 4).

APPLICATION   Drug trials.

BIBLIOGRAPHY

1 Bargheon (J.): Etude en double insu de l'Hydergine chez le sujet âgé. *Nouvelle Presse Médicale*, 1973, 2, 2053-2055.

2 Boismare (F.), Paux (G.), Delaunay (P.): Etude en double aveugle de l'Hydergine chez le sujet âgé. *Nouvelle Presse Médicale*, 1975, 4, 2529.

3 Georges (D.), Lallemand (A.), Coustenoble (J.), Loria (Y.): Validation par l'analyse factorielle d'une échelle d'évaluation clinique des troubles de la sénescence cérébrale: application à l'essai thérapeutique. *Thérapie*, 1977, 32, 173-180.

4 Henry (J.F.), Loria (Y.), Lallemand (A.), Georges (D.), Berthaux (P.): Etude de la fiabilité inter-juges d'une échelle d'évaluation clinique des troubles de la sénescence cérébrale. *La Revue de Gériatrie*, février 1978, tome 3, n° 1, 20-22.

5 Israël (L.), Georges (D.), Lallemand (A.), Loria (Y.): Echelle d'appréciation clinique et tests psychométriques en gériatrie: recherche de corrélation. *Thérapie*, 1979, 34, 585-590.

6 Marchal (G.): Etude de l'Hydergine en gériatrie. *Thér. Prat.*, 1974, 3, 61-64.

7 Maurer (M.), Bour (J.): Etude de l'Hydergine en gériatrie. *J. Méd. Nord. Est.*, 1976, 6, 26-27.

8 Shader (R.I.), Harmatz (J.S.), Salzman (C.): A new scale for clinical assessment in geriatric populations: Sandoz clinical assessment – geriatric (SCAG). *Journal of the American Geriatrics Society*, 1974, 22, 107-113.

COMPREHENSIVE ASSESSMENT AND REFERRAL EVALUATION (C.A.R.E.)

SPECIFICITY

* * *

TYPE OF INSTRUMENT

Questionnaire of
600 items

REFERENCE	**Gurland (B.J.), Kuriansky (J.), Sharpe (L.), Simon (R.), Stiller, (P.), Birkett (P.)** · – The comprehensive assessment and referral evaluation (CARE): rationale, development, and reliability. *International Journal of Aging and Human Development,* 1977-1978, 8, 1, 9-41.

Language: Original version published in English and translated into Spanish.
U.S.A.

Location: See ref. biblio nº 15

For all information concerning the instrument write to the author at the following address:

Barry Gurland,
Columbia University
Center for Geriatrics and Gerontology
100 Haven Avenue
Tower 3-29 F
New York, New York 10032, U.S.A.

ORIGIN

This questionnaire was developed on the basis of previous works of the author, the Mental Schedule by **Spitzer** (ref. 16), the Present State Examination by **Wing** (ref. 18) and statistical analysis of results of the preliminary version obtained on a sample of elderly persons. The instrument resulted from comparative study of health and social problems carried out on populations of elderly persons in New York and London.

PURPOSE

This instrument was conceived to enable joint medical, mental and social assessment of problems of elderly persons from the multidimensional, clinical and research point of view, providing the most essential information for medical personnel.

POPULATION

Elderly community residents. Other versions of the instrument are applicable to institutionalised populations.

ADMINISTRATION

Rater: Nurses aide.

Time required: 45 minutes to an hour and a half, depending on the version used.

Training: Training is necessary.

Scoring: Depends on the items and depends on the version.
Based on semi-standardised interview.

VARIABLES

Three groups of variables are assessed:
· Medical: Cardio-vascular disorders, cerebrovascular disorders, cancer, diabetes, activity limitation.
· Mental: Depression, dementia.
· Social: Criminal problems, social isolation, neighbourhood problems.

VALIDATION

The C.A.R.E. was originally developed and normed on samples of 396 community resident elderly in Great Britain (London) and 445 in the United States (New York). They were both probability samples (ref. 15):
Face validity
Predictive validity concerning morbidity, mortality after 1 year.
Inter-rater reliability, internal consistency.

APPLICATION

Clinical
    Diagnosis
    Outcome studies
    Programming treatment

Research
    Epidemiological studies
    Drug trials
    Care planning

1 Bennett (R.), Cook (D.): Isolation of the aged in the New York City. In: "Planning for the elderly in New York City": Community Council of Greater New York, April 1980, 26-42.

2 Dean (L.), Teresi (J.), Wilder (D.): The human element in survey research. *International Journal of Aging and Human Development*, 1977, 8, 83-92.

3 Golden (R.R.), Teresi (J.A.), Gurland (B.J.): Detection of dementia and depression cases with the Comprehensive Assessment and Referral Evaluation Interview Schedule. *Int. J. Aging Hum. Dev.*, 1982, 16, 4, 241-254.

4 Gurland (B.J.): A broad clinical assessment of psychopathology in the aged. In: Eisdorfer (C.), Lawton (M.P.) Eds.: "The psychology of adult development and aging". Washington: American Psychological Association, 1973, 343-377.

5 Gurland (B.J.): The assessment of the mental health status of older adults. In: Birren (J.E.), Sloane (R.) Eds.: "Handbook of mental health and aging". Englewood Cliffs, N.J.: Prentice Hall, Inc., 1980, 671-700.

6 Gurland (B.J.): The borderlands of dementia: the influence of socio-cultural characteristics on rates of dementia occurring in the senium. In: Miller (N.E.), Cohen (G.) Eds.: "Clinical aspects of Alzheimer's disease". New York: Raven Press, 1981, 61-84.

7 Gurland (B.J.), Copeland (J.R.M.), Sharpe (L.), Kelleher (M.J.), Kuriansky (J.B.), Simon (R.): Assessment of the older person in the community. *International Journal of Aging and Human Development*, 1977, 8, 1-8.

8 Gurland (B.J.), Cross (P.): Epidemiology of psychopathology in old age. Some implications for clinical services. *Psychiatr. Clin. North Am.*, 1982, 5, 1, 11-26.

9 Gurland (B.J.), Cross (P.), Defiguerido (J.), Shannon (M.), Mann (A.H.), Jenkins (R.), Bennett (R.), Wilder (D.H.), Killeffer (E.), Godlove (C.): A cross-national comparison of the institutionalized elderly in the cities of New York and London. *Psychological Medicine*, 1979, 9, 781-788.

10 Gurland (B.J.), Dean (L.), Copeland (J.R.M.), Gurland (R.), Golden (R.): Criteria for the diagnosis of dementia in the community elderly. *Gerontologist*, 1982, 22, 2, 180-186.

11 Gurland (B.J.), Dean (L.), Cross (P.), Golden (R.): The epidemiology of depression and dementia in the elderly: the use of multiple indicators of these conditions. In: Cole (J.O.), Barrett (J.E.) Eds.: "Psychopathology in the aged". New York: Raven Press, 1980, 37-60.

12 Gurland (B.J.), Dean (L.), Gurland (R.), Cook (D.): Personal time dependency in the elderly of New York City. In: "Dependency in the elderly of New York City": Community Council of Greater New York, October 1978.

13 Gurland (B.J.), Golden (R.R.), Challop (J.): Unidimensional and multidimensional approaches to the differentiation of depression and dementia in the elderly. In: Corkin (S.), Davis (K.L.), Growden (J.H.), Usdin (E.), Wurtman (R.J.), Eds.: "Alzheimer's disease: a report of progress in research". New York: Raven Press, 1981.

14 Gurland (B.J.), Golden (R.), Dean (L.): Depression and dementia in the elderly of New York City. In: "Planning for the elderly in New York City": Community Council of Greater New York, April 1980, 9-24.

15 Gurland (B.J.), Kuriansky (J.B.), Sharpe (L.), Simon (R.), Stiller (P.), Berkett (P.): The Comprehensive Assessment and Referral Evaluation (CARE): rationale, development and reliability. *International Journal of Aging and Human Development*, 1977-1978, 8, 1, 9-42.

16 Spitzer (R.L.), Fleiss (J.L.), Burdock (E.L.), Hardesty (A.S.): The Mental Status Schedule: Rationale, reliability and validity. *Comprehensive Psychiatry*, 1964, 5, n° 6, 384-395.

17 Wilder (D.E.): The assessment of chronicity: results of a longitudinal study. In: "Planning for the elderly in New York City": Community Council of Greater New York, April 1980, 43-50.

18 Wing (J.K.), Cooper (J.E.), Sartorius (N.): Measurement and classification of psychiatric symptoms: an instruction manual for the PSE and CATEGO Program. London: Cambridge University Press, 1974.

P.M.S. | IV.12

MULTIDIMENSIONAL FUNCTIONAL ASSESSMENT QUESTIONNAIRE (OARS)

SPECIFICITY

$* \quad * \quad *$

TYPE OF INSTRUMENT

Questionnaire,
101 Questions

REFERENCE	**Center for the Study of Aging and Human Development. Duke University** · − Multidimensional functional assessment: the OARS methodology. 2nd edition. Duke University: Center for the Study of Aging and Human Development, 1978.

Language: Original in English. Spanish language version available.
U.S.A.

Location: Summary enclosed in volume two page 67
See ref. biblio nº 1

For all information concerning the instrument write to:

Center for Study of Aging and Human Development
Duke University, Box 3003
Durham, North Carolina 27710, U.S.A.

ORIGIN

The Older Americans Resources and Services (OARS) instrument was developed in response to a need to investigate alternatives to institutionalization among older persons. It is developed from two earlier versions, the OARS Clinical Instrument and the OARS Community Survey Questionnaire, from which the most discriminatory items were selected.

PURPOSE

This questionnaire aims primarily to measure, in a detailed but simple and concise manner, functional status in five minimally correlated domains: social, economic, mental health, physical health, and self-care capacity (ADL). Further, it assesses the impact of alternative services. This evaluation can be used at both an individual and populational level.

POPULATION

Aged persons in general.

ADMINISTRATION

Rater: Intended for use by physicians, psychiatrists, social workers, researchers, policy makers.

Time required: 45 minutes, of which 30 minutes is for the first section (A).

Training: Training sessions offered monthly. There is a training manual (ref. 1).

Scoring: Each item can be scored individually. Scores in each dimension can be summarized on a 6 point rating scale ranging from 1 (level of functioning excellent) to 6 (level of functioning totally impaired). These 5 dimension ratings can be used to develop a functional status profile (ref. 1).

VARIABLES

Physical health: illnesses and chronic disorders, medication, self-assessed health, medical treatment.
Mental health: organicity, psychiatric impairment, self-assessed mental health.
Activities of daily living.
Social: amount and adequacy of contact with family and friends, extent of help available.
Economic: specific income by source, self-assessed income adequacy.

VALIDATION

The following validity studies have been carried out (ref. 1, 6).
Content validity.
Discriminant validity (to ensure minimal overlap among the five dimensions).
Criterion validity (comparison with ratings made after personal examination by geropsychiatrists, physicians'assistants, physical therapists).
Sensitivity (ability to discriminate among groups of persons known to differ in functional status).
Reliability: Inter-rater agreement among raters of different disciplines, rater self-agreement over time, response reliability (response with self over time).

OTHER WORKS
cited by author

Many studies have been done using the questionnaire (ref. 2, 3, 4, 5, 12).

APPLICATION

Epidemiological surveys, individual clinical evaluations, assessment of needs, assessment of services required, assessment of service impact, public policy issues

1 Center for the Study of Aging and Human Development. Duke University: Multidimensional functional assessment: the OARS methodology. 2nd edition. Duke University: Center for the Study of Aging and Human Development, 1978.

2 Comptroller General of the U.S.: The well-being of older people in Cleveland, Ohio. Washington: General Accounting Office (HRD 77-70), April 1977.

3 Comptroller General of the U.S.: Home-health: the need for a national policy to better provide for the elderly. Washington: General Accounting Office (HRD 78-19), December 1977.

4 Comptroller General of the U.S.: Conditions of older people: national information system needed. Washington: General Accounting Office (HRD 79-95), September 1979.

5 Fillenbaum (G.G.), Maddox (G.L.): Assessing the functional status of LRHS participants: Technique, findings, implications. Technical report 2. Data Archives for Aging and Adulthood. Duke University, Durham, NC: Center for the Study of Aging and Human Development, 1979.

6 Fillenbaum (G.G.), Smyer (M.A.): The Development, validity, and reliability of the OARS multidimensional functional assessment questionnaire. *Journal of Gerontology*, 1981, vol. 36, n° 4, 428-434.

7 Fiske (D.W.): Measuring the concepts of personality. Chicago: Adline Publ.Co., 1971.

8 Gurland (B.), Kuriansky (J.), Sharpe (L.), Simon (R.), Stiller (P.), Birkett (P.): The Comprehensive assessment and referral evaluation (CARE): Rationale, development and reliability. *International Journal of Aging and Human Development*, 1977, 8, 9-42.

9 Gurland (B.), Yorkston (N.J.), Goldberg (K.), Fleiss (J.L.), Sloane (R.B.), Cristol (A.H.): The Structured and Sealed Interview to Assess Maladjustment (SSIAM): Factor analysis, reliability and validity. *Archives of General Psychiatry*, 1972, 27, 264-267.

10 Haberman (P.W.): Appendix. The Reliability and validity of the data. In: Kosa (J.), Antonovsky (A.), Zola (I.K.) Eds.: "Poverty and health". Cambridge, MA: Harvard Univ. Press, 1969.

11 Sherwood (S.): Ed.: Long-term care: a handbook for researchers, planners and providers. New York: Spectrum Publ. Inc. 1975.

12 Smyer (M.A.): The Differential usage of services by impaired elderly. *Journal of Gerontology*, 1980, 35, 249-255.

13 Srole (L.), Langner (T.S.), Michael (S.T.), Opler (M.K.), Rennie (T.A.C.): Mental health in the metropolis: the midtown Manhattan Study. Vol. 1. New York: McGraw-Hill, 1962.

GERIATRIC RESIDENT GOALS SCALE (G.R.G.S.)

SPECIFICITY

* * *

TYPE OF INSTRUMENT

Check-list of
86 items in 6 groups

REFERENCE	**Cornbleth (T.)** · – Evaluation of goal attainment in geriatric settings. *Journal of the American Geriatrics Society*, 1978, 26, 9, 404-407.
	Language: Original version published in English. **U.S.A.**
	Location: Enclosed in volume two page 90 See ref. biblio n° 2
	For all information concerning the instrument write to the author at the following address:
	Terry Cornbleth, 426, Morewood Avenue Pittsburgh, Pennsylvania 15213, U.S.A.

ORIGIN

The instrument was developed in 2 stages.
During the first stage members of the nursing team identified the objectives of therapy being applied to elderly persons, especially those relating to the **Stockton** Geriatric Rating Scale (ref. 5), and the **Plutchik** Rating Scale (ref. 6).
On the basis of their conclusions, certain items were modified, and others developed so that each would correspond to the behavior observed and could be measured without ambiguity.

PURPOSE

To establish a precise and attainable list of objectives, permitting individual and group assessment, applicable to different programmes of care. To determine the impact of programmes designed to enhance the functional independence of the geriatric residents.

POPULATION

Elderly persons living in residential homes.

ADMINISTRATION

Rater: Nurse responsible for patient.

Time required: 1 hour.

Training: Not necessary.

Scoring: The 86 questions are scored as answers of the yes-no type. An affirmative answer always indicates independence in relation to the item considered.

VARIABLES

- · Eating activities
- · Dressing activities
- · Grooming activities
- · Communication
- · Locomotor activities
- · Other activities

VALIDATION

Was completed on the whole male population of residents of the "Veteran's Administration Nursing Home Care Unit".
Concurrent validity based on classification of degree of dependence in 4 levels.
Discriminative sensitivity based on scoring obtained with a questionnaire consisting of 30 items relating to cognitive functioning (ref. 2).
Studies on reliability: **Internal consistency, test-retest** and **inter-rater reliability**.

APPLICATION

Clinical: On the individual level in defining therapeutic goals depending on the resident's status, and evaluating programmes effectiveness.
On group level to elaborate programmes of care (treatment-planning), for resource allocation.
For staff training, to make staff more aware of the functional status of the patients, to facilitate communication between team members concerning the patient.
Research: To serve as a model for the design of similar instruments.

IV.13

1 Cornbleth (T.): A Psychosocial problem catalogue. JSAS Catalog of selected documents in Psychology, 1975, 5, 194. (MS. n° 863).

2 Cornbleth (T.): Evaluation of goal attainment in geriatric settings *Journal of the American Geriatrics Society*, 1978, vol. 26, n° 9, 404-407.

3 Cornbleth (T.), Cornbleth (C.): Reality orientation for the elderly. JSAS Catalog of selected documents in Psychology, 1977, 7, 80. (MS. n° 1539).

4 Goga (J.A.), Hambacher (W.O.): Psychologic and behavioral assessment of geriatric patients: a review. *Journal of the American Geriatrics Society*, 1977, 23, 232.

5 Meer (B.), Baker (J.A.): The Stockton geriatric rating scale. *Journal of Gerontology*, 1966, 21, 392.

6 Plutchik (R.), Conte (H.), Lieberman (M.), et al: Reliability and validity of a scale for assessing the functioning of geriatric patients. *Journal of the American Geriatrics Society*, 1970, 18, 491.

LONDON PSYCHOGERIATRIC RATING SCALE (L.P.R.S.)

SPECIFICITY

* * *

TYPE OF INSTRUMENT

Ordinal rating scale
36 items, 3 grades

REFERENCE   **Hersch (E.L.), Kral (V.A.), Palmer (R.B.)** · – Clinical value of the London Psychogeriatric Rating Scale. *Journal of the American Geriatrics Society*, 1978, 26, 8, 348-354.

Language: Original version published in English.
Canada.

Location: Enclosed in volume two page 169
See ref. biblio № 4

For all information concerning the instrument write to the author at the following address:

Edwin Hersch,
Dpt of Education and Researchp
London Psychiatric Hospital
850 Highbury Avenue
London, Ontario N0A 4H1, Canada

ORIGIN   Numerous analyses from special publications, especially those American and Canadian articles on research, processed by Medlars.

PURPOSE   To provide a rapid and precise global assessment of a psychogeriatric patient's level of functioning, for clinical and research purposes.

POPULATION   All categories of geriatric inpatients.

ADMINISTRATION   *Rater:* One or two nurses per patient.

Time required: 15 minutes, if the rater is familiar with the instrument.

Training: Brief training is necessary. Journal articles concerning the use of most parts of this scale, and a manual, are available.

Scoring: Each item is coded 0,1 or 2. The higher the score, the greater the degree of disability in the patient's functioning. The scoring for all 4 parts of the scales is expressed as a percentage.

VARIABLES   The global level of disability is assessed using 4 "sub-scales".
· Mental disorganisation/confusion   · Socially irritating behavior
· Physical disability   · Disengagement

VALIDATION   Was done on a psychogeriatric inpatient population, based on the global score and the score obtained for each of the 4 "sub-scales".
Factor analyis
External validity based on placement of patients in different care units, depending on their degree of disability.
Predictive validity on following outcome (discharge, transfer to nursing home, long-term hospitalisation, death), 1 or 2 years after initial assessment, and to predict the likely result of group psychotherapy.
Discriminative validity between clinical diagnoses (dementia, schizophrenia, manic depressive psychosis) (ref. 4).
Inter-rater reliability and **test-retest** reliability.

OTHER WORKS
cited by author
Selection of 5 scale items differentiating patients who will or will not be discharged during the following 6 months.
Studies on the predictive validity of this LPRS prognosis index (ref. 5).

APPLICATION   **Clinical** Permits assessment of deterioration or improvement of a patient over time.
Research Studies on the correlation between the level of functioning and electroencephalogram or scanner examination results.
Drug trials
Evaluation of programmes of care.

1 Goga (J.A.), Hambacher (W.O.): Psychologic and behavioral assessment of geriatric patients: a review.
Journal of the American Geriatrics Society, 1977, 25,
232.

2 Gurel (L.), Linn (M.W.), Linn (B.S.): Physical and
mental impairment-of-function evaluation in the
aged: the Pamie scale. *Journal of Gerontology*, 1972,
27, 83.

3 Hersch (E.L.), Csapo (K.G.), Palmer (R.B.): Development of the London Psychogeriatric Rating Scale (an
extension and statistical reevaluation of the Stockton
geriatric rating scale). *London Psychiat. Hosp. Res.
Bull.*, 1978, 1, 3-21.

4 Hersch (E.L.), Kral (V.A.), Palmer (R.B.): Clinical value of the London Psychogeriatric Rating Scale. *Journal of the American Geriatrics Society*, 1978, vol. 26, n°
8, 348-354.

5 Hersch (E.L.), Merskey (H.), Palmer (R.B.): Prediction of discharge from a psychogeriatric unit. *Canadian Journal of Psychiatry*, april 1980, vol. 25, n° 3, 234-
241.

6 Meer (B.), Baker (J.A.): The Stockton geriatric rating
scale. *Journal of Gerontology*, 1966, 21, 392.

ORIGINE DE LA DEPENDENCE
SOURCE OF DEPENDENCY

SPECIFICITY

* * *

TYPE OF INSTRUMENT

Ordinal rating scale
13 items, 5 grades

REFERENCE

Israël (L.), Ohlmann (Th.), Hugonot (L.) · – Techniques psychométriques particulières adaptées aux personnes âgées. Application aux essais cliniques contrôlés. In: "Recherche expérimentale et investigations cliniques dans la sénescence cérébrale". Symposium Bâle, 5-6 Juin 1978. Paris: Sandoz , 1978, 185-189.

Language: Original version published in French.
France.

Location: Enclosed in volume two page 172
See ref. biblio nº 1

For all information concerning the instrument write to the author at the following address:

Liliane Israël,
Pavillon Chissé, C.H.R.U.
38700 La Tronche
Grenoble, France

ORIGIN
This instrument was inspired by numerous works from the literature: **Plutchik** (ref. 7), **Stockton** (ref. 6), **Lawton** (ref. 4), **Linn** (ref. 5), **Gurel** (ref. 3), **Crichton** (ref. 8).

PURPOSE
To determine origin and intensity of dependency in relation to the personality of the patient.

POPULATION
Institutionalized elderly persons.

ADMINISTRATION
Rater: Physician, psychologist, nurse's aide.

Time required: 5 minutes.

Training: Not necessary.

Scoring: Double scoring (quantitative and qualitative), quantitative score varies from 13 to 65. Less than 13: autonomy without difficulties
　　　13-25: autonomy with effort
　　　26-39: compensated dependency
　　　40-52: needs occasional assistance
　　　53-65: total dependency, needs permanent assistance.
Additional appreciation of etiology is introduced by adding to the quantitative score a qualitative appreciation which is coded:
　　　· O (Organic) if the defined disorder is of organic etiology
　　　· P (Psychological) if the disorder is of psychological etiology.
　　　· S (Social) if it directly depends on social environment (institution or surroundings).
Score can also be transformed into a global profile. It gives a synopsis of the patient's characteristics and facilitates longitudinal assessment.

VARIABLES
Five groups of variables:
　　　· Sensory functions (eyesight and hearing)
　　　· Rudimentary functions (sleep-appetite)
　　　· Communication and expression (language, expression, voice and gesture)
　　　· Dependency for vital functions (motor and feeding)
　　　· Dependency for self-care (dressing and toileting).

VALIDATION
Inter-rater and **test-retest reliability** (ref. 2).

APPLICATION
Impact of institution on the degree of patient's dependency.
Evaluation of autonomy and indications for remaining in or discharge from the institution.
To evaluate needs for equipment.

IV.15

1 Israel (L.), Ohlmann (Th.), Hugonot (L.): Techniques psychométriques particulières adaptées aux personnes âgées: Application aux essais cliniques contrôlés. In: «Recherche expérimentale et investigations cliniques dans la sénescence cérébrale». Symposium Bâle, juin 1978. Paris: Sandoz, 1978, 185-189.

2 Israêl (L.), Ohlmann (Th.), Hugonot (R.): Application des statistiques et de l'informatique à l'étude de l'efficacité des médicaments à visée cérébrale. Communication présentée à la journée inter-régionale de gérontologie, Avignon, 19-11-1977.

3 Gurel (L.), Linn (M.W.), Linn (B.S.): Physical and mental impairment of function evaluation in the aged: the PAMIE scale. *Journal of Gerontology*, 1972, 27, 1, 83-90.

4 Lawton (M.P.), Brody (E.): Assessment for older people: self maintaining and instrumental activities of daily living. *Gerontologist*, 1969, 9, 179-196.

5 Linn (M.W.): A rapid disability rating scale. *Journal of the American Geriatrics Society*, 1967, vol. 15, n° 2, 211-214.

6 Meer (B.), Baker (J.A.): The Stockton geriatric rating scale. *Journal of Gerontology*, 1966, 21, 392-403.

7 Plutchik (R.), Conte (H.), Lieberman (M.), Bakur (M.) et al.: Reliability and validity of a scale for assessing the functioning of geriatric patients. *Journal of the American Geriatrics Society*, 1970, vol. 18, n° 6, 491-500.

8 Robinson (R.A.): Some problems of clinical trials in elderly people. *Gerontologia Clinica*, 1961, 3, 247-257.

GERIATRIC RAPID DIAGNOSTIC BATTERY (G.R.D.B.)

SPECIFICITY

* * *

TYPE OF INSTRUMENT

Compound instrument: Psychometric test Rating scales Questionnaire Inventory

---

REFERENCE **Murkofsky (C.), Conte (H.), Plutchik (R.), Karasu (T.)** · − Clinical utility of a rapid diagnostic test series for elderly psychiatric outpatients. *Journal of the American Geriatrics Society*, 1978, 26, 1, 22-26.

Language: Original version in English.
U.S.A..

Location: See ref. biblio nº 2

For all information concerning the instrument write to the author at the following address:

Robert Plutchik,
Department of Psychiatry
Albert Einstein College of Medicine of Yeshiva University
1300 Morris Park Avenue
Bronx, New York 10461, U.S.A.

ORIGIN   This composite battery consists of 7 instruments; 2 of the instruments are from other authors: A Self Rating Depression Scale from **Zung** (ref. 7), and A Scale for Assessment of Cognitive and Perceptual Functioning in Geriatric Patients from **Plutchik et al.** (ref. 6).
The other 5 instruments are original.

PURPOSE   The instrument was designed to assist psychiatrists in the process of diagnosing the elderly, and in assessing the level of functioning.

POPULATION   Elderly out-patients suffering from psychiatric disorders

ADMINISTRATION   *Rater:* The instruments are self-completed with the exception of Plutchik geriatric scale.

Time required: 20 – 40 minutes.

Training: Not necessary for applying the instruments, but necessary for interpretation of results.

Scoring: Depends on the instrument concerned.

VARIABLES   This compound instrument covers a wide variety of areas:
· Problem check list
· Depression (ref. 7)
· Daily Life Problems (Activities of Daily Living)
· Social interaction
· Cognitive, perceptual and motor functioning (ref. 5)
· Questionnaire on information concerning previous diseases
· Drugs, medication and alcohol consumption.

VALIDATION   Was completed on a population of elderly out-patients suffering from organic brain syndrome or depression, or both, mean age 60 years, and on a control group of elderly persons in good health, mean age 70,8 years (ref. 2):
Discriminative sensitivity for each instrument tested on sick population and control group.
Reliability: internal consistency of instruments forming the compound instrument

APPLICATION   **Clinical:**   · As a basis for diagnosis, taking into account medical, physiological, social and emotional aspects. Prognosis
Research: · For etiological research in dysfunctions
Therapeutic: · As a guide determining therapy, adapted to the patient's specific disorder.

1 Goldfarb (A.I.): Aging and organic syndrome. Bloomfield, New Jersey: Health Learning Systems Inc., 1974.

2 Murkofsky (C.), Conte (H.R.), Plutchik (R.), Karasu (T.B.): Clinical utility of a rapid diagnostic test series for elderly psychiatric outpatients. *Journal of the American Geriatrics Society*, 1978, vol. 26, n° 1, 22-26.

3 Nunnally (J.C.): Psychometric theory. New York: Mc Graw-Hill Book Company, 1967, 196-198, 210-211.

4 Pfeiffer (E.) Ed.: OARS Multidimensional functional assessment questionnaire. Durham, NC: Duke University, Center for the Study of Aging and Human Development, 1975.

5 Plutchik (R.): Conceptual and practical issues in the assessment of the elderly. In: Raskin (A.), Jarvik (L.F.) Eds: "Psychiatric symptoms and cognitive loss in the elderly". New-York: Halstead Press, 1979, 19-38.

6 Plutchik (R.), Conte (H.), Lieberman (M.): Development of a scale (GIES) for assessment of cognitive and perceptual functioning in geriatric patients. *Journal of the American Geriatrics Society*, 1971, vol. 19, 614.

7 Zung (W.W.): A self-rating depression scale. *Arch. Gen. Psychiat.*, 1965, 13, 63.

8 Zung (W.W.): Factors influencing the self-rating depression scale. *Arch. Gen. Psychiat.*, 1967, 16, 543.

9 Zung (W.W.): Depression in the normal aged. *Psychosomatics*, 1967, 8, 287.

10 Zung (W.W.), Richards (C.B.), Short (M.J.): Self-rating depression scale. *Arch. Gen. Psychiat.*, 1965, 13, 508.

BATTERIE DE FICHES D'EVALUATION
EVALUATION FORMS BATTERY

SPECIFICITY

* * *

TYPE OF INSTRUMENT

Several rating scales, check-list, combined clinical observations

REFERENCE	**Zay (N.), Boily-Sirois (H.)** · − Indicateurs sociaux et système statistique pour les services aux personnes âgées. III: Le système d'information. Université Laval, Québec: Laboratoire de Gérontologie sociale, 1978. Instrument not published.
	Language: Will be published in French. **Canada**
	For all information concerning the instrument or bibliographies write to the author at the following address:
	Nicolas Zay, Laboratoire de Recherche en Gérontologie Sociale Faculté des Sciences Sociales Université Laval Québec, G1K 7P4, Canada

ORIGIN

The instrument has 3 principal sources:
· Technical works and articles dealing with collection of data for statistical use, with the aim of elaborating the social indicators for devising and evaluating polices on aging.
· Specific works dealing with the inventories and the assessment of pathological states, functional capacities (rating scale A.D.L.), the ability to accomplish everyday tasks (rating scale from the geriatric Center from Philadelphia), etc.
· Documents reporting on the distribution of health care and social services in Quebec.

PURPOSE

This battery of assessment instruments was developed with the aim of establishing an information system before developing an integrated system of data for planning purposes.

POPULATION

Out-patients requiring care either in an institution or at home. Inpatients.

ADMINISTRATION

Rater: Physician, nurse, psychologist, social worker, any other trained person.

Time required: Varies according to the type of instrument.

Training: Is desirable. Discussions may precede or follow assessment. They can last from half an hour up to 4 hours depending on previous professional training.

Scoring: Each type of variable can be scored from 0-10. The total score, with 50 as the maximum value, corresponds to the level of disability of the subjects:
· Less than 15 points: needs assistance.
· From 15-24 points: programme of care and home help in the day center.
· From 25-32 points: dependency requires institutional care.
· From 33-40 points: severe disability.
· From 40-50 points: total dependency.

VARIABLES

This battery comprises a number of instruments whose aim is to provide a global assessment of the elderly person.
· Requirements expressed by the patient.　　· Functional ability
· Mental state　　· Social resources
· Sensory, psychological and emotional state　　· Material resources

VALIDATION

A "multiple purpose system" was used. It was possible to complete validation only on the basis of certain categories of problem or according to purpose. Therefore, it was not systematically done, certain categories being under-represented. However, global validation was completed on a sample of 800 subjects by approximately sixty professionals in Quebec.

OTHER WORKS
cited by author

Certain parts of the instrument were used for the assessment of residents of a residential home. The complete instrument is in regular use in some centers for social services in Quebec. A shortened version of this instrument was used by the CRSS of Quebec to assess patients frequently and to develop a resources inventory in the day centers and residential homes of the region.

APPLICATION

Planning, management, care and research.

DISABILITY ASSESSMENT SCHEDULE (D.A.S.)

SPECIFICITY

* *

TYPE OF INSTRUMENT

Rating scale of
97 items

REFERENCE	**World Health Organization** · − Disability Assessment Schedule (D.A.S.). Geneva: World Health Organization, October 1979. Unpublished.

Language: English, Turkish, German, Bulgarian, Arabic, Italian, Czechoslovakian, Serbo-Croate, Chinese, French.

Location: Enclosed in volume two page 173
See ref. biblio nº 7

For all information concerning the instrument write to the author at the following address:

A. Jablensky,
World Health Organization
Division of Mental Health
1211 Geneva 27, Switzerland

ORIGIN

W.H.O. Collaborative Study on the Assessment and Reduction of Psychiatric Disability

PURPOSE

The instrument was designed for a standardized assessment of the social behavior and social functioning of the psychiatric patient within his own cultural and social context. Disability is conceived here in terms of disturbances in the performance of social roles as a result of a mental disorder.

POPULATION

Psychiatric patients in hospital and psychiatric out-patients

ADMINISTRATION

Rater: Psychologist, psychiatrist, social worker, clinician.

Time required: 30 – 45 minutes.

Training: Necessary. Practical training in the use of the instrument is desirable. The experience of the interviewer should permit him to compare his observations of the patient's functioning with that of someone with presumed normal or average functioning of the same age, sex and socio-cultural environment.

Description: 97 items divided into five sections. The information is collected by means of an interview with a key informant (someone close to the patient such as a member of the family, a good friend) and from the patient himself. There is a manual for use with the instrument.

VARIABLES

Five aspects are assessed:
· Overall behavior
· Social role performance
· Behavior in hospital (if applicable)
· Modifying factors that might influence social adjustment
· Global evaluation of patient's social adjustment.

VALIDATION

Discussed in various papers and publications.

APPLICATION

Clinical:
Evaluation of care, prognosis

Research:
Epidemiological studies, treatment and management programmes.

1 Assessment and reduction of psychiatric disability. Report of an exchange of visits of collaborating investigators, Zagreb 14-20 September 1975.

2 Assessment and reduction of psychiatric disability. Report of an exchange of visits of collaborating investigators, Mannheim 31 March – 2 April 1977.

3 Assessment and reduction of psychiatric disability. Report of an exchange of visits of collaborating investigators, Varna 9-12 October 1978.

4 Assessment and reduction of psychiatric disability. Report of an exchange of visits of collaborating investigators, Ankara 8-11 October 1979.

5 Assessment and reduction of psychiatric disability. Report of an exchange of visits of collaborating investigators, Groningen 6-10 October 1980.

6 Jablensky (A.), Schwarz (R.), Tomow (T.): WHO collaborative study on impairments and disabilities associated with schizophrenic disorders. A preliminary communication: objectives and methods. In: "Epidemiology research as a basis to the organization of extramural psychiatry": proceedings of the Second European Symposium on Social Psychiatry. *Acta Psychiat. Scand.*, 1980, Suppl. 285, 62.

7 World Health Organization: Disability Assessment Schedule (D.A.S.). Geneva: World Health Organization, October 1979. Unpublished.

8 World Health Organization: International classification of impairments, disabilities and handicaps. A manual of classification relating to the consequences of disease. Geneva: World Health Organization, 1980.

ECHELLE DE DEPENDANCE – AUTONOMIE (E.D.A.)
SCALE OF DEPENDENCY – AUTONOMY

SPECIFICITY

☐ * * * ☐

TYPE OF INSTRUMENT

Ordinal rating scale
25 items in 5 groups

REFERENCE	**Delcros (M.), Lanoë (R.)** · – Une nouvelle échelle d'évaluation de la dépendance des patients dans les établissements de long séjour. *La Revue de Gériatrie*, 1980, tome 5, n° 8, 395-400.

Language: Published in French.
France.

Location: Enclosed in volume two page 174
See ref biblio n° 1

For all information concerning the instrument write to the authors at the following addresses:

Renée Lanoë,
Hôpital Paul Brousse
14, avenue P.V. Couturier
94804 Villejuif Cedex, France

Michel Delcros,
Hôpital Corentin Celton
37 Bd Gambetta
92133 Issy Les Moulineaux, France

ORIGIN

Personalized rating scale, developed in two institutions in Paris according to their respective needs. It was inspired by the **Stockton** geriatric rating scale (ref. 4), the S.C.A.G. (ref. 6), **Crichton** (ref. 5) **Exton-Smith** (ref. 2) and **Hugonot** (ref. 3).

PURPOSE

Is twofold: clinical and practical aims.
This instrument was devised, first, to assess individual dependency in accordance with the institution with the aim of personalising the types of care and involving the nurse's aide, and second, to establish precisely and to appraise the different types of nursing care which are mentioned in the instrument, for the benefit of management.

POPULATION

Long-term inpatients.

ADMINISTRATION

Rater: Nursing staff, nurse's aide, nurse.

Time required: 2-3 minutes.

Training: Rapid.

Scoring: 25 items scored from 1-4. The score varies from 25 to 100.
   Slightly dependent: less than 30.
   Average dependent: from 30 to 65.
   Very dependent: over 65.

VARIABLES

Five aspects of a person's activities were studied
· Motor activities (4 items)
· Activities of daily living (5 items)
· Frequency of paramedical care (4 items)
· Perception, orientation, memory (6 items)
· Relations with others (6 items)

VALIDATION

Studies of **inter-rater reliability** (ref. 1); **Test-retest reliability**.

OTHER WORKS
cited by author

Studies of the respective burdens of staff by different categories of nursing.
Current and daily clinical use.

APPLICATION

Institutional interest: to achieve unity of scoring and to promote team work.
Diagnosis of dependency, and its development.
Prognosis for reestablishment of independence.

1 Delcros (M.), Lanoe (R.), Une nouvelle échelle d'évaluation de la dépendance des patients dans les établissements de Long Séjour. *Revue de Gériatrie*, 1980,
tome 5, 8, 395-400.

2 Exton-Smith (A.N.), Norton (D.), Mc Laren (R.): An
investigation of geriatric nursing problems in hospital.
London: National Corporation for the Care of Old
People, 1962.

3 Hugonot (L.): Contribution à l'étude des échelles de
dépendance en gériatrie. Thèse de doctorat en médecine, Grenoble, 1977.

4 Meer (B.), Baker (J.A.): The Stockcon geriatric rating
scale. *Journal of Gerontology*, 1966, 21, 392-403.

5 Robinson (R.A.): Some problems of clinical trials in
elderly people. *Geront. Clin.*, 1961, 3, 247-257.

6 Shader (R.I.), Harmatz (J.S.), Salzman (C.). A new
scale for clinical assessment in geriatric population:
Sandoz clinical assessment geriatric (SCAG). *Journal
of the American Geriatrics Society*, 1974, 22, 3, 107-113.

COMPREHENSIVE HEALTH QUESTIONNAIRE (C.H.Q.)

SPECIFICITY

* * *

TYPE OF INSTRUMENT

Questionnaire
102 questions

REFERENCE	**Kozarević (D.), Milicević (L.), Vojvodić (N.)** · – Health status and health care system of war veterans in Yugoslavia. Beograd, Yugoslavia, 1980.

Language: Original version published in Serbo-Croat. Translated into English.
Yugoslavia

Location: English version enclosed in volume two page 68
See ref. biblio nº 9

For all information concerning the instrument and the translation write to the author at the following address:

Djordje Kozarević,
Institute of Chronic Diseases and Gerontology
Slobodana Penezica 35
11000 Beograd, Yugoslavia

ORIGIN
The main source in the instrument's conception was the questionnaire of the Yugoslavia Cardiovascular and Respiratory Diseases Study (ref. 11), as well as the WHO cooperative study "Health Care of the Elderly" (ref. 14).

PURPOSE
The purpose of this instrument was to assess health status (in terms of subjective feelings and objective findings) and to measure functional abilities as well as use of different health care services.

POPULATION
Adult out-patients over 60 years of age.

ADMINISTRATION
Rater: Physician and nurse.

Time required: 50 minutes.

Training: Brief training is necessary.

VARIABLES
Seven groups of variables are assessed:
· Personal and group characteristics and habits (occupation, formal education, physical activity, alcohol consumption and smoking) including complaints for the last 2 weeks.
· History of infectious and chronic diseases and conditions.
· Impairments of different organs and systems (cardiovascular, respiratory, etc) and disability for work, recreation and personal care during the past 3 months.
· Results of physical examination of major systems and blood pressure levels.
· Final diagnostic summary of leading diseases according to I.C.D.-WHO.
· Utilisation of health care services during the past year (out-patient clinic, hospital, home care, rehabilitation centers, etc).
· Check-list of measures undertaken after interview and physical examination.

VALIDATION
Different parts of the questionnaire were validated separately.

OTHER WORKS
cited by author
The instrument is used in the routine systematic evaluation of the health and social status of 25.000 war veterans in Belgrade and other regions of Yugoslavia (ref. 6, 7, 9, 14). The baseline information is to be used for determination of main risk factors in the development of various diseases, disabilities, premature death, and consequences of aging (ref. 13).

APPLICATION
The instrument is for clinical and psychosocial uses, for longitudinal and cross-sectional epidemiological studies, permitting systematic evaluation of health status and use of health services aimed at assessing the needs and demands of the elderly population and for early diagnosis and planning.

1 Grundy (F.), Reinike (W.A.): Healthy practice research and formalized. Managerial methods. Public Health Papers 51, Genève: WHO, 1973.

2 Hrabac (T.), Pirc (B.), Kozarevic (Dj.): Needs and demands for medical care with special emphases on chronic diseases. Sarajevo: Institute of Public Health of Bosnia and Hercegovina, 1974.

3 Josipovic (V.), Kozarevic (Dj.), Thurm (R.): Epidemiology of essential hypertension among various ethnic groups in Yugoslavia: methodology. Beograd: Institute of Chronic Diseases and Gerontology-Center of Hypertension, 1977.

4 Knox (E.G.) Ed.: Epidemiology in health care planning. WHO-IEA. Oxford: Oxford University Press, 1979.

5 Kostrzewski (J.) Ed.: Measurement of levels of health. WHO Reg. Publ., European Series 7. Copenhagen: WHO, 1979.

6 Kozarević (Dj.): Risk factors epidemiology: importance for prevention of pathologic ageing. Hamburg, 1981.

7 Kozarević (Dj.): Health status and performance in activities of daily living in old age. Prepared for: Working group to define means of prevention of disability in the elderly. Cologne, Nov. 16-19, 1981.

8 Kozarević (Dj.), Mc Gee (D.), Vojvodić (N.), Racic (Z.), Dawber (T.), Gordon (T.), Zukel (W.): Frequency of alcohol consumption and morbidity and mortalita. *Lancet*, March 22 1980.

9 Kozarević (Dj.), Milicević (L.J.), Vojvodić (N.): Health status and health care system of war veterans in Yugoslavia. Beograd, 1980.

10 Kozarević (Dj.), Pirc (B.), Dawber (Th.), Kahn (H.), Zukel (W.): Prevalence and incidence of coronary disease in a population study: the Yugoslavia cardiovascular disease study. *Journal of Chronic Diseases*, 1971, vol. 24, 495-505.

11 Kozarević (Dj), Roberts (A.): Respiratory diseases: investigation of etiologic and risk factors: methodology. Beograd: Post-graduate Medical Institute, 1973.

12 Kozarević (Dj.), Vuković (Z.), Racić (Z.), Vojvodic (N.): Process of ageing and coronary heart disease incidence: The yugoslav epidemiologic study of 11, 121 men. Xth World congress of gerontology, Jerusalem, Israël, 1975.

13 Mc Gee (D.): Homogeneity of the effect of risk factors on the incidence of cardiovascular diseases. Baltimore, Maryland: School of Hygiene and Public Health of the Johns Hopkins University, 1977.

14 Protocol of the study on health care of the elderly. Second meeting of the investigators participating in the study on Health care of elderly, ICP/SPM 004 (3), 1978.

15 Roemer (M.J.): Evaluation of community health centers. Public health papers 48. Genève: WHO, 1972.

16 World Health Organization: Measurement of levels of health. The community needs for rehabilitation and social adaptation services. European series n° 7, IEA. Genève: WHO, 1979.

17 World Health Organization: International classification of impairments, disabilities, and handicaps. Genève: WHO, 1980.

EVALUATION GLOBALE DE L'AUTONOMIE
GLOBAL EVALUATION OF AUTONOMY

SPECIFICITY

* * *

TYPE OF INSTRUMENT

Nominal rating scale
13 items, 4 grades

REFERENCE **Patron (C.)** · − L'évaluation de l'autonomie dans le cadre du maintien à domicile de la personne âgée. *La Revue de Gériatrie*, 1980, tome 5, nº 8, 381-386.

Language: Published in French.
France

Location: Enclosed in volume two page 176

For all information concerning the instrument write to the author at the following address:

Christine Patron,
Secrétariat d'Etat chargé des Personnes Agées
61, rue Dutot
75732 Paris Cedex 15, France

ORIGIN This instrument is original. It consists of a personal assessment of the consequences of disease on levels of functioning and activities of daily living.

PURPOSE The instrument was developed to evaluate whether the work of the home help services facilitates the reestablishment of independence and integration of social changes, or alternatively intensifies isolation and dependency.

POPULATION All elderly dependant persons who are living at home.

ADMINISTRATION *Rater:* Social worker, people close to the elderly person, nurse, home help service staff.

Rater required: 10 minutes.

Training: Familiarisation with the scoring system.

Scoring: The frequency of visits to day centers or the use of home health care is scored according to half-day units, with 10 for day centers and home help, 14 for home health care, 7 for meals and services provided once a day.
Initial scoring is graphically presented as dark lines, and after 4 weeks as dashes.

VARIABLES Three groups of variables are assessed:
· Independence: Washing, dressing, feeding, motor activities, health state, mental state.
· Resources in surroundings: House, family, neighbours, integration.
· Social and health services: day centers, home care, provision of meals at home, home help.

VALIDATION Experimental scale was applied in Montargis, France.

APPLICATION This instrument can be used as a means to follow-up sick persons and as a guide for those providing care. Its primary purpose is to establish whether the services provided permit the reestablishment of independence or whether they induce in the elderly person an even greater degree of dependency.

EDINBURGH PSYCHOGERIATRIC DEPENDENCY RATING SCALE (P.G.D.R.S.)

SPECIFICITY

* * *

TYPE OF INSTRUMENT

Ordinal rating scale
36 items, grades
vary from 2 to 6

REFERENCE	**Wilkinson (I.M.), Graham-White (J.)** · − Psychogeriatric Dependency Rating Scales (PGDRS). A method of assessment for use by nurses. *British Journal of Psychiatry*, 1980, 137, 558-565.

Language: Original version published in English.
Great Britain

Location: Enclosed in volume two page 198
See ref. biblio № 13

For further information concerning the guidebook of instructions for the use of this instrument write to the author at the following address:

Ian Wilkinson,
Dpt of Clinical Psychology
Memorial Hospital
Hollyhurst Road
Darlington DL3 8BR, Great Britain

ORIGIN
This scale was developed by a team of nurses from the work of **Plutchik** (ref. 10), **Gurel** (ref. 4), **Ferm** (ref. 1), **Grauer** (ref. 2) and from the Stockton Geriatric Rating Scale (ref. 8). These sources added to the personal observations of the nursing team responsible for the development of the scale.

PURPOSE
The primary aim is to provide a brief clinical assessment of the overall level and type of nursing care demanded, in terms of the degree of dependency upon nursing staff. This can be particularly useful to indicate appropriate placement for a particular patient.

POPULATION
The assessment was developed on a population of elderly people who were within, or were likely to require, institutional care. (Norms are available for groups in hospital, residential homes, and living in the community with or without support).
N.B. The assessment is not recommended for those who are functioning quite well in terms of orientation, physical ability, and behavioural disturbance.

ADMINISTRATION
Rater: Nurse.

Time required: 5 minutes.

Training: One day of training by a psychologist.

Scoring: A manual of instructions assists the rater to assign a specific score to each item.

VARIABLES
All variables attempt to measure "Dependency" defined operationally for the purposes of this study as "nursing time demanded by patients".
Items are grouped into three dimensions which are assessed concurrently:
· Orientation (10 items, all with 2 rating points)
· Behaviour (16 items, all with 3 rating points)
· Physical (16 items, varying from 3-6 rating points)
A separate score is then calculated for each dimension. These scores can be used to indicate the absolute and relative level of problems in each of these dimensions.

VALIDATION
Was carried out on an elderly population, and consisted of (ref. 14):
Face validity
Concurrent validity
Predictive validity
Inter-rater reliability: poorly associated items were eliminated.

APPLICATION
The test has three areas of application:
Clinical: to define conditions for admission to hospital and other services;
to define the criteria for the placement of patients to the appropriate department;
to provide a clear view of important nursing problems.
Research: to compare the characteristics of different populations.
Management: to determine the need for nursing staff.

1 Ferm (L.): Behavioural activities in demented geriatric patients. *Gerontologia Clinica*, 1974, 16, 185-194.

2 Grauer (H.), Birnbaum (F.): A geriatric functional rating scale to determine the need for institutional care. *Journal of the American Geriatrics Society*, 1975, vol. 23, n° 10, 472-476.

3 Guilford (J.P.): Fundamental statistics in psychology and education. 3rd ed. New York: Mc Graw-Hill, 1956.

4 Gurel (L.), Linn (M.W.), Linn (B.S.): Physical and mental impairment of function evaluation in the aged: the PAMIE scale. *Journal of Gerontology*, 1972, 83-90.

5 Hall (J.): Inter-rater reliability of ward rating scales. *British Journal of Psychiatry*, 1974, 125, 248-255.

6 Isaacs (B.), Walkey (F.): Measurement of mental impairment in geriatric practice. *Gerontologia Clinica*, 1964, vol. 6, 114-123.

7 Klingner (A.), Kachanoff (R.), Dastoor (D.P.), Worenklein (A.), Charlton (S.), Gutbrodt (E.), Muller (H.F.): A psychogeriatric assessment program. III: Clinical and experimental psychological aspects. *Journal of the American Geriatrics Society*, 1976, vol. 24, 17-24.

8 Meer (B.), Baker (J.): The Stockton geriatric rating scale. *Journal of Gerontology*, 1966, vol. 21, 392-403.

9 Milne (J.S.), Maule (M.M.) Cormack (S.), Williamson (J.): The design and testing of a questionnaire and examination to assess physical and mental health in older people using a staff nurse as an observer. *Journal of Chronic Diseases*, 1972, vol. 25, 385-405.

10 Plutchik (R.), Conte (H.), Lieberman (M.), Bakur (M.), Grossman (J.), Lehrman (N.): The reliability and validity of a scale for assessing the functioning of geriatric patients. *Journal of the American Geriatrics Society*, 1970, vol. 18, 491.

11 Salzman (C.), Kochansky (G.), Shader (R.): Rating scales for geriatric psychopharmacology-a review. *Journal of the American Geriatrics Society*, 1973, vol. 21, 3-50.

12 Silver (C.P.): Simple methods of testing ability in geriatric patients. *Gerontologia Clinica*, 1972, 14, 110-122.

13 Wilkinson (I.M.), Graham –White (J.): Psychogeriatric dependency rating scales (PGDRS): a method of assessment for use by nurses. *British J. Psychiat.*, 1980, vol. 137, 558-565.

14 Wilkinson (I.M.), Graham-White (J.): Dependency rating scales for use in psychogeriatric nursing. *Health Bulletin*, 1980, vol. 38, 36-42.

15 Wilson (L.A.), Brass (W.): Brief assessment of the mental state in geriatric domiciliary practice: the usefulness of the mental state questionnaire. *Age and Ageing*, 1973, vol. 2, 92-101.

SYSTEME D'INFORMATION (C.T.M.S.P.)

INFORMATION SYSTEM (C.T.M.S.P.)

SPECIFICITY

* * *

TYPE OF INSTRUMENT

Compound instrument

REFERENCE	**Equipe de Recherche Opérationnelle en Santé (E.R.O.S.)** · – C.T.M.S.P.: un système d'information pour un réseau de services prolongés. L'évaluation des services requis et la mesure des ressources requises par le bénéficiaire. Montréal: E.R.O.S., 1981. Not published

Language: Written in French.
Canada

Location: Enclosed in volume two page 201

For all information concerning the instrument write to the author at the following address:

Charles Tilquin,
Equipe E.R.O.S.
Université de Montréal
3535 Reine Marie, suite 501
Montréal, Québec H3V 1H8, Canada

ORIGIN

This original system permits the establishment of a data bank reflecting the needs of the population which can serve as a basis for future planning.

PURPOSE

The system was devised to produce indicators permitting the management to reach optimal decisions, taking into account the needs of the assessed person, and to ensure harmony between these needs and an appropriate programme of care. The system aids the professional staff management in deciding to which programme a patient must be admitted, taking into account his needs.

POPULATION

Elderly out-patients or inpatients

ADMINISTRATION

Rater: Nurse or social worker, multidisciplinary team: social worker, nurse, psychotherapist, physician, occupational therapist.

Time required: 1 hour in the first phase. 20 minutes in the second phase.

Training: Is necessary.

Scoring: Grades used vary.

DESCRIPTION

There are 3 phases.

1. The system collects necessary information for an exact assessment of the subject. It is necessary to have a form for the assessment of independence and a form for medical information.

2. A multidisciplinary team identifies, on the basis of information acquired in phase one, all services required (in terms of time) the assessed person. It is also necessary to have: a form for service allocation which has the following 6 components: supporting services, nursing care, medical services, social services, physiotherapy and occupational therapy.

3. According to the levels of the services required it is necessary to choose the most adequate programme which will fulfill the needs identified. A fourth form is necessary: a scheme establishing the links between different levels of required services and the existing programmes available in the area in question.

VARIABLES

Physical characteristics:
· Sensory capacity
· Mobility
· Functional autonomy (ADL)

Habits:
· Feeding
· Chewing
· Smoking

Relationships within the family and
social relationships:
· Contact with those living nearby
· Management and regulation

Impression and observation of the
rater and those providing care:
· Orientation
· Memory
· Concentration, comprehension, adaptation
· Questionnaire – autonomy

· Sleeping
· Individual activities
· Group activities
· Managing finances

· Personal characteristics
· Attitude towards receiving help
· Reliability and source of information

VALIDATION — Was not published. Is currently in progress.

OTHER WORKS
cited by author

Two fields of current use:
· Orientation-admission. From 1979: Territory of the Public Health Department (D.S.C. of Verdun). From 1981: the Quebec-metropolitain (3 territories of the D.S.C.) From 1983: Laurentides-Lanaudire region, region of Montreal-Metropolitain.
· Planning. 1981-1983: Planning the institutional resources of Quebec. A sample of 1519 subjects from 37 establishments (different publications and reports-contact P. Lamarche, WHO Copenhagen), 1982-83: Planning the institutional resources of the Laurentides-Lanaudiere region (data currently collected from the complete inpatient population: 2875 persons).
· Numerous other applications.

APPLICATION — Planning and indications for placement into appropriate institutions.

1 Chagnon (M.), Audette (L.M.), Lebrun (L.), Tilquin (C.): Seeking a methodology for the development of a patient classification. Proceedings of the AIIE/ORSA/HMSS Joint National Conference on Health System Productivity Improvement, 1976, 44-60.

2 Chagnon (M.), Audette (L.M.), Lebrun (L.), Tilquin (C.): Validation of patient classification by level of nursing resources requirements. *Medical Care*, 1978, 16, 6, 465-475.

3 Chagnon (M.), Audette (L.M.), Lebrun (L.), Tilquin (C.): Construction and implementation of a patient classification by level of nursing resources requirements. *Nursing Research*, 1978, 27, 2, 107-112.

4 Chagnon (M.), Audette (L.M.), Tilquin (C.): Patient classification by care required. *Dimensions in Health Services*, 1977, 54, 9, 32-37.

5 Cléroux (R.), Dubuc (S.), Tilquin (C.): The age replacement problem with minimal repair and random repair costs. *Operations Research*, 1979, 27, 6, 1158-1167.

6 Florian (M.), Tilquin (C.), Vanderstraeten (G.): An implicit enumeration algorithm for complex scheduling problems. *The International Journal of Production Research*, 1975, 13, 1, 25-40.

7 Lebeau (A.), Sicotte (C.), Tilquin (C.), Tremblay (L.): Le concept d'autonomie, indicateur synthétique et opérationnel du mode de vieillissement: une approche systémique. *Santé mentale au Québec*, 1980, 5, 2, 70-90.

8 Sicotte (C.), Tilquin (C.), Hirbour (F.): The planning process in providing care for the aged. Proceedings of the Seminar: Care for the aged – The new majority. Ottawa: University of Ottawa, 1978, 252-278.

9 Tilquin (C.): On scheduling with earliest starts and due dates on a group of identical machines. *Naval Research Logistics Quarterly*, 1975, 22, 4, 777-785.

10 Tilquin (C.): La classification des patients pédiatriques de l'hôpital Ste-Justine: innovations et critiques. Actes du Colloque sur la Théorie des Systèmes et la Gestion Scientifique des Services Publics. HEC and Univ. de Montréal 1975, 34-41.

11 Tilquin (C.): Patient classification does work. *Dimensions in Health Services*, Janvier 1976, 12-16.

12 Tilquin (C.): Modeling health services systems. *Medical Care*, 1976, 14, 3, 223-240.

13 Tilquin (C.): Un cadre conceptuel et méthodologique pour les classifications de malades selon leurs besoins et soins infirmiers. Actes de la Conférence sur la Science des Systèmes dans le domaine de santé, Paris, 1976. London: Taylor and Francis, 1977, 289-296.

14 Tilquin (C.): The schizophrenia of patient classification. *Dimensions in Health Services*, 1977, 54, 9, 26-28.

15 Tilquin (C.): Client classification systems by health resources requirements. Proceedings of the MEDINFO 1977 Conference, North Holland, Amsterdam, 1977, 1045.

16 Tilquin (C.): Le système PRN 76: pour une approche plus scientifique en gestion des soins infirmiers. *L'Administrateur Hospitalier*, 1980, 3, 2, 21-24.

17 Tilquin (C.): Le système PRN 76: pour une approche plus scientifique de gestion des soins infirmiers – seconde partie. *L'Administrateur Hospitalier*, 1980, 3, 3, 21-25.

18 Tilquin (C.): Complexité, cybernétique et recherche opérationnelle. Actes du 17e Congrès de l'AHQ. Montréal: AHQ, 1980, 75-79.

19 Tilquin (C.) Ed.: Programme de la seconde Conférence Internationale sur la Science des Systèmes dans le domaine de la Santé. Montréal: I.N.S.A., 1980, 242.

20 Tilquin (C.) Ed.: Actes de la seconde Conférence Internationale sur la Science des Systèmes dans le domaine de la Santé – Vol. I: volet communautaire. Oxford: Pergamon Press International, 1981, 947.

21 Tilquin (C.) Ed.: Actes de la seconde Conférence Internationale sur la Science des Systèmes dans le domaine de la Santé – Vol. II: volet hospitalier. Oxford: Pergamon Press International, 1981, 924.

22 Tilquin (C.) et al.: CTMSP 81 – L'évaluation des services requis et la mesure des ressources requises par le bénéficiaire. Abstract. Montréal: I.N.S.A., 1981, 114.

23 Tilquin (C.), Audette (L.M.), Carle (J.), Lambert (P.), Sicotte (C.): Quantification of nursing care requirements in view of nursing management. Actes du Congrès of the World Association for Medical Informatics. Paris: W.A.M.I., 1978, 127-144.

24 Tilquin (C.), Audette (L.M.), Carle (J.), Simard (A.), Lambert (P.): Determining nursing team size and composition. *Dimensions in Health Services*, 1978, 55, 12, 12-16.

25 Tilquin (C.), Audette (L.M.), Carle (J.), Simard (A.), Lambert (P.): Evaluation quantitative en soins infirmiers. *Administration Hospitalière et Sociale*, 1978, 25, 2, 42-54.

26 Tilquin (C.), Carle (J.), Saulnier (D.), Lambert (P.): PRN 80 – La mesure du niveau des soins infirmiers requis par le bénéficiaire. Montréal: I.N.S.A., 1981, 259.

27 Tilquin (C.), Carle (J.), Saulnier (D.), Lambert (P.): PRN 80 – Measuring nursing care required. Montréal: I.N.S.A. 1981, 270.

28 Tilquin (C.), Carle (J.), Saulnier (D.), Lambert (P.): la dotation du personnel soignant en fonction des volumes de soins requis dans les différents services – le système PRN 76. In: Gremy (F.) et al. Eds.: "Medical informatics, Europe 81". Springer Verlag, 1981, 429-435.

29 Tilquin (C.), Cléroux (R.): The block replacement model with inactivity periods and general cost structure. *The Canadian Journal of Statistics*, 1974, 2, 2, 197-214.

30 Tilquin (C.), Cléroux (R.): Periodic replacement with minimal repair at failure and adjustments costs. *Naval Research Logistics Quarterly*, 1975, 22, 2, 243-253.

31 Tilquin (C.), Cléroux (R.): Block replacement policies with general cost structures. *Technometrics*, 1975, 17, 3, 291-298.

32 Tilquin (C.), Cléroux (R.): Periodic replacement with minimal repair at failure and general cost function. *The Journal of Statistical Computation and Simulation*, 1975, 4, 63-67.

33 Tilquin (C.), Houde (C.): L'Hôpital de jour: alternative à l'hôpital traditionnel. *Le Médecin du Québec*, 1979, 14, 12, 93-97.

34 Tilquin (C.), Lambert (P.), Vanderstraeten (G.): A conceptual framework for planning paramedical manpower – two cases studies. *OGEP Gestioni Pubbliche, Supplemento* 3/81, 1981, 55-70.

35 Tilquin (C.), Pineault (R.), Sicotte (C.), Audette (L.M.): Administration d'un réseau de services socio-sanitaires pour les personnes âgées. *Administration Hospitalière et Sociale*, 1977, 23, 4, 26-32.

36 Tilquin (C.), Pineault (R.), Sicotte (C.), Audette (L.M.): Services socio-sanitaires pour les personnes âgées: un système de classification des individus par type de besoins en ressources socio-sanitaires. In: "Modélisation et maîtrise des systèmes techniques, économiques et sociaux – tome I: Hommes et techniques". Paris, 1977, 419-427.

37 Tilquin (C.), Pineault (R.), Sicotte (C.), Lambert (P.), Hirbour (F.), Audette (L.M.), Carle (J.): An information system for administration and planning of long term care for the aged. Actes du Congrès of the World Association for Medical Informatics. Paris: W.A.M.I., 1978, 71-78.

38 Tilquin (C.), Saulnier (D.), Vanderstraeten (G.): Planning and measuring nursing care required: an integrated approach. In: Barber (B.) Ed.: "The impact of computer in nursing". In press.

39 Tilquin (C.), Sicotte (C.): L'évaluation des besoins des personnes âgées dans la perspective de la gestion du système de soins et services prolongés. In: Gremy (F.) et al. Eds.: "Medical informatics, Europe 81". Springer Verlag, 1981, 799-805.

40 Tilquin (C.), Sicotte (C.), Pineault (R.): Un système d'information pour la gestion et la planification dans le domaine des soins prolongés aux personnes âgées. Actes du Congrès de l'Association en Santé Publique du Québec. Montréal: ASPQ, 1978, 112-125.

41 Tilquin (C.), Sicotte (C.), Tousignant (F.), Gagnon (G.), Cloutier (F.), Urbanski (E.), Lambert (P.): C.T.M.S.P. 81: l'évaluation des services requis et la mesure des ressources requises par le bénéficiare. Montréal: I.N.S.A., 1981, 281.

42 Tilquin (C.), Sicotte (C.), Tousignant (F.), Gagnon (G.), Cloutier (F.), Urbanski (E.), Lebeau (A.), D'Amour (D.), Paradis (C.), Paradis (M.), Poirier (L.), Mallette (L.): C.T.M.S.P. 81: L'orientation du bénéficiaire dans le réseau. Montréal: I.N.S.A., 1982, 160.

43 Tilquin (C.), Sicotte (C.), Tousignant (F.), Gagnon (G.), Lebeau (A.), D'Amour (D.), Paradis (M.), Fournier (J.), Lambert (P.): C.T.M.S.P. 81: L'évaluation de l'autonomie et l'évaluation médicale du bénéficiaire. Montréal: I.N.S.A., 1982, 132.

44 Tilquin (C.), Sicotte (C.), Tousignant (F.), Pineault (R.): Un système d'évaluation des besoins des services sociosanitaires pour les personnes âgées. Actes du premier congrès francophone de Gérontologie. Paris: Masson, 1981, 620-624.

45 Tilquin (C.), Sicotte (C.), Vallée (G.), Tousignant (F.), Lambert (P.), Paquin (T.): The physical, emotional and social condition of an aged population in Quebec. In: Marshall (V.W.) Ed.: "Aging in Canada: Social perspectives". Toronto: Fitzhenry and Whiteside, 1980, 222-231.

ECHELLE D'EXPRESSION DE L'AUTONOMIE: GERONTE
EXPRESSION OF AUTONOMY SCALE: GERONTE

SPECIFICITY

* * *

TYPE OF INSTRUMENT

Visual rating scale
27 items 3 grades
(to be processed
by computer)

REFERENCE	**Leroux (R.), Viau (G.), Fournier (M.), Bergeot (R.), Attalli (G.)** · – Visualisation d'une échelle simple d'autonomie: Géronte. *La Revue de Gériatrie*, 1981, tome 6, nᵒ 9, 433-436.

Language: Published in French
France

Location: Enclosed in volume two page 177
See ref biblio nᵒ 16

For all information concerning the instrument write to the authors at the following addresses:

Robert Leroux,
Service de Gériatrie
Hôpital de Vierzon
18100 Vierzon, France

Georget Attalli,
7, rue du Professeur Florence
69003 Lyon, France

The film "Géronte" can be obtained from: "Société de Gérontologie de l'Ouest et du Centre, Le Mans, France".

ORIGIN	The original scale is based on the concept of visual presentation in multi-dimensional space.
PURPOSE	For practical purposes. Enables assessment and synopsis follow-up of independence.
POPULATION	Elderly persons living in a residential home or elderly out-patients.
ADMINISTRATION	*Rater:* Physician, nurse's aide, social worker. *Time required:* 2-3 minutes. *Training:* 3-4 hours. *Scoring:* Visual presentation on a figure: 3 grades. White: Bedridden – Gray: Partially disabled – Black: Able

VARIABLES

Six types of activities:
Locomotor activities:
· Global independence
· Needs help in achieving independence
· Independence indoors
· Independence outdoors
Self care activities:
· Continence
· Feeding
· Dressing
· Washing

Activities outside of home:
· Leisure
· Shopping
· Using buses
· Visit

Sensory functioning:
· Speech
· Vision
· Hearing
Mental handicap

Domestic activities:
· Communication
· Housekeeping
· Preparation of meals
· Handling objects

VALIDATION	Standardisation was done on a sample of 350 inpatients and on elderly living at home (ref. 18).
OTHER WORKS cited by author	Twelve geriatric services use Geronte on the basis of 4 contracts with INSERM. They are all equipped with a micro-computer system. A geronte computer programme permits the visualising of Geronte Groupe, after the factor loading for each item is calculated. This Geronte Groupe enables comparisons of different population groups.
APPLICATION	Diagnosis, prognosis and development of independence. Epidemiological studies, rehabilitation procedures, drug trials.

IV.24

1   Attalli (G.): Informatisation de Géronte. Journées de Gériatrie, Le Mans 23-24 mai 1981. *Symbiose, Revue des Professions de Santé*, 1981, n° 20.

2   Attalli (G.), Bergeot (R.), Fournier (M.), Viau (G.), Leroux (R.): Quantification des handicaps des personnes âgées. *Revue de Médecine de Tours*, 1980, tome 14, n° 9-1, 1521-1524.

3   Attalli (G.), Guyotat (J.), Mounier (B.), Rastello (J.), Darnoud (G.), Pollet (F.): Etude longitudinale des facteurs de risque de décompensation psychiatrique chez les personnes âgées. *Psychologie Médicale*, 1982, 14, 3, 467-475.

4   Attalli (G.), Leroux (R.): Programme d'informatique dans un service de gériatrie. *Revue de Gériatrie*, 1979, tome 4, n° 3, 95-103.

5   Attalli (G.), Leroux (R.): Un outil pour l'évaluation des handicaps: Géronte. In: Henrard (J.C.) Ed.: "Santé publique et vieillissement". Les Colloques de l'Inserm. Paris: INSERM, 1981, vol. 101, 147-154.

6   Attalli (G.), Leroux (R.): Informatisation d'un service de gériatrie. Relation entre la logistique, l'autonomie (Géronte) et les diagnostics. *Revue de Gériatrie*, 1982, tome 7, n° 1, 5-8.

7   Dubos (G.), Hugonot (R.): Evaluation de la dépendance des personnes âgées. *Revue de Gériatrie*, 1980, tome 5, n° 8, 367-370.

8   Gitz (A.M.), Etheve (M.), Kissel (C.), Rucher (M.F.), Niederger (M.P.), Charras (D.), Kuntzmann (F.): L'évaluation de l'autonomie des vieillards en unité de long séjour, facteur de communication et d'information de l'équipe soignante. A propos d'une technique d'évaluation. *Revue de Gériatrie*, 1980, tome 5, n° 9, 423-424.

9   Godon (M.): Géronte, un élément du dossier de soins. Journées de Gériatrie, Le Mans, 23-24 mai 1981. *Symbiose, Revue des Professions de Santé*, 1981, n° 20.

10 Hamilton (M.): A rating scale for depression. *J. Neurol. Neurosurg. Psychiatry*, 1960, 23-56.

11 Henrard (J.C.), Cassou (B.), Colvez (A.), Lazar (P.): Perte d'autonomie ou handicap, problèmes conceptuels. *Revue de Gériatrie*, 1980, tome 5, n° 8, 375-378.

12 Leroux (R.): Visualisation des handicaps: Géronte. Journées de Gériatrie, Le Mans, 23-24 mai 1981. *Symbiose, Revue des Professions de Santé*, 1981, n° 20.

13 Leroux (R.), Attalli (G.): L'informatique dans un service de Gériatrie. *Revue de Médecine de Tours*, 1982, tome 16, n° 2-1, 177-182.

14 Leroux (R.), Attalli (G.), Abonnat (Y.), Noël (J.L.), Pinot (P.): Détermination des besoins d'hébergement, d'hospitalisation, de maintien à domicile des personnes âgées. In: "Accidents vasculaires cérébraux. Recherche épidémiologique". Premier Congrès Francophone de Gérontologie, Paris, 17-18 septembre 1979. Paris: Masson, 1981, 590-593.

15 Leroux (R.), Attalli (G.), Abonnat (Y.), Noël (J.L.), Pinot (P.): Etude par enquête des limites d'une politique de maintien à domicile pour les personnes âgées. *Revue de Gériatrie*, 1982, tome 7, n° 1, 27-30.

16 Leroux (R.), Viau (G.), Fournier (M.), Bergeot (R.), Attalli (G.): Visualisation d'une échelle simple d'autonomie: Géronte. *Revue de Gériatrie*, 1981, tome 6, n° 9, 433-436.

17 Parish (J.G.), James (D.W.): A method for evaluating the level of independence during the rehabilitation of the disabled. *Rhumatology and Rehabilitation*, 1982, 21, 107-114.

18 Saft (M.): Visualisation d'une échelle de handicap pour personnes âgées. Thèse Med. Tours, 1981, 149.

19 Viau (G.): Géronte et la rééducation fonctionnelle. Journées de Gériatrie, Le Mans, 23-24 mai 1981. *Symbiose, Revue des Professions de Santé*, 1981, n° 20.

20 Windley (P.G.), Arch (D.), Scheiot (R.J.): An ecological model of mental health among small-town rural elderly. *Journal of Gerontology*, 1982, vol. 37, n° 2, 235-242.

CLIFTON ASSESSMENT PROCEDURES FOR ELDERLY (C.A.P.E.)

SPECIFICITY

* * *

TYPE OF INSTRUMENT

Rating scale
Questionnaire, Test

REFERENCE

Pattie (A.H.) · − A survey version of the Clifton assessment procedures for the elderly (C.A.P.E.). *British Journal of Clinical Psychology*, 1981, 20, 173-178.

Pattie (A.H.), Gilleard (C.J.) · − Manual of the Clifton assessment procedures for the elderly (C.A.P.E.). Kent: Hodder and Stoughton, 1979.

Language: Original version published in English, translations in Polish and French. **Great Britain**

Location: Enclosed in volume two page 202
See ref biblio nº 12, 18

For all information concerning the instrument and the translations write to the publisher or the author at the following addresses:

Hodder and Stoughton Educational
P.O. Box 702, Mill Road
Dunton Green
Sevenoaks, Kent, TN13 2YD, Great Britain

A.H. Pattie
York Psychology Services
Clifton Hospital
York, YO3, 6RD, G.B.

ORIGIN
The C.A.P.E. is based on **Clifton's** "Cognitive Assessment Scale" (ref. 13) which, together with the "Behavioural Rating Scale" (ref. 7) was inspired by the "Stockton Geriatric Rating Scale" (ref. 10).

PURPOSE
The instrument was devised with the aim of evaluating the degree of disablement of the elderly on the cognitive and behavioural level, and to assess the degree of their dependency.

POPULATION
Elderly out-patients and inpatients.

ADMINISTRATION
Rater: Physician, psychologist, non-specialist medical personnel.
The "Behavioural Rating Scale" should always be applied by those who are close to the subject.
Time required: 15-25 minutes in all. (10-15 minutes for the "Cognitive Assessment Scale", 5-10 minutes for the "Behavioural Rating Scale").
Training: Familiarisation with the instrument

DESCRIPTION
The C.A.P.E. is composed of 2 instruments: the "Cognitive Assessment Scale" and the "Behavioural Rating Scale". The "Cognitive Assessment Scale" is divided into 3 parts:
· The first is a verbal questionnaire exploring information and orientation (12 questions).
· The second is comprised of 4 sub-tests investigating mental abilities: counting, saying the alphabet, writing and reading.
· The third part is a psychomotor test.
The "Behavioural Rating Scale" is a rating scale with 3 grades assessing the possibilities for physical and social independence for the patient through 18 items. Scoring is done on the back of the summary sheet where a classification of 5 classes establishes the degree of dependency.

VARIABLES
Seven variables in two fields:
Cognitive functioning:
· Information-orientation
· Mental abilities
· Psychomotor ability

Behavioural disability:
· Physical disability
· Apathy
· Communication difficulties
· Social disturbance

VALIDATION
A factor analysis of principal components established a general factor of dependency (41-60% of the explained variance). Norming was done for each variable as well as for all enabling the differentiation of 5 grades of dependency (see the above mentioned manual).
Concurrent validity and **test-retest reliability** were completed (ref. 13, 14, 15).

OTHER WORKS
cited by author
A shortened "survey version" was developed (ref. 12) together with a number of other studies (ref. 11, 16, 17, 19).

APPLICATION
This instrument has diagnostic and prognostic value for clinical and experimental purposes. It can also contribute to the establishment of indications for placement which form a part of research done for epidemiological studies.

1 Bergman (K.), Foster (E.M.), Justice (A.W.), Mathews (V.): Management of the demented elderly patient in the community. *British Journal of Psychiatry*, 1978, 132, 441-449.

2 Boyd (W.D.): Psychiatric illness in the elderly. In: Forrest (A.D.), Affleck (J.W.), Zeally (A.K.). Eds: "Companion to psychiatric studies". Edinburgh: Churchill Livingstone, 1978.

3 Cattell (R.B.), Balcar (K.R.), Horn (J.L.), Nesselroade (J.R.): Factor matching procedures: an improvement on the S index; with tables. *Educational and Psychological Measurement*, 1969, 29, 781-792.

4 Donaldson (L.J.), Clayton (D.G.), Clarke (M.): The elderly in residential care: mortality in relation to functional capacity. *Journal of Epidemiology and Community Health*, 1980, 34, 96-101.

5 Gibson (A.J.), Moyes (I.C.), Kendrick (D.C.): Cognitive assessment of the elderly long-stay patient. *British Journal of Psychiatry*, 1980, 137, 551-557.

6 Gilleard (C.J.), Pattie (A.H.): The Stockton geriatric rating scale: a shortened version with British normative data. *British Journal of Psychiatry*, 1977, 131, 90-94.

7 Gilleard (C.J.), Pattie (A.H.): The effect of location on the elderly mentally infirm: relationship to mortality and behavioural deterioration. *Age and Ageing*, 1978, vol. 7, n° 1, 1-6.

8 Gilleard (C.J.), Pattie (A.H.), Dearman (G.): Behavioural disabilities in psychogeriatric patients and residents of old people homes. *J. of Epidemiology and Community Health*, 1980, vol. 34, n° 2, 106-110.

9 Kay (D.W.K.), Beamish (P.), Roth (M.): Old age mental disorders in Newcastle-Upon-Tyne. *British Journal of Psychiatry*, 1964, 110, 146-158.

10 Meer (B.), Baker (J.A.): The Stockton geriatric rating scale. *Journal of Gerontology*, 1966, 21, 392-403.

11 Pattie (A.H.): Disability in the elderly and patterns of care: a psychological study. Unpublished. D. Phil. Thesis, University of York, 1980.

12 Pattie (A.H.): A survey version of the Clifton assessment procedures for the elderly (CAPE). *Brit. J. of Clinical Psychology*, 1981, 20, 173-178.

13 Pattie (A.H.), Gilleard (C.J.): A brief psychogeriatric assessment schedule: validation against psychiatric diagnosis and discharge from hospital. *British Journal of Psychiatry*, 1975, 127, 489-493.

14 Pattie (A.H.), Gilleard (C.J.): The Clifton assessment schedule: further validation of a psychogeriatric assessment schedule. *British J. of Psychiatry*, 1976, 129, 68-72.

15 Pattie (A.H.), Gilleard (C.J.): The two-year predictive validity of the Clifton assessment schedule and the shortened Stockton geriatric rating scale. *British Journal of Psychiatry*, 1978, 133, 457-460.

16 Pattie (A.H.), Gilleard (C.J.): Admission and adjustment of residents in homes for the elderly. *J. of Epidemiology and Community Health*, 1978, vol. 32, 212-214.

17 Pattie (A.H.), Gilleard (C.J.): Psychological assessment and the care of the elderly. *Social Work Today*, 1979, vol. 10, n° 46.

18 Pattie (A.H.), Gilleard (C.J.): Manual of the Clifton assessment procedures for the elderly (C.A.P.E.). Kent: Hodder and Stoughton, 1979.

19 Pattie (A.H.), Gilleard (C.J.), Bell (J.): The Relationship of the intellectual and behavioural competence of the elderly to their present and future needs from community, residential and hospital services. Report for Yorkshire R.H.A., Research Grant Committee, 1979.

20 Pattie (A.H.), Williams (A.), Emery (D.): Helping the chronic patient in an industrial therapy setting: an experiment in inter-disciplinary cooperation. *Brit. J. of Psychiatry*, 1975, 126, 30-33.

21 Robinson (R.A.): Some applications of rating scales in dementia. In: Glen (A.I.M.), Wheeley (L.J.) Eds: "Alzheimer's disease". Edinburgh: Churchill Livingstone, 1979.

22 Sanford (J.R.A.): Tolerance of debility in elderly dependents by supporters at home: its significance for hospital practice. *British Medical Journal*, 1975, 3, 471-473.

QUESTIONNAIRE D'ENQUETE POUR ETUDE EPIDEMIOLOGIQUE
QUESTIONNAIRE FOR EPIDEMIOLOGICAL STUDIES

SPECIFICITY

* * *

TYPE OF INSTRUMENT

Questionnaire
18 principal headings
Rating scales

REFERENCE	Vignat (J.P.), Israël (L.), Broutchoux (F.) · – Recueil des données psychologiques et psychiatriques dans les enquêtes épidémiologiques chez les personnes âgées. In: "Accidents vasculaires cérébraux. Recherche épidémiologique". Premier congrès francophone de gérontologie, Paris, 17-18 septembre 1979. Paris: Masson, 1981, 421-441.

Language: Original version published in French.
France

Location: Enclosed in volume two page 205
See ref biblio nº 15

For all information concerning the instrument write to the author at the following address:

Liliane Israël,
Pavillon Chissé, C.H.R.U.
38700 La Tronche
Grenoble, France

ORIGIN   Numerous instruments and studies from the literature (ref. 10, 11, 12, 13, 14, 15, 16, 17).
Presentation and structure are original.

PURPOSE   The instrument is designed as a "canvas" or "model" which can be a source of inspiration for epidemiological surveys concerning defined somatic disorders when there is a need to evaluate psychological or psychopathological factors.

POPULATION   Elderly over 60 years, inpatients or out-patients.

ADMINISTRATION   *Rater:* Psychologist, physician, social worker.

Time required: 1 hour.

Training: Necessary.

Scoring: The instrument is composed of rating scales (5 points) and questions suitable for scoring.

VARIABLES
Past history:
· Genealogy and family history
· Previous experiences
· Attitudes toward the past
· Attitudes toward the present
· Attitudes toward the future
· Ecological data

Psychiatric data:
· Symptoms
· Defence mechanisms
· Communication
· Other elements of evaluation.

Psychological data:
· Appearance
· Emotional dependency
· Behavior and character
· Attitudes toward others
· Dependency
· Intellectual attitudes
· Attitudes toward drugs

Comments and global impression

These different variables are scored on two levels: investigative and comprehensive, which alternate through the administration. Comprehensive attitude requires two levels of empathic responding that are to be recorded on each occasion.

VALIDATION   Experimental questionnaire not yet used.

APPLICATION   Epidemiological surveys concerned with medical variables, where additional psychological and psychiatric information is needed.

1 Berthaux (P.): La mesure du vieillissement. *Gazette Médicale de France*, 1974, 81, 20, 2591-2602.

2 Durand (Y.): La formulation expérimentale de l'Imaginaire et ses modèles. *Circé*, 1969, 1, 151-248.

3 Georges (D.), Lallemand (A.), Coustenoble (J.), Loria (Y.): Validation pour l'analyse factorielle d'une échelle d'évaluation clinique des troubles de la sénescence cérébrale. Application à l'essai thérapeutique. *Thérapie*, 1977, 32, 173-180.

4 Hamilton (M.): General problems of psychiatric rating scales especially for depression. In: Pichot (P.) ed: "Psycological measurements in psychopharmacology. Mod. Probl. Pharmacopsychiat". Basel: Karger, 1974, 7, 125-138.

5 Israel (L.), Ohlmann (Th.), Hugonot (L.): Techniques particulières adaptées aux personnes âgées: leur validation par analyse factorielle en gériatrie. In: «Recherche expérimentale et investigation clinique de la sénescence cérébrale. Bâle: Sandoz, 1978.

6 Israel (L.), Ohlmann (Th.), Hugonot (R.), Drouet D'Aubigny (G.): Echelle clinique d'évaluation de la personnalité. Validation par analyse factorielle en gériatrie. *Encéphale*, 1980, tome VI, 81-91.

7 Moor (L.): Détérioration cérébrale ou vieillissement normal? Comment apprécier objectivement le fonctionnement intellectuel. *Ouest Médical*, 1977, 21, 1479-1484.

8 Plutchik (R.), Conte (H.), Lieberman (M.): Development of a scale (GIES) for assessment of cognitive and perceptual functioning in geriatric patients. *J. Am. Geriatrics Soc.*, 1971, vol. 19, n° 7, 614-623.

9 Poitrenaud (J.): Les modifications psychologiques liées à l'âge. *Gazette Méd.France*, 1968, 75, n° 16, 3359-3368.

10 Poitrenaud (J.), Barrère (H.): La mesure des déficits intellectuels pathologiques chez le sujet âgé. *Gazette Méd. France*, 1968, 75 n° 16, 3371-3394.

11 Rey (A.): L'examen clinique en psychologie. 2e édition. Paris: P.U.F., 1964.

12 Rorschach (H.): Psychodiagnostic. Paris: P.U.F., 1953.

13 Rosensweig (L.): Le test de Rosensweig. Picture Frustration Reaction Study. Paris: Editions du Centre de Psychologie Appliqueé, 1948.

14 Salzman (C.), Shader (R.), Kochansky (G.), Grenier (D.): Rating scales for psychotropic drug research with geriatric patients – Behaviour ratings. *J. Am. Geriatrics Society*, 1972, 20, 209-214.

15 Vignat (J.P.), Israel (L.), Broutchoux (F.): Recueil des données psychologiques et psychiatriques dans les enquêtes épidémiologiques chez les personnes âgées. In: "Accidents vasculaires cérébraux. Recherche épidémiologique". Premier congrés francophone de gérontologie, Paris, 17-18 Septembre 1979. Paris: Masson, 1981, 421-441.

16 Wechsler (D.): La mesure de l'intelligence chez l'adulte. 4e ed. Paris: P.U.F., 1973 , 291 p.

17 Wittenborn (J.R.): Wittenborn psychiatric rating scales. New York: Psychological Corporation, 1955.

SELF-ASSESSMENT SCALE – GERIATRIC (S.A.S.G.)

SPECIFICITY

* * *

TYPE OF INSTRUMENT

Ordinal rating scale
19 items, 7 grades

REFERENCE	**Yesavage (J.A.), Adey (M.), Werner (P.D.)** · – Development of a geriatric behavioral self-assessment scale. *Journal of the American Geriatrics Society*, 1981, 29, 6, 285-288.

Language: Original version published in English. Translated by the author into French and German.
U.S.A.

Location: Enclosed in volume two page 178
See ref biblio nº 9

For all information concerning the instrument or translations, write to the author at the following address:

Jerome Yesavage,
Department of Psychiatry and Behavioral Sciences,
Stanford University, Medical Center
P.O. Box 3832
Stanford, California 94305, U.S.A.

ORIGIN   The instrument is a self rating version of Sandoz Clinical Geriatric S.C.A.G. (ref. 7, 8).

PURPOSE   To develop a self-rating version of the commonly used existing scale (SCAG).

POPULATION   Elderly persons in good health or those suffering from mild dementia or moderate forms of dementia.

ADMINISTRATION *Rater:* The instrument is self completed.

Time required: 10-15 minutes.

Training: Not necessary.

Scoring: Each item is scored according to a scale of increasing frequency, from 1 (never) to 7 (several times a day). The global score varies from 19 to 133.

VARIABLES   The instrument consists of 18 items assessing four categories: mood, cognition, sociability and self-care:

· Confusion   · Hostility
· Loss of recent memory   · Indifference
· Loss of attention   · Obstructive behavior
· Disorientation   · Unsociability
· Depression   · Láck of cooperation
· Emotional lability   · Fatigue
· Lack of cleanliness   · Loss of appetite
· Anxiety   · Loss of initiative
· Irritability   · Global impression

VALIDATION   On a population of elderly subjects, mean age 66, all of whom were included in drug trials (ref. 9):
Concurrent validity: studies on the correlation of each item of the S.A.S.G. with corresponding items from the S.C.A.G.; applied by a rater-experimenter.
Reliability: Test-retest with one-week interval.

APPLICATION   Assessing treatment effects (drug trials or other trials). Programming care. May serve:
· for locating persons not seeking help, but who may benefit from treatment;
· as a means for evaluating the degree of disability in populations who are not regularly seen in health care settings;
· to assess the impact of projects aimed to improve the quality of life of the elderly.

1 Blackburn (R.): Personality in relation to extreme aggression in psychiatric offenders. *British Journal of Psychiatry*, 1968, 114, 821.

2 Carroll (B.J.), Fielding (J.M.), Blashki (T.G.): Depression rating scales: a critical review. *Arch. Gen. Psychiat.*, 1973, 28, 361.

3 Crook (Th.): Psychometric assessment in the elderly. In: Raskin (A.), Jarvik (L.) Eds: "Psychiatric symptoms and cognitive loss in the elderly". Washington, DC: Hemisphere Publ., 1978, 207-220.

4 Gottschalk (L.A.), Gleser (G.C.), Springer (K.J.): Three hostility scales applicable to verbal samples. *Arch. Gen. Psychiat.*, 1963, 18, 88.

5 Hughes (J.R.), Williams (J.G.), Currier (R.D.): An ergot alkaloid preparation (Hydergine) in the treatment of dementia: critical review of the clinical literature. *Journal of the American Geriatrics Society*, 1976, 24, 490.

6 Kochansky (G.E.): Psychiatric rating scales for assessing psychopathology in the elderly: critical review. In: Raskin (A.), Jarvik (L.), pathology in the elderly: critical review. In: Raskin (A.), Jarvik (L.), Eds: "Psychiatric symptoms and cognitive loss in the elderly". Washington, DC: Hemisphere Publ., 1978, 125-156.

7 Sandoz Clinical Assessment-Geriatric manual. East Hanover, N.J.: Sandoz Pharmaceuticals, 1979.

8 Shader (R.I.), Harmatz (J.S.), Salzman (C.): A new scale for clinical assessment in geriatric populations: Sandoz Clinical Assessment-Geriatric (SCAG). *Journal of the American Geriatrics Society*, 1974, vol. 22, 107.

9 Yesavage (J.A.), Adey (M.), Werner (P.D.): Development of a geriatric behavioral self-assessment scale. *Journal of the American Geriatrics Society*, 1981, vol. 29, n° 6, 285-288.

MULTILEVEL ASSESSMENT INSTRUMENT (M.A.I.)

SPECIFICITY

* * *

TYPE OF INSTRUMENT

Questionnaire of
216 items

REFERENCE	**Lawton (M.P.), Moss (M.), Fulcomer (M.), Kleban (M.)** · – A research and service oriented multilevel assessment instrument. *Journal of Gerontology*, 1982, 37, 1, 91-99.

Language: Original version published in English
U.S.A.

Location: See ref biblio n° 17

For all information concerning the instrument write to the author at the following address:

M. Powell Lawton,
Philadelphia Geriatric Center
5301 Old York Road
Philadelphia, Pennsylvania 19141, U.S.A.

ORIGIN
The instrument is inspired by the OARS (ref. 5), the CARE (ref. 9) and the author's own concepts related to levels of functioning and levels of competence (ref. 13).

PURPOSE
The instrument was conceived to meet the needs of a prospective, experimental survey measuring the well-being of the aged in different areas: physical, mental, social, economic.

POPULATION
Elderly out-patients or elderly persons living in residential homes.

ADMINISTRATION
Rater: Nurse. The majority may also be answered by an informant.
Time required: 50 minutes
Training: Necessary. Takes 3 days.

VARIABLES
Seven fields are assessed:
· Activities of daily living
· Cognition
· Time use
· Social interaction
· Physical health
· Personal adjustment
· Perception of the environment

VALIDATION
Was completed on a population of 590 elderly persons living in a residential home or in the community (ref. 17):
Construct validity
Concurrent validity
External validity
Inter-rater reliability
Test-retest reliability

APPLICATION
Research:
Epidemiological studies
Assessment of change occuring in patients receiving nursing care.

1 Andrews (F.M.), Withey (S.B.): Social indicators of well-being. New York, Plenum Press, 1976.

2 Bradburn (N.M.): The structure of psychological well-being. Chicago: Adline, 1969.

3 Campbell (A.), Converse (P.E.), Rodgers (W.L.): The quality of American life: perceptions, evaluations, and satisfaction. New York: Russell Sage, 1976.

4 Craik (K.H.): The comprehension of the everyday physical environment. *Journal of the American Institute of Planners*, 1968, 34, 29-37

5 Duke University. Center for the Study of Aging: Multidimensional functional assessment: The OARS methodology. 2nd ed. Durham, NC: Duke University, 1978.

6 Fillenbaum (G.), Pfeiffer (E.): The Mini-Mult: a cautionary note. *Journal of Consulting and Clinical Psychology*, 1976, 44, 698-703.

7 George (L.K.), Bearon (L.B.): Quality of life in older persons. New York: Human Sciences Press, 1980.

8 Gerard (R.): Aging and levels of organization. In: Birren (J.E.) Ed.: "Handbook of aging and the individual". Chicago: Univ.of Chicago Press, 1959.

9 Gurland (B.J.), Kuriansky (J.), Sharpe (L.), Simon (R.), Stiller (P.), Birkett (P.): The comprehensive assessment and referral evaluation (CARE): rationale, development, and reliability. *International Journal of Aging and Human Development*, 1977-1978, 8, 9-41.

10 Havens (B.), Thompson (E.): Aging needs assessment schedule. Winnipeg, Province of Manitoba, Canada: Department of Health and Community Services, 1976.

11 Kahn (R.L.), Goldfarb (A.I.), Pollack (M.), Peck (A.): Brief objective measures for the determination of mental status in the aged. *American Journal of Psychiatry*, 1960, 107, 326-328.

12 Katz (S.), Downs (T.D.), Cash (H.R.), Grotz (R.C.): Progress in development of the index of ADL. *Gerontologist*, 1970, 10, 20-30.

13 Lawton (M.P.): Assessing the competence of older people. In: Kent (D.), Kastenbaum (R.), Sherwood (S.) Eds.: "Research, planning and action for the elderly". New York: Behavioral Publications, 1972.

14 Lawton (M.P.): The Philadelphia Geriatric Center Morale Scale: a revision. *Journal of Gerontology*, 1975, 30, 85-89.

15 Lawton (M.P.), Brody (E.M.): Assessment of older people: self maintaining and instrumental activities of daily living. *Gerontologist*, 1969, 9, 179-186.

16 Lawton (M.P.), Cohen (J.): The generality of housing impact on the wellbeing of older people. *Journal of Gerontology*, 1974, 29, 194-204.

17 Lawton (M.P.), Moss (M.), Fulcomer (M.), Kleban (M.H.): A research and service oriented multilevel assessment instrument. *Journal of Gerontology*, 1982, vol. 37, n° 1, 91-99.

18 Lawton (M.P.), Ward (M.), Yaffe (S.): Indices of health in an aging population. *Journal of Gerontology*, 1967, 22, 334-342.

19 Lowenthal (M.): Lives in distress. New York: Basic Books, 1964.

20 National Center for Health Statistics: Health interview survey procedure, 1957-1974. Vital and Health Statistics, Series 1, n° 11. Rockville, MD: U.S. Dept. of Health, Education and Welfare, 1975.

21 Nydegger (C.) Ed.: Measuring morale: a guide to effective assessment. Washington, DC: Gerontological Society, 1977.

22 Pfeiffer (E.): A short portable mental status questionnaire for the assessment of organic brain deficit in elderly patients. *Journal of the American Geriatrics Society*, 1975, 23, 433-441.

NÜRNBERGER – ALTERS – INVENTAR (N.A.I.)
NUREMBERG GERONTOPSYCHOLOGICAL INVENTORY

SPECIFICITY

* * *

TYPE OF INSTRUMENT

Compound instrument including:
· 6 performance measures, 1 observation scale (15 items)
· 1 rating scale to be done by the investigator (9 items)
· 2 self-assessments (12 and 15 items resp.)

REFERENCE **Oswald (W.D.), Fleischmann (U.M.)** · – Nürnberger-Alters-Inventar: N.A.I. (The Nüremberg Gerontopsychological Inventory): Test instructions, materials and standard scores. Nuremberg, 1982.

Language: Original version published in German.
Translated into English, French version in preparation.
F.R.G.

Location: English version enclosed in volume two page 208
See ref. bilbio nº 15

For all information concerning the instrument or translations write to the author at the following address:

Wolf Oswald,
Universität Erlangen-Nürnberg
Regensburger Strasse 160
D – 8500 Nürnberg 30, FRG, RFA

ORIGIN Five performance measures by **Wechsler** (ref. 17, 18), **Chapuis** (ref. 3), **Benton** (ref. 1). One performance test, ratings and questionnaires by the authors.

PURPOSE Assessment and evaluation of age specific and therapeutically induced changes according to psychometric standards.

POPULATION Elderly (60 years and older), institutionalized and in private dwelling.

ADMINISTRATION *Rater:* Observer-rating has to be done by a nurse or close family members, rating has to be done by the psychologist, self evaluations with 2 separate scales. Performance tests and NAR have to be done by a psychologist, NAB has to be done by a nurse or relatives of the subject.
Time required: Performance tests take 30 minutes. It is recommended to do pretests of all test procedures.
Scoring: See the manual (ref. 15).

DESCRIPTION Performance measures:
· Digit Span (Wechsler)   · Maze Test (Chapuis)
· Digit Symbol (Wechsler)   · Benton Test (Benton)
· Block Design (Wechsler)   · Zahlen-Verbindungs-Test G (Oswald & Fleischmann)

Rating scales and questionnaires:
· A gerontopsychological personality rating, (NAR).
· A gerontopsychological observation scale for activities-of-daily-living, (NAB).
· A gerontopsychological self-rating scale, (NAS).
· A gerontopsychological questionnaire for life satisfaction, (NAF).

VARIABLES Performance measures: factor analyses reveal a "speed" / "power" distinction including memory rating scales and questionnaires; factor analyses depict the dimensions – activity/passivity:
· Mood; – anxiety for the NAR   · Self rated physical sphere; – activity
· Physical well-being; – instrumental activities   · Mood for the NAF
· Speech communication for the NAB

Norm scores are available for all test procedures for aged 55-69 years, 70-79 years and 80 – 95 years:

VALIDATION **Factor analyses** of the performance test and questionnaires
Interrelations between all assessment levels;
Correlation with independent physician's evaluation; and with EEG parameters;
Drug sensitivity;
Cross validations.

APPLICATION Drug trials.

1 Benton (A.L.): Der Benton-test. Bern, Stuttgart, 1968.

2 Cattell (R.B.): Personality and motivation, structure and measurement. New York, 1957.

3 Chapuis (F.): Der Labyrinth – Test. Bern, Stuttgart, 1959.

4 Fleischmann (U.M.): A differential-gerontological investigation of the speed/power dimensions in test performance. Paper presented at the XII International Congress of Gerontology, Hamburg, July 1981.

5 Herzfeld (U.), Christian (W.), Oswald (W.D.), Ronge (J.), Wittgen (M.): Zur Wirkungsanalyse von Hydergine im Langzeitversuch. Eine interdisziplinäre Studie. *Medizinische Klinik*, 1972, 67, 1118-1125.

6 Oswald (W.D.): Psychometrics as a method of testing drugs. *Sandorama*, 1979, 4, 26-31.

7 Oswald (W.D.): Psychometrische Verfahren und Fragebogen für gerontopsychologische Untersuchungen. *Zeitschrift für Gerontologie*, 1979, 12, 341-350.

8 Oswald (W.D.): Das Nürnberger-Alters-Inventar (NAI) als psychometrische Methode der klinischen Pharmakologie. In: Platt (D.) Hrsg.: "Funktionsstörungen des Gehirns im Alter". Stuttgart: Schattauer Verlag, 1981, 129-136.

9 Oswald (W.D.): Der Zahlen-Verbindungs-Test (ZVT-G) und Zusammenhänge mit Selbstbewertung, Alltagsaktivitäten und Persönlichkeitsmerkmalen bei N=50 Probanden zwischen 63 und 84 Jahren. In: Oswald (W.D.), Fleischmann (U.M.) Eds: "Experimentelle Gerontopsychologie". Weinheim: Beltz, 1981.

10 Oswald (W.D.): Psychometrics as a method in the framework of rehabilitation. Paper presented at the IVth World Congress of IRMA, April 1982.

11 Oswald (W.D.): Activities of daily living on the speed/power components in test performance. *Zeitschrift für Gerontologie*, 1982, 15.

12 Oswald (W.D.), Dennler (H.J.): Psychometric testing of elderly patients in the framework of clinical pharmacology. In: S.I.R.: Scientific International Research, Ed.: Proceedings of the International Symposium on experimental and clinical methodologies for study of acute and chronic cerebrovascular diseases, March 24-26 1980. Paris, New York: Pergamon Press, 1981, 351-357.

13 Oswald (W.D.), Fleischmann (U.M.): Psychometrics-problems and possibilities in clinical research. Paper presented at the XII International Congress of Gerontology, Hamburg, July 1981.

14 Oswald (W.D.), Fleischmann (U.M.): The Nuremberg Gerontopsychological Inventory as a psychometric assessment in aging brain. Paper presented at the International Symposium "Aging brain and ergot alkaloids", Roma, Oct. 28-30, 1981.

15 Oswald (W.D.), Fleischmann (U.M.): Nürnberger-Alters-Inventar (NAI), The Nuremberg Gerontopsychological Inventory: Test Instructions, materials and standard scores. Nuremberg, 1982.

16 Oswald (W.D.), Roth (E.): Der Zahlen – Verbindungs-Test (Z.V.T) Göttingen, 1978.

17 Wechsler (D.): A standardized memory scale for clinical use. *Journal of Psychology*, 1945, 19, 87-95.

18 Wechsler (D.): The measurement and appraisal of adult intelligence. Baltimore: Williams and Wilkins, 1939.

FUNCTIONAL ACTIVITIES QUESTIONNAIRE

SPECIFICITY

* * *

TYPE OF INSTRUMENT

Ordinal rating scale
10 items, 7 grades

REFERENCE	**Pfeffer (R.I.), Kurosaki (T.T.), Harrah (C.H.), Chance (J.M.), Filos (S.)** · – Measurement of functional activities in older adults in the community. *Journal of Gerontology,* 1982, vol. 37, 3, 323-329.

Language: Original version published in English.
U.S.A.

Location: See ref. biblio nº 9

For all information concerning the instrument write to the author at the following address:

Robert Pfeffer,
Department of Neurology
UCI Medical Center
101 City Drive South
Orange, California 92668, U.S.A.

ORIGIN
The original concept of the instrument is based on previous studies done by the author concerning instruments for assessing activities of daily living (ref. 8).

PURPOSE
The instrument was devised as a means for distinguishing functional impairments and resulting states of dependency.

POPULATION
Elderly out-patients or elderly persons living in residential homes or those living at home.

ADMINISTRATION
Rater: Nurse, social worker, patient's family or relatives.
Time required: 10-15 minutes.
Training: Brief training is necessary.
Scoring: Each of the 10 items is scored from 0 to 3 depending on the degree of severity.

VARIABLES
Functional activities of daily living assessed by clinical tests done by the patient.

VALIDATION
Was completed on a population of elderly persons (ref. 9):
Concurrent validity with the IADL from Lawton (ref. 7), Folstein's Scale (ref. 1), Smith's tests (ref. 13) and Raven (ref. 11).
External validity.

APPLICATION

Clinical:
Differential diagnosis
Prognosis
Evaluation of therapy

Research:
Epidemiological studies

1 Folstein (M.F.), Folstein (S.W.), Mc Hugh (P.R.): «Mini-mental state»: a practical method for grading the cognitive state of patients for the clinician. *Journal of Psychiatric Research*, 1975, 12, 189-198.

2 Gallagher (D.), Thompson (L.W.), Levy (S.M.): Clinical psychological assessment of older adults. In: Poon (L.W.) Ed.: "Aging in 1980's". Washington, DC: American Psychological Association, 1980.

3 Gilleard (C.J.), Pattie (A.H.): The Stockton geriatric rating scale: a shortened version with British normative data. *British Journal of Psychiatry*, 1977 131, 90-94.

4 Kahn (R.L.), Goldfarb (A.I.), Pollack (M.), Peck (A.): Brief objective measures for the determination of mental status in the aged. *American Journal of Psychiatry*, 1960, 117, 326-328.

5 Kleban (M.), Lawton (M.P.), Brody (E.M.), Moss (M.): Behavioral observations of mentally impaired aged: those who decline and those who do not. *Journal of Gerontology*, 1976, 31, 333-339.

6 Kuriansky (J.), Gurland (B.J.): The performance test of activities of daily living. *International Journal of Aging and Human Development*, 1976, 7, 343-352.

7 Lawton (M.P.), Brody (E.M.): Assessment of older people: self-maintaining and instrumental activities of daily living. *Gerontologist*, 1969, 9, 179-186.

8 Pfeffer (R.I.), Kurosaki (T.T.), Harrah (C.), Chance (J.M.), Bates (D.), Detels (R.), Filos (S.), Butzke (C.): A survey diagnostic tool for senile dementia. *American Journal of Epidemiology*, 1981, 114, 515-527.

9 Pfeffer (R.I.), Kurosaki (T.T.), Harrah (C.H.), Chance (J.M.), Filos (S.): Measurement of functional activities in older adults in the community. *Journal of Gerontology*, 1982, vol. 37, n° 3, 323-329.

10 Plutchik (R.), Conte (H.), Lieberman (M.), Bakur (M.), Grossman (J.), Lehrman (N.): Reliability and validity of a scale for assessing the functioning of geriatric patients. *Journal of the American Geriatrics Society*, 1970, 18, 491-500.

11 Raven (J.C.): Guide to using the coloured progressive matrices. London: H.K. Lewis and Company Ltd, 1956.

12 Remington (M.), Tyre (P.G.): The social functioning schedule: a brief semi-structured interview. *Social Psychiatry*, 1979, 14, 151-157.

13 Smith (A.): Symbol digit modalities test. Los Angeles, California: Western Psychological Services, 1973.

14 Spitzer (R.L.), Endicott (J.): Medical and mental disorder: proposed definition and criteria. In: Spitzer (R.L.), Klein (D.F.) Eds.: "Critical issues in psychiatric diagnosis". New York: Raven Press, 1978.

15 Weissman (M.M.), Sholomskas (D.), Pottinger (M.), Prusoff (B.A.), Locke (B.Z.): Assessing depressive symptoms in five psychiatric populations: a validation study. *American Journal of Epidemiology*, 1977, 106, 203-214.

GRILLE POUR L'EVALUATION DU DEGRÉ DE DEPENDANCE
DEPENDENCY FRAME FOR ELDERLY LIVING IN RESIDENTIAL HOMES

SPECIFICITY

* * *

TYPE OF INSTRUMENT

Ordinal rating scale
14 items, 6 grades

REFERENCE	The instrument was not published.
	Language: Written in French. **Switzerland**
	Location: Enclosed in volume two page 179
	For all information concerning the instrument write to the following address:
	Centre d'Information et Coordination pour Personnes Agées C.I.C.P.A. 6, rue du Nant 1207 Geneva, Switzerland

ORIGIN

The instrument is original, and was developed by the C.I.C.P.A. (Information and Coordination Center for the Elderly).

PURPOSE

To establish the amount of retirement pensions depending on the degree of handicap of elderly persons living in a home for the aged. The instrument also has the aim to establish a common language between various homes for the aged.

POPULATION

Elderly persons whose troubles are of somatic origin living in a home for the aged.

ADMINISTRATION

Rater: Nursing and paramedical staff in contact with the elderly person, the team responsible for programming treatment.

Time required: 15 minutes.

Training: Is carried out by a nurse adviser who is at the disposal of those raters having difficulties in applying the instrument.

Scoring: The questions were scored according to severity; one denotes independence and six dependency. Three categories were defined:
- A. – Pensioners completely independent (14 to 20)
- B. – Semi-dependent pensioners   (21 to 40)
- C. – Pensioners completely dependent   (41 to 80)

VARIABLES

Fourteen items cover assessment of dependency:

- Mobility
- Washing-dressing
- Feeding
- Continence
- Sleeping (resting)
- Mental state
- Orientation

- Communication
- Cooperation
- Care-Administration of drugs
- Preventive care
- Therapeutic care
- Physical rehabilitation
- Social therapy

VALIDATION

The instrument was developed by a nurse tutor. It was then tested and applied by a group of nurses employed in different homes for the aged.

OTHER WORKS
cited by author

The instrument is in current use in 7 institutions with approximately 1000 beds.

APPLICATION

Clinical: Can be used for survey and also to define goals for programming treatment for the elderly.

1 Colvez (A.), Henrard (J.C.): Evaluation des Centres de jour pour personnes âgées. *Gérontologie et société*, 1978, cahier n° 7, 33-42.

2 Dastoor (D.P.), Norton (S.), Boillat (J.), Minty (J.): A psychogeriatric assessment program. I: Social functioning and ward behavior. *Journal of the American Geriatrics Society*, 1975, vol. 23, n° 10, 465-471.

3 Garrad (J.), Bennett (A.E.): A validated interview schedule for use in population surveys of chronic disease and disability. *Brit. J. prev. soc. Med.*, 1971, 97-104.

4 Grauer (H.), Birnbom (F.): A geriatric functional rating scale to determine the need for institutional care. *Journal of the American Geriatrics Society*, 1975, vol. 23, n° 10, 472-476.

5 Katz (S.), Downs (T.D.), Cash (H.R.), Grotz (R.C.): Progress in development of the index of ADL. *The Gerontologist*, Spring 1970, part I, 20-30.

6 Plutchik (R.), Conte (H.), Lieberman (M.), Bakur M.) et al: Reliability and validity of a scale for assessing the functioning of geriatric patients. *Journal of the American Geriatrics Society*, 1970, vol. 18, n° 6, 491-500.

7 Williams (R.G.A.), Johnston (M.), Willis (L.A.), Bennett (A.E.): Disability: a model and measurement technique. *Brit. J. prev. soc. Med.*, 1976, 71-79.

GRILLE DE DEPENDANCE
DEPENDENCY ASSESSMENT SCALE

SPECIFICITY

$$* \quad * \quad *$$

TYPE OF INSTRUMENT

Ordinal rating scale
11 items, 3-6 grades

REFERENCE	**Centre de Gériatrie. Genève** · – Appréciation du degré d'autonomie-dépendance dans les activités de la vie quotidienne au Foyer de Jour, à domicile. The instrument was not published.

Language: Written in French.
Switzerland

Location: Enclosed in volume two page 180

For all information concerning the instrument write to the following address:

Italo Simeone,
Centre de Gériatrie
Rue du Nant, 8
12007 Geneva, Switzerland

ORIGIN

This instrument was inspired by the works of **Dastoor** (ref. 1), **Garrard** (ref. 2), **Grauer** (ref. 3), **Williams** (ref. 5), **Paillard** (ref. 4).

PURPOSE

The instrument was developed to establish a psychological profile and to give a better definition of the elderly population frequenting the Day Center in Geneva.

POPULATION

The instrument is to be applied on an out-patient population which is physically handicapped (vascular diseases, arthritis) and, above all, psychiatrically handicapped, (depression, loneliness, social isolation).

ADMINISTRATION

Rater: Nurse's aide.

Time required: 20-45 minutes depending on the type of handicap.

Training: Being closely familiar with the elderly person is necessary.

Scoring: The scale has 6 items with 5 grades. The 5 items assessing the activities of daily living are divided into different grades.

VARIABLES

Two groups of variables:
1. **Activities of daily living:**
   Self-care
   Feeding
   Therapeutic care
   Domestic activities
   Orientation
   Mobility

2. **Means of communication:**
   Vision
   Hearing
   Communication
   Leisure activities
   Relations with nursing staff

OTHER WORKS
cited by author

Medical studies concerning the Day Centers sponsored by the Department for Social Care and Public Health of the Canton of Geneva. Day centres receiving elderly persons with chronic diseases and mental disorders, where efforts are made to prevent their hospitalisation.

APPLICATION

· Medico-social profile of the population frequenting the day centres.
· Evaluation of treatment programming.
· Training for nurse's aides.

1   Dastoor (D.P.), Norton (S.), Boillat (J.), Minty (J.), Papadopoulou (F.), Muller (H.F.) A psychogeriatric assessment program. I: Social functioning and ward behavior. *J. of the Amer. Geriatr. Soc.*, 1975, 23, 10, 465-471.

2   Garrad (J.), Bennett (A.E.): A validated interview schedule for use in population surveys of chronic disease and disability. *Brit. J. Prevent. Soc. Med.*, 1971, 25, 95-104.

3   Grauer (H.), Birnbom (F.): A geriatric functional rating scale to determine the need for institutional care. *J. of the Amer. Geriat. Soc.*, 1975, 23, 10, 472-476.

4   Paillard (L.): Grille d'évaluation du degré de dépendance des pensionnaires d'une pension de personnes âgées. Genève: Ecole le Bon Secours.

5   Williams (R.G.A.), Johnston (M.), Willis (L.A.), Bennett (A.E.): Disability: a model and measurement technique. *Brit J. Prevent. Soc. Med.*, 1976, 30, 71-78.

SPECIFICITY

* * *

BILANS DE BEL AIR
SCHEDULE OF BEL AIR

By J. de Ajuriaguerra, J. Richard, R. Tissot, J. Constantinidis.

Was developed under the direction of **J. de Ajuriaguerra**, whose works, since 1960 have served to introduce new concepts in Geriatric Psychiatry.

Two models were used: Genetic Psychology (Piaget) and Neuropsychology which were best suited to therapeutic goals of adapting and developing attainable and necessary aspects of functioning.

The authors have pointed out the importance of studying not only impairments but also the best remaining abilities, in a qualitative, structural, contemporary and longitudinal analysis of behaviour. They consider this as a necessary first stage in any quantitative assessment. It is also necessary to reach an understanding of the mechanisms underlying this behavior. They insist on the biasis of observing and scoring behavior, as they insist that these cannot be considered as having the best approach to assess the patient's potential.

They introduce a normative approach which seeks to guard against preconceptions in categorising observations.

The following bibliography permits a more extensive review and a deeper appreciation of the development of their work in the period 1960-1982.

1 Ajuriaguerra (J. de), Boehme (M.), Richard (J.), Sinclair (H.), Tissot (R.): Désintégration des notions de temps dans les démences dégénératives du grand âge. *Encéphale*, 1967, 56, 385-438.

2 Ajuriaguerra (J. de), Dias Cordeiro (J.), Steeb (U.), Fot (K.), Tissot (R.), Richard (J.): A propos de la désintégration des capacités d'anticipation des déments dégénératifs du grand âge. *Neuropsychologia*, 1969, 7, 301-311.

3 Ajuriaguerra (J. de), Gauthier (G.): Etude de la désorganisation motrice dans un groupe de déments séniles «alzheimérisés». *Méd. et Hyg.*, 1964, 22, 409-410.

4 Ajuriaguerra (J. de), Kluser (J.P.) et al.: Praxies idéatoires et permanence de l'objet. Quelques aspects de leur désintégration conjointe dans les syndromes du grand âge. *Psychiat. Neurol.*, 1965, 150, 306-319.

5 Ajuriaguerra (J. de), Muller (M.), Tissot (R.): A propos de quelques problèmes posés par l'apraxie dans la démence. *Rev. Neurol.*, 1960, 102, 640-642.

6 Ajuriaguerra (J. de), Rego (A.), Richard (J.), Tissot (R.): De quelques aspects des troubles de l'habillage dans des démences tardives dégénératives ou à lésions vasculaires diffuses. *Ann. Méd. Psychol.*, 1967, 125, 189-218.

7 Ajuriaguerra (J. de), Rego (A.), Richard (J.), Tissot (R.): Psychologie et psychométrie du vieillard. *Confront. Psychiat*, 1970, 5, 27-37.

8 Ajuriaguerra (J. de), Rego (A.), Tissot (R.): Activités motrices stéréotypées dans les démences du grand âge. *Ann. Méd. Psychol.*, 1963, 121, 641-664.

9 Ajuriaguerra (J. de), Rego (A.), Tissot (R.): Le réflexe oral et quelques activités orales dans les syndromes démentiels du grand âge. Leur signification dans la désintégration psycho-motrice. *Encéphale*, 1963, 52, 189-219.

10 Ajuriaguerra (J. de), Rey Bellet-Muller (M.), Tissot (R.): A propos de quelques problèmes posés par le déficit opératoire de vieillards atteints de démence dégénérative en début d'évolution. *Cortex*, 1964, 1, 232-256.

11 Ajuriaguerra (J. de), Richard (J.), Tissot (R.): De l'application des méthodes de la psychologie génétique à l'étude de l'évolution des fonctions cognitives dans l'âge avancé. *Revue de Gérontologie d'expression française*, Juin 1972, 3, 17-24.

12 Ajuriaguerra (J. de), Richard (J.), Tissot (R.), Vengos (P.), Luke (A.), Raboud (A.M.): Les conduites alimentaires dans les démences dégénératives ou mixtes à prédominance dégénérative du grand âge. *Annales Médico-Psychologiques*, 1976, 2, 2, 213-241.

13 Ajuriaguerra (J. de), Steeb (U.), Richard (J.), Tissot (R.): Processus d'induction dans les démences dégénératives du grand âge. *Encéphale*, 1970, 59, 239-268.

14 Ajuriaguerra (J. de), Stretilevitch (M.), Tissot (R.): A propos de quelques conduites devant le miroir de sujets atteints de syndromes démentiels du grand âge. *Neuropsychologia*, 1963, 1, 59-73.

15 Ajuriaguerra (J. de), Tissot (R.): Application clinique de la psychologie génétique. In: "Psychologie et épistémologie génétique". Thèmes piagétiens. Paris: Dunod, 1966, 333-338.

16 Ajuriaguerra (J. de), Tissot (R.): Some aspects of psycho-neurologic disintegration in senile dementia. In: Muller (C.), Ciompi (L.) Eds.: "Senile dementia". Berne: Huber, 1968, 69-79.

17 Burnand (Y.), Richard (J.), Tissot (R.), Ajuriaguerra (J. de): Nature du déficit opératoire des vieillards atteints de démence dégénérative: conservation des quantités physiques, épreuves de causalité et de transitivité. *Encéphale*, 1972, 61, 5-31.

18 Burnand (Y.), Richard (J.), Tissot (R.), Ajuriaguerra (J. de): Acquisition d'un schème sensori-moteur par des sujets atteints d'amnésie de fixation. Mémoire au sens strict. Mémoire au sens large selon J. Piaget. *Annales Médico-Psychologiques*, 1977, 1, 3, 427-441.

19 Duval (F.): Désintégration du langage au cours des démences séniles dégénératives. Ses rapports avec les données de l'acquisition chez l'enfant. Thèse Méd., Paris, 1966.

20 Fot (K.), Richard (J.), Tissot (R.), Ajuriaguerra (J. de): Le phénomène de l'extinction dans la double stimulation tactile de la face et de la main chez les déments dégénératifs du grand âge. *Neuropsychologia*, 1970, 8 493-500.

21 Gaillard (J.M.): Désintégration du schéma corporel dans les états démentiels du grand âge. *J. Psychol. Norm. Path.*, 1970, 67, 443-472.

22 Gainotti (G.): Deterioramento intellettivo e desintegrazione psico-motrice nelle demenze. *Acta Neurol. Napoli*, 1970, 25, 607-627.

23 Guilleminault (C.): Désintégration de la perception stéréognosique dans les démences dégénératives du grand âge. Thèse Méd., Paris, 1968.

24 Richard (J.): De quelques aspects de la désintégration des fonctions supérieures du système nerveux central dans les démences tardives. *Médecine et Hygiène*, 1964, 22, 411-412.

25 Richard (J.): Démences séniles et comportements. *Fortbildungskurse schweiz. Ges. Psych.*, 1971, 4, 85-100.

26 Richard (J.): Neuro-psychologie et gériatrie. *Médecine et Hygiène*, 1974, 32, 1189-1193.

27 Richard (J.): De l'application et de l'intérêt des méthodes de la psychologie génétique en gériatrie avec un exemple sur la désintégration de la stéréognosie dans les démences dégénératives du grand âge. *Psychol. Med.*, 1975, 7, 9.

28 Richard (J.): Algunos problemas metodologicos propuestos para el estudia de la cognicion del paciente anciano. *Revista Española de Gerontologıa y Geriatria*, 1978, 13, 1, 59-74.

29 Richard (J.): Assessment modalities of cognitive functions of the aged patient: proceedings of the tenth congress of the Collegium International Neuro-Psychopharmacologicum, Québec, July 1976. In: Deniker (P.), Radouco-Thomas (C.), Villeneuve (A.) Eds.: "Neuro-psychopharmacology". Oxford, New York: Pergamon Press, 1978, 33-38.

30 Richard (J.): La prise en charge (pharmacologique et psycho-sociale) des états déficitaires cérébraux liés à l'âge: Symposium Bel-Air VI, Evian, Septembre 1979. In: Tissot (R.) Dir.: "Etats déficitaires cérébraux liés à l'âge". Genève: Ed. Georg., 1980, 355-366.

31 Richard (J.): Le vieillard, pierre de touche de la psychologie et de la psychiatrie. *La Revue Française de Santé Publique*, 1981, 16, 31-40.

32 Richard (J.): De la cognition dans la psychopathologie de l'âge avancé. In: Gilmore (A.J.M.), Svanborg (A.), Marois (A.), Battie (W.M.), Piotrowski (J.) Eds.: "Aging: a challenge to science and society. Vol. 2: Medicine and social science". Oxford: Oxford University Press, 1981, 117-128.

33 Richard (J.): Troubles majeurs du comportement: confusion et démence. In: Bourlière (F.): "Gérontologie: Biologie et clinique". Paris: Flammarion, 1982, 273-288.

34 Richard (J.), Bizzini (L.): Du caractère ontogénétique de l'épreuve de Pierre Marie-Behague et de son utilisation dans l'étude de l'orientation spatiale des démences de l'âge avancé. *Acta Psychiatrica Belgica*, 1979, 79, 3, 33-253.

35 Richard (J.), Bizzini (L.): Des procédures d'étude de la cognition dans les démences de l'âge avancé (de la structure à la fonction). Archives Piaget de Lisbonne, sous presse.

36 Richard (J.), Bizzini (L.), Arrazola (L.), Palas (C.): De l'actualisation des structures cognitives dans les démences à (ou à prédominance de) plaques séniles (PS) et dégénérescences neuro-fibrillaires (DNF). *Médecine et Hygiène*, 1981, 39, 4027-4036.

37 Richard (J.), Bizzini (L.), Boglietti (T.): De la réalisation d'itinéraires dans les démences de l'âge avancé. *Médecine et Hygiène*, 1979, 37, 3839-3842.

38 Richard (J.), Bizzini (L.), Boglietti (T.): De l'orientation spatiale et du sens de direction dans les démences à plaques séniles et à dégénérescences neuro-fibrillaires. *Revue de l'Université de Moncton (Nouveau-Brunswig)*, 1982, 14, 3, 149-162.

39 Richard (J.), Constantinidis (J.): Les démences de la vieillesse. *Confrontations Psychiatriques*, 1970, 5, 39-61.

40 Richard (J.), Constantinidis (J.): Les démences organiques de l'adulte. In: Pequignot (H.) Ed.: "Pathologie médicale". Paris: Masson, 1975, 1354-1369.

41 Richard (J.), Tissot (R.): Mémoire et intelligence dans les syndromes démentiels dégénératifs de l'âge avancé. *Rev. Méd. Dijon*, 1974, 9, 475-479.

42 Richard (J.), Tissot (R.), Engelberts (P.): Le signe de la main accompagnée vers le visage (note de séméiologie neurogériatrique). *Revue Médicale de Suisse Romande*, 1978, 98, 567-568.

43 Tissot (R.): Démences et mémoire. *Encéphale*, 1973, 62, 491-505.

44 Tissot (R.), Joannides (A.), Richard (J.), Ajuriaguerra (J. de): Activités perceptives visuelles dans les démences dégénératives du grand âge. *Rev. oto-neuro-ophtal.*, 1972, 44, 205-212.

45 Tissot (R.), Richard (J.), Duval (F.), Ajuriaguerra (J. de): Quelques aspects du langage des démences dégénératives du grand âge. *Acta neurol. belg.*, 1967, 67, 911-923.

2 - SUMMARY TABLES OF INSTRUMENTS INCLUDED

TITLE	YEAR	AUTHOR Country	SPECIFICITY FORM	LANGUAGE	ORIGIN	POPULATION
1. Depression Adjective Check List	1965	LUBIN United States	* * Check list	English Spanish, Dutch, Hebrew, Chinese	Original	All persons able to rea and understand Out-patient Inpatient
2. Self Rating Depression Scale	1965	ZUNG United States	* * Ordinal rating scale	30 languages	Grinker Overall Friedman	All depressed patient Out-patient Inpatient
3. Hamilton Rating Scale for Depression	1967	HAMILTON Great Britain	* * Ordinal rating scale	English French, German, Italian, Spanish, Japanese, Korean,	Original psychiatric texts	Out-patient Inpatient
4. New Physician's Rating List	1969	FREE United States	* * Ordinal rating scale	English	Lorr Overall	Out-patient
5. Psychotic Inpatient Profile	1969	LORR United States	* Ordinal rating scale Check list	English	Original	Inpatient Hospitalized
6. Measurement of Morale in Elderly	1973	PIERCE United States	* * * Check list	English	Srole Thompson	Inpatient Out-patient
7. Beck Depression Inventory	1974	BECK United States	* * Ordinal rating scale	English and other languages	Original	Inpatient Out-patient (psychiatric)
8. Echelle d'Observation Clinique	1974	CROCQ France	* Ordinal rating scale	French, English, Spanish, Arabic	Hamilton Wittenborn	Out-patient Inpatient
9. Philadelphia Geriatric Center Morale Scale	1975	LAWTON United States	* * * Check list	English Japanese	PGC Morale Scale	Inpatient Out-patient
10. Brief Anxiety Rating Scale	1976	WANG United States	* * Ordinal rating scale	English	Symptomatology of anxiety form Hamilton, Zung	Out-patient Inpatient
11. Standardized Assessment of Patients with Depressive Disorders	1977	W.H.O. Switzerland	* Nominal rating scale	English, French, Japanese, Polish, Bulgarian, German, Hindu	W.H.O. Cooperative study	Inpatient
12. Mania Rating Scale	1978	BECH Denmark	* Ordinal rating scale	Danish, French, English, German	Biegel Petterson	All ages with mania
13. Irritability-Depression -Anxiety Scale	1978	SNAITH Great Britain	* Ordinal rating scale	English, German French, Italian	Caine, Duke Hamilton	Inpatient Out-patient
14. Montgomery and Asberg Depression Rating Scale	1979	MONTGOMERY Great Britain	* * Ordinal rating scale	English and european languages, Chinese	C.P.R.S.	Depressed patients Out-patient Inpatient
15. W.H.O. Depression Scale	1980	BECH Denmark	* Mixed rating scale	English	WHO depression rating scale. Two Newcastle rating scales	
16. Self Rating Anxiety Scale	1980	ZUNG United States	* Ordinal rating scale	English, French, German, Italian, Siamese, Chinese, Dutch	Hamilton Feighner F.D.A.	Out-patient Inpatient
17. Carroll Rating Scale	1981	CARROLL United States	* * Check list	English	Hamilton	Depressed patients Out-patient Inpatient
18. Melancholia Rating Scale	1982	BECH Denmark	* Ordinal rating scale	Dutch, English, German, Spanish, Italian, French	Hamilton Cronholm Ottosson	Out-patient Inpatient
19. Geriatric Depression Scale	1982	YESAVAGE BRINK United States	* * * Check list	English, French, Spanish, German	Original	Depressed patients Out-patient Inpatient

RATER	N° OF ITEMS GRADES	TIME REQUIRED *Training*	APPLICATIONS	VARIABLES
Self- administered	7 check lists 32 adjectives	2 minutes *Light*	Diagnosis, screening, epidemiology, drug trials	Depressive mood
Self- administered	20 items 4 grades	3 minutes *Light*	Diagnosis, screening, research, drug trials	Anxiety, feeling of emptiness, disturbed mood, general and specific somatic symptoms, psycho-motor symptoms, suicidal thoughts, irritability
Psychiatrist, all trained persons	21 items 3-5 grades	20-30 minutes *Intensive*	Drug trials	Symptoms of melancholia
Physician	19 items 6 grades	5 minutes *Light*	Clinical, diagnosis, research, drug trials	Anxiety, depression, somatisation
Physician, nurse's aide, all persons acquainted with the patient	96 items 4-2 grades	10-15 minutes *Light*	Diagnosis, prognosis, research, drug trials	Behavior: mobility, withdrawal anxious depression, belligerence, need for care, observational data; perceptual disorganisation, disorientation
Psychologist, physician	45 items	2-4 hours *Medium or intensive*	Clinical practice, research	Depression, satisfaction, equanimity, will to live, social difficulties, physical health, sociability, perception positive or negative of ageing
Psychiatrist, psychologist, self-administered	21 items 4 grades	5 minutes *Light*	Outcome, screening	Intensity of depression
Physician	20 items 6 grades	20 minutes *No*	Drug trials	Intellectual efficiency, reaction time, neurotic symptoms, cooperation
Self- administered	17 items	10 minutes *No*	Clinical, research, rating of changes	Morale, psychological well-being
Physician, qualified staff	12 items 4 grades	10 minutes *Intensive*	Clinical, diagnosis, rating of changes, drug trials	Psychosomatic symptomatology of anxiety
Physician, psychologist, nurse's aide	60 items 5 grades	40 minutes *Yes*	Research, drug trials, epidemiology, care planning	Depression, psychiatric disorders
Psychiatrist, psychologist, skilled observer	11 items 5 grades	15-30 minutes *training course in psychiatry*	Drug trials, research	Symptoms of mania
Self- administered	18 items 4 grades	5 minutes *No*	Rating of changes	Irritability, depression, anxiety
Psychiatrist, psychologist, nurse, physician	10 items 7 grades	20 minutes 1-2 sessions	Drug trials, evaluation of treatment	Depression
Physician, psychologist, skilled observer	17 items	20 minutes *Intensive*	Clinic, diagnosis, drug trials, research	Depressive syndromes
Self-administered	20 items 4 grades	3 minutes *Light*	Clinic, diagnosis, drug trials, screening	Psycho-affective symptoms, anxiety
Self-administered	52 items	10 minutes *No*	Prognosis, screening, drug trials, longitudinal studies,	Depression
Psychiatrist, psychologist, trained staff	11 items 5 grades	15-30 minutes	Research, drug trials, screening	Symptomatology of melancholia
Self- administered	30 items	5-10 minutes *Light*	Drug trials, screening, diagnosis	Depression

TITLE	YEAR	AUTHOR Country	SPECIFICITY FORM	LANGUAGE	ORIGIN	POPULATION
1. Histoire du Lion	1965	BARBIZET France	** Psychometric test	French English	Modified Lesage's test	Out-patient Inpatient
2. Visual Retention Test	1965	BENTON United States	** Psychometric test	English, French, other languages	Original, Jacobs, Thurstone	Inpatient Out-patient
3. Shaw-Blocks Test	1967	LESTER United States	** Non verbal test	English	Bromley, Heim, Howson	Children, adults Inpatient Out-patient
4. Memory Battery	1968	BARBIZET France	** Psychometric test	English	Original	Out-patient Inpatient (adults with cerebral lesions)
5. Three Dimensional Constructional Praxis Test	1968	BENTON United States	** Non verbal test	English, French, other languages	Critchley, Fogel	Out-patient Inpatient
6. Information-Memory- Concentration Test	1968	BLESSED Great Britain	*** Psychometric test	English	Original	Inpatient Out-patient
7. Dementia Scale	1968	BLESSED-ROTH Great Britain	*** Rating scale	English	Original	Inpatient Out-patient
8. Scale for the Measurement of Memory	1968	WILLIAMS Great Britain	** Psychometric test	English	Wechsler, Rey & Davis, Walton	Out-patient Inpatient
9. Praxies Grapho-Motrices	1969	ANDREY France	** Non verbal test	French	Bender	Out-patient Inpatient
10. Simple Non-Language Test of New Learning	1969	FOWLER United States	** Non verbal test	English	Wechsler	Inpatient Out-patient
11. Short Term Memory Test	1970	DANA United States	*** Psychometric test	English	Original, Cameron, Gilbert Kamin, Maxwell Pelz, Wechsler	Inpatient (patients with psychiatric disorders)
12. Screening Test for Organic Brain Disease	1970	NAHOR United States	** Non verbal test	English	Numerous works	Inpatient Out-patient
13. Wechsler Adult Intelligence Scale	1970	WECHSLER United States	** Psychometric test	English, French, Italian, other languages	Wechsler- Bellevue Intelligence rating scale	Inpatient Out-patient
14. Geriatric Inter- personal Evaluation Scale	1971	PLUTCHIK United States	*** Psychometric test	English	Kahn, Wilson Dinoff	Inpatient
15. Embedded Figures Test	1971	WITKIN United States	** Non verbal test	English	Gottschaldt	Inpatient Out-patient (patient with psycho-motor and visual disorders)
16. Mental Test Score	1972	HODKINSON Great Britain	*** Questionnaire	English	Blessed Roth	Inpatient
17. Set Test	1972	ISAACS Great Britain	*** Psychometric test	English	Not specified	Out-patient Inpatient

MENTAL - COGNITIVE FUNCTIONS

...TER	N° OF ITEMS GRADES	TIME REQUIRED *Training*	APPLICATIONS	VARIABLES
...ychologist, ...ysician	22 items	3 minutes *Light*	Clinical practice, diagnosis, prognosis, research, drug trials	Immediate memory, recall, capacity for synthesis, forgetfulness, attention, language
...ychologist	10 items	5 minutes *Intensive*	Clinical practice, diagnosis, research	Visual and immediate memory, visuo-spatial ability
...ychologist, ...ysician		10-15 minutes *Light*	Clinical practice, Research	Logical reasoning, creativity, rigidity
...ychologist, ...eech-therapist	6 sub-tests	25 minutes *Intensive*	Clinical practice, diagnosis	Immediate memory recall, learning, retention
...ychologist	3 sub-tests	16 minutes *Learning the method*	Clinical practice, diagnosis	Three dimensional constructional ability, visuo-spatial ability
...ysician, ...ychologist, ...rse's aide, ...cial worker	27 questions	30 minutes *Light*	Clinical practice, research, diagnosis	Dementia, orientation, memory, concentration, cognitive performance
...ychologist, ...ysician, ...rse's aide	11 items 4 grades	35-40 minutes *Light*	Differential diagnosis, research	Dementia, change in activities of daily living, habits, personality
...ychologist, ...ysician	5 sub-tests	10 minutes *Light*	Clinical practice, diagnosis	Immediate memory, medium term memory, long term memory, recognition, verbal and non verbal learning
...ychologist	10 figures	10 minutes *No*	Diagnosis, research	Somatic pathology, eye-hand coordination
...ychologist, ...ysician	10 items	20 minutes *Light*	Clinical practice, diagnosis	Short term recognition, learning
...ychologist, ...ysician, ...rse's aide	5 items	15 minutes *Light*	Clinical practice, diagnosis	Spatial memory recall
...ychologist, ...ysician	8 items	10 minutes *No*	Clinical practice, diagnosis	Eye-hand coordination
...ychologist	11 sub-tests	75 minutes *Intensive*	Clinical practice, diagnosis, prognosis, research, epidemiology	Verbal performance, intelligence, attention, concentration, visuo-spatial ability
...ychologist, ...erapist	16 items	25 minutes *Training technique*	Clinical practice, therapeutic evaluation	Perception, memory, intelligence
...ychologist	12 items	20 minutes *Learning the method*	Clinical practice, research	Perceptual and logical analysis, visuo-spatial ability, field-dependance, independance, cognitive style
...ychologist, ...ysician, ...rse's aide	10 questions	3 minutes *No*	Clinical, screening	Memory, orientation, general information
...ychologist, ...ysician, ...rse's aide, ...n-specialist ...re staff	4 sub-tests	5 minutes *Minimum*	Clinical practice, screening of dementia, epidemiology	Mental agility, recall, irritability

TITLE	YEAR	AUTHOR Country	SPECIFICITY FORM	LANGUAGE	ORIGIN	POPULATION
18. Simple Methods of Testing Ability	1972	SILVER Great Britain	* * * Psychometric test	English	Original	Inpatient
19. Dementia Screening Scale	1974	HASEGAWA Japan	* * * Questionnaire	Japanese English French	Kaneko, Shinfuku, Roth, Blessed Guttman	Out-patient Inpatient
20. Echelle de Dévelop- pement de la Pensée Logique	1974	LONGEOT France	* * Non verbal test	French	Piaget, Inhelder	All aged persons understanding orders
21. Abbreviated Mental Test	1974	QURESHI Great Britain	* * * Questionnaire	English	Roth, Hopkins	Inpatient
22. Mini Mental State	1975	FOLSTEIN United States	* * * Psychometric test	English Spanish Portuguese	Kirby, Meyer	Out-patient Inpatient
23. Ischemia Score	1975	HACHINSKI Canada	* * Check list	English	Original Mayer-Gross Rosen	Out-patient Inpatient
24. Short Portable Mental Status Questionnaire	1975	PFEIFFER United States	* * * Questionnaire	English	Wechsler, Kahn	Out-patient Inpatient
25. Batterie de Vigilance en Institution	1976	ISRAEL France	* * * Psychometric test	French	Zazzo, Wechsler, Rey, Thurstone	Inpatient
26. Philadelphia Geriatric Center Mental Status Questionnaire	1977	FISHBACK United States	* * * Questionnaire	English	Kahn, Pfeiffer	Out-patient Inpatient
27. Cognitive Capacity Screening Examination	1977	JACOBS United States	* * Questionnaire	English	Numerous authors	Out-patient Inpatient
28. Confusion Assessment Schedule	1977	SLATER Great Britain	* * * Questionnaire	English	Slater, Roth	Demented patients Out-patient Inpatient
29. Modified Tooting Bec Questionnaire	1978	DENHAM Great Britain	* * * Questionnaire	English French	Roth, Blessed Isaacs, Doust	Inpatient
30. Echelle d'Efficience Intellectuelle	1978	JANIN France	* * * Psychometric test	French	Benton, Bender Wechsler	Out-patient Inpatient

TER	N° OF ITEMS GRADES	TIME REQUIRED *Training*	APPLICATIONS	VARIABLES
ysician, psychologist, rse's aide (ecialised or not)	16 items	15 minutes *No*	Clinical practice, estimation of discharge-readiness	Memory, orientation, speech, praxia, sight and hearing
ysician, psychologist	11 questions 4 grades	15 minutes *No*	Diagnosis, research, epidemiological studies	Orientation, memory, general information, arithmetic
ychologist	5 sub-tests	75 minutes *To get familiar with technique*	Clinical practice, research	9 factors of intelligence, cognitive deficit
ysician, psychologist, rse's aide	10 items	3 minutes *No*	Clinical practice, diagnosis	Orientation for time, place and persons, dementia
ysician, psychologist, rse's aide (non spe-lised), social worker	11 sub-tests	10 minutes *Light*	Clinical practice, screening of functional disorders, diagnosis, prognosis, training	Orientation, recent memory, attention-concentration, arithmetic, speech, motor activities
ysician	9 or 13 items	5 minutes *Intensive*	Clinical, etiological diagnosis of dementia, drug trials	Evolution and history of the disease, neuro-psychiatric status, previous medical history
ysician, psychologist, rse's aide, cial worker	10 questions	2 minutes *No*	Functional diagnosis, prognosis, drug trials, surveys	Recent and remote memory, orientation in time and place, mental agility
ychologist	7 sub-tests	25 minutes *Psychological training*	Clinical practice, drug trials	Awareness, memory, mental agility, psychomotor ability
ysician, nurse, rse's aide	35 items	10 minutes *No*	Clinical diagnosis, organicity	Orientation in time and place, memory, intelligence, independence
ysician, psychologist, ental health ofessional	30 items	5 minutes *To get familiar with technique*	Clinical practice, diagnosis	Orientation, recent and medium memory recall, attention, concentration, mental agility, logical thought process, arithmetic
on qualified rsonnel	21 items	10 minutes *No*	Clinical, functional diagnosis	Orientation, memory
ychologist, physician, rse's aide	16 items	3 minutes *No*	Clinical prognosis, care planning	Orientation for time, place and persons, general information
ysician, ychologist	5 tests	30 minutes *Training in psychometric testing*	Clinical practice, diagnosis, research	Visuo-spatial perception, recent and remote memory attention, concentration, logical thought process

MENTAL - COGNITIVE FUNCTIONS

TITLE	YEAR	AUTHOR Country	SPECIFICITY FORM	LANGUAGE	ORIGIN	POPULATION
31. Stimulus Recognition Test	1979	BRINK United States	*** Psychometric test	English	Mental Status Questionnaire, Face Hand test	Out-patient Inpatient
32. Misplaced Objects Task	1979	CROOK United States	*** Non verbal test	English	Original	Out-patient Inpatient
33. Extended Scale for Dementia	1979	HERSCH Canada	*** Psychometric test	English	Mattis, Dementia scale, W.A.I.S.	Demented elderly persons
34. Kendrick Battery for the Detection of Dementia in the Elderly	1979	KENDRICK Great Britain	*** Psychometric test	English, Spanish	Synonym Learning Test, Walton Black Test	Out-patient Inpatient (over 55 years)
35. Galveston Orientation and Amnesia Test	1979	LEVIN United States	** Questionnaire	English	Pattie, Shapiro, Plutchik, Roth, Kahn, Kay, Folstein, Pfeiffer	Out-patient Inpatient (Elderly with head injury)
36. Check List Differentiating Pseudodementia from Dementia	1979	WELLS United States	** Check list	English	Original	Inpatient
37. Orientation Scale for Geriatric Patients	1980	BERG Sweden	*** Questionnaire	Swedish, English	Kahn, Qureshi, Lifshitz, others	Inpatient
38. Hierarchic Dementia Scale	1980	COLE Canada	*** Rating scale Check-list	English	Luria, Piaget, Constantinidis, Ajuriaguerra	Out-patient Inpatient (demented)
39. Batterie de Vigilance en Ambulatoire	1980	ISRAEL France	*** Psychometric test	French	Zazzo, Wechsler, Rey, Thurstone	Out-patient
40. Echelle Clinique d'Aptitudes Intellectuelles	1980	ISRAEL France	*** Ordinal rating scale	French	Original	Out-patient
41. Batterie de Fluidité à l'Usage des Généralistes	1980	ISRAEL France	*** Psychometric test	French	Original	Out-patient
42. Batterie de Mémoire en Ambulatoire	1980	ISRAEL France	*** Psychometric test	French	Original Literature	Out-patient
43. Examen Psychologique pour Personnes Agées Hospitalisées	1980	ISRAEL France	*** Psychometric test	French	Zazzo, Clement, Wechsler, Rey, Thurstone	Inpatient
44. Guild Memory Test	1981	GILBERT United States	** Psychometric test	English	Babcock, Benton, Wechsler	Out-patient Inpatient (without mental and physical disorders)
45. Shopping List Task	1981	MAC CARTHY United States	*** Psychometric test	English	Various authors	Out-patient Inpatient (memory disorders)
46. Memory Activity Scale	1982	SIGNORET France	** Psychometric test	English French	Original	Out-patient Inpatient
47. Bilan d'évaluation du Syndrome Démentiel	1982	ISRAEL France	*** Questionnaire Tests	French	Ajuriaguerra, Longeot	Out-patient Inpatient

ATER	N° OF ITEMS GRADES	TIME REQUIRED *Training*	APPLICATIONS	VARIABLES
sychologist	10 items	12 minutes *To get familiar with the technique*	Clinical practice, diagnosis, research	Dementia, recognition, recent memory
hysician, sychologist, urse's aide	Clinical approval	6 (3+3) minutes +20 pauses	Clinical practice, diagnosis, prognosis,	Memory recall
sychologist	23 sub-tests	60 minutes *Light*	Clinical practice, research, drug trials, diagnosis	Dementia, cognitive variables
hysician, sychologist, urse's aide, ocial worker	2 sub-tests	15 minutes *1/2 day regular repeating*	Clinical practice, diagnosis, prognosis, drug trials, research, screening for dementia	Visual memory for recent events, speed of performance
hysician, sychologist, urse	10 items	5 minutes *Light*	Clinical prognosis, drug trials	Orientation in time and place, recent memory anterograde and retrograde amnesia
hysician	22 items	15 minutes *Intensive*	Clinical, research	Behavior, symptoms of pseudo-dementia
hysician, sychologist, urse's aide, ocial worker	10 questions	5 minutes *No*	Clinical, diagnosis, research, drug trials, prognosis	Dementia, orientation for time, place and toward persons
hysician, sychologist, urse's aide	20 rating scales 5-10 items per rating scale	30 minutes *Light*	Drug. trials, diagnosis, prognosis	Praxia, memory, orientation, recognition
sychologist	7 sub-tests	15 minutes *Psychological training*	Clinical practice, research, drug trials, diagnosis	Awareness, memory, psychomotor ability, mental agility
hysician, sychologist	9 items 5 grades	5 minutes *No*	Drug trials, clinic	Awareness, attention, dynamism, verbal fluency, orientation, memory, fatigability
hysician sychologist, urse's aide	5 sub-tests	20 minutes *1 period 2-3 hours*	Clinical practice, drug trials	Memory, attention, mental agility
sychologist	7 sub-tests	10-20 minutes *Necessary*	Epidemiology, drug trials	Memory, immediate recall, learning, inhibition
sychologist	7 sub-tests	20-25 minutes *Necessary*	Clinical practice,	Memory, mental agility, psychomotor ability
sychologist	8 sub-tests	20-30 minutes *Psychometric training*	Clinical practice, research, differential diagnosis	Immediate recall, attention concentration, associative memory
hysician, sychologist	10 items (5 tests)	10 minutes *To get familiar with the technique*	Clinical practice (memory disorders)	Recent and medium term memory, retention, recall, recognition, learning
hysician, sychologist	14 sub-tests	45 minutes *Intensive*	Clinical diagnosis	Memory
sychologist, hysician, ccupational erapist	Clinical approach	25 minutes *Necessary*	Clinical care planning	Memory, gnosis, operational mechanism spatial structuration

TITLE	YEAR	AUTHOR Country	SPECIFICITY FORM	LANGUAGE	ORIGIN	POPULATION
1. Nurse's Observation Scale for Inpatient Evaluation	1965	HONIGFELD United States	** NOSIE 80 * NOSIE 30 Ordinal rating scale	English, German, Italian, French, Spanish, Swedish	Various	Inpatient
2. Discharge Readiness Inventory	1966	HOGARTY United States	** Ordinal rating scale	English	Original	Psychiatric adults, chronics
3. Archétype Test à 9 Éléments	1967	DURAND France	** Test Questionnaire	French, Portuguese, English	Original Durand	Out-patient Inpatient
4. Short Scale for the Assessment of Mental Health	1967	SAVAGE United States	*** Check list	English	M.M.P.I.	Out.-patient Inpatient
5. Patient Activity Check List	1969	AUMACK United States	* Inventory Check list	English	Higg's works of schizophrenics	Psychiatric Inpatients
6. Viro Orientation Scale	1972	KASTENBAUM United States	*** Nominal rating scale	English	Original	Out-patient Inpatient
7. Adult Personality Rating Schedule	1972	KLEBAN-BRODY United States	*** Ordinal rating scale	English	Philadelphia Geriatric Centre Brody	Out-patient Inpatient (Deteriorated)
8. Senior Apperception Technique	1973	BELLAK United States	*** Projective test	English	Murray's T.A.T. Wolk's G.A.T.	Out-patient Inpatient
9. Behavior Rating Scale	1973	WILLIAMS United States	*** Rating scale	English	Original Kankakee hospital	Inpatient (disabled and hospitalized)
10. Present State Examination	1973	WING SARTORIUS Great Britain	* Questionnaire	English 30 languages	Various tests Lorr, Spitzer, Wittenborn	Out-patient Inpatient (not demented)
11. D - Test	1974	FERM Finland	*** Ordinal rating scale	Finnish English	Isaacs, Walkey, Grauer, Kahn, Pfeiffer, Inglis, Wechsler	Out-patient Inpatient (psychogeriatric patients)
12. Geriatric Mental State Schedule	1976	COPELAND Great Britain	*** Questionnaire	English, German, French, Danish, Dutch	Wing, Spitzer	Out-patient Inpatient (before all)
13. Hypochondriasis Scale Institutional Geriatric	1978	BRINK United States	*** Check list	English, Spanish	M.M.P.I. Rating scale of Pilowski	Out-patient Inpatient
14. Short Psychiatric Evaluation Schedule	1979	PFEIFFER United States	*** Check list	English	M.M.P.I. Kincannon, Savage, Britton	Out-patient Inpatient
15. Survey Psychiatric Assessment Schedule	1980	BOND Great Britain	*** Questionnaire	English	Copeland	Out-patient Inpatient (hospitalized)
16. Evaluation Clinique de la Personnalité	1980	ISRAEL France	*** Ordinal rating scale	French, English	Numerous rating scales from English literature	Out-patient (over 65 years)
17. M. Test	1981	MEZZENA Italy	* Projective test	Italian	T.A.T. Rorschach	Whole population
18. Behavioural and Mood Disturbance Scale	1982	GREENE Great Britain	*** Ordinal rating scale	English	Gurel, Lawton, Meer, Pattie Bergmann, Wilkinson	Demented, at home

ATER	N° OF ITEMS GRADES	TIME REQUIRED *Training*	APPLICATIONS	VARIABLES
urse, nurse's aide	80 or 30 items 5 grades	20 minutes *Light*	Research, clinical drug trials	Social competence, social interests, tidiness, irritability, psychosis, depression, cooperation
ocial worker	45 items 9 grades	30 minutes	Clinical practice, research	Psychosocial adaptation, adaptability, aggressive attitude, psychopathological symptoms
sychiatrist, psychologist	27 answers open ended	1 hour to 1 hour and 30 minutes *Intensive*	Clinical research, diagnosis, prognosis, psychotherapy	Symbolic structures, nervousness, debility, psychosis, psychosomatic disorders
hysician, psychologist, urse, social worker	15 items	5 minutes *Necessary*	Clinical practice, prognosis, drug trials	Mental health, somatic status, sleeping, perceiving health activities, anxiety
urse's aide	24 items	Very short *Light*	Clinical and sociological practice	Appropiate and inappropiate behavior
hysician, psychologist, urse's aide, ocial worker	4 grades	5 minutes *Intensive*	Clinical practice, diagnosis, prognosis, research, drug trials, training in behavioral observation	Vigor, integration of cognitive functions, sociability, orientation
ocial worker, elatives	50 items 5 grades	15-30 minutes *No*	Prognosis and clinical practice (evaluative prognosis for deterioration)	Aggressivity, emotional, v investment, negativism, anxiety, social integration
sychologist	16 blanks	5 minutes by blank *Yes*	Psychodiagnosis	Family and social relationships, perception of environment
urse's aide	50 items 10 points	30 minutes *Necessary*	Clinical practice, evaluation of progress and needs	Adaptability, expressiveness, psysical appearance, self-care, mental alertness, responsibility, attitude
sychiatris, ained lay nterviewer	20 items	45-60 minutes *a week's training necessary*	Epidemiology, drug trials, research, prognosis, screening of mental pathology	Psychiatric symptoms, mood
hysician, psychologist, urse's aide	13 items 6 grades	30 minutes	Rating of changes, research, drug trials, epidemiological studies	Activities of daily living, orientation, family and social relationships, behavior
hysician, psychologist, urse, social worker	600 items	30-40 minutes *Intensive*	Research, diagnosis, prognosis, epidemiological studies, follow-up	Psychiatric symptoms
hysician	6 items	1 minute *Light*	Diagnosis, research, clinical practice	Hypochondrial attitudes
hysician, psychologist, urse's aide, ocial worker	15 questions	7 minutes *Brief*	Drug trials, diagnosis, prognosis, psychogeriatric research	Depression, hypochondria, anguish, dissatisfaction, anti-social behavior
hysician, psychologist, urse's aide, nurse	51 items 2-3 grades	10-25 minutes *Necessary (by film)*	Longitudinal epidemiological studies, determination of needs and public services	Somatic pathology, mood nervousness, schizophrenia and delirium
hysician, psychologist,	26 bi-polar items, 5 grades	10 minutes *Necessary*	Clinical trials, research, drug trials, diagnosis of emotional maladjustment	Balance and imbalance, social adaptation, emotionality
hsycian, psychologist,	20 blanks	20 minutes *Necessary*	Psychodiagnostic evaluation, drug trials	Life style, personality, behavior
elative	31 items 5 grades	15-20 minutes *No*	Prognosis, indications for placement care planning, therapeutic studies	Mood, behavior, apathy

MENTAL

YEARS	AUTHORS	Type of instrument*	VALIDITY					RELIABILITY			SENSITIVITY			Other
			Face	Construct	Concurrent	External	Predictive	Inter-rater	Test-Retest	Split half, Parallel forms, Int. consistency	Inter Individual	Intra Individual	Scoring	
MOOD														
1965	LUBIN	CL			X					X				X
1965	ZUNG	Ro		X	X	X				X	X			X
1967	HAMILTON	Ro		X	X			X						
1969	FREE	Ro		X	X	X				X				
1969	LORR	Ro.CL		X				X	X		X	X		X
1973	PIERCE	CL		X							X			
1974	BECK	Ro				X	X	X		X	X	X		
1974	CROCQ	Ro												
1975	LAWTON	CL		X						X				
1976	WANG	Ro			X	X				X		X		
1977	SARTORIUS	Rn												X
1978	BECH	Ro						X						X
1978	SNAITH	Ro		X	X					X	X			X
1979	MONTGOMERY	Ro		X	X			X				X		X
1980	BECH	Rmix						X						X
1980	ZUNG	Ro	X		X					X	X			X
1981	CARROLL	CL			X	X			X	X	X			
1982	BECH	Ro			X			X		X				X
1982	YESAVAGE BRINK	CL			X				X	X	X	X		
BEHAVIOR														
1965	HONIGFELD	Ro		X		X		X			X	X		
1966	HOGARTY	Ro	X					X						
1967	DURAND	T		X	X	X								
1967	SAVAGE	CL				X					X			X
1969	AUMACK	CL				X	X	X	X	X	X			
1972	KASTENBAUM	Rn		X				X						
1972	KLEBAN	Ro		X			X							X
1973	BELLAK	T												X
1973	WILLIAMS	R						X					X	
1974	WING	Q				X		X						
1974	FERM	R				X	X	X	X	X				
1976	COPELAND	Q		X	X	X		X	X					
1978	BRINK	CL									X			X
1979	PFEIFFER	CL			X						X			X
1980	BOND	Q.CL			X									X
1980	ISRAEL	Ro		X				X						
1981	MEZZENA	T												
1982	GREENE	Ro		X							X			

*Type of instrument:

CL	: Check list	R	: Rating scale
Q	: Questionnaire	Ro	: Ordinal rating scale
T	: Test	Rn	: Nominal rating scale
		Rmix	: Mixed rating scale

MENTAL

COGNITIVE FUNCTIONS

YEARS	AUTHORS	Type of instrument*	VALIDITY					RELIABILITY			SENSITIVITY			Distribution norms Standardization
			Face	Construct	Concurrent	External	Predictive	Inter-rater	Test-Retest	Split half, Parallel forms, Int. consistency	Inter Individual	Intra Individual	Scoring Other	
1965	BARBIZET	T				X					X			X
1965	BENTON	T		X							X	X		X
1967	LESTER	T			X				X					
1968	BARBIZET	T												X
1968	BENTON	T						X	X					X
1968	BLESSED-ROTH	T			X									
1968	BLESSED-ROTH	E				X		X	X					
1968	WILLIAMS	T									X			X
1969	ANDREY	T												X
1969	FOWLER	T			X									X
1970	DANA	T							X					
1970	NAHOR	T				X					X			
1970	WECHSLER	T							X					X
1971	PLUTCHIK	T							X		X			
1971	WITKIN	T		X	X	X			X		X			
1972	HODKINSON	Q			X				X		X			
1972	ISAACS	T			X									X
1972	SILVER	T						X						
1974	HASEGAWA	Q		X	X	X					X			X
1974	LONGEOT	T		X										X
1974	QURESHI	Q			X				X					
1975	FOLSTEIN	T			X				X		X			
1975	HACHINSKI	CL			X	X					X			
1975	PFEIFFER	Q			X	X			X					
1976	ISRAEL	T		X										X
1977	FISHBACK	Q				X								
1977	JACOBS	Q			X			X						
1977	SLATER	Q				X								
1978	DENHAM	Q				X								
1978	JANIN	T												X
1979	BRINK	T			X	X					X			
1979	CROOK	T			X				X					
1979	HERSCH	T		X	X				X	X	X			
1979	KENDRICK	T		X		X	X		X	X	X			X
1979	LEVIN	Q			X		X	X			X			
1979	WELLS	CL			X	X	X							
1980	BERG	Q		X					X	X				
1980	COLE	Rn			X			X						
1980	ISRAEL	T		X										X
1980	ISRAEL	Ro		X				X				X		
1980	ISRAEL	T		X										X
1980	ISRAEL	T		X										X
1981	GILBERT	T			X					X				X
1981	MAC CARTHY	T												X
1982	SIGNORET	T												X
1982	ISRAEL	T				X								

TITLE	YEAR	AUTHOR Country	SPECIFICITY FORM	LANGUAGE	ORIGIN	POPULATION
1. Self Perception Questionnaire	1966	PRESTON United States	* * * Questionnaire	English	Thesis of Sytman, Concept of Myamoto	Out-patient
2. Social Dysfunction Rating Scale	1969	LINN United States	* * * Ordinal rating scale	English	Original and various works from literature	Out-patient Inpatient
3. Interview for Recent Life Events	1971	PAYKEL Great Britain	* Interview	English	Works from Holmes and Rahe	Adults all ages (not memory-impaired) Out-patient Inpatient
4. Personal Habits, Environment and Psychosocial Factors	1973	KOZAREVIĆ Yugoslavia	* * Nominal rating scale	Serbo-Croat, English	Original	Adults 45-74 years Out-patient Inpatient
5. Attitudes et Perceptions Mutuelles des Médecins-Malades-Familles	1976	ISRAEL France	* * * Questionnaire	French	Works of S. Pacaud	Inpatient
6. Psychodiagnostic Test	1976	RORSCHACH F.R.G.	* * Projective test	German, French, English and most of the european languages	Original	Out-patient
7. Life Events Inventory	1976	TENNANT Australia	* Questionnaire	English	Works of Paykel Holmes	Out-patient Inpatient
8. Test Projectif	1977	LAFORESTRIE France	* * * Projective test	French	Original	Out-patient Inpatient
9. Aspects Psychologiques et Sociaux du Vieillissement	1978	ISRAEL France	* * * Questionnaire	French	Works of Paillat, other question-naires	Out-patient
10. Relatives' Stress Scale	1982	GREENE Great Britain	*** (to family) Ordinal rating scale	English	Original, inspired by various works from literature	Family of demented person living with him

RATER	N° OF ITEMS GRADES	TIME REQUIRED *Training*	APPLICATIONS	VARIABLES
Self-administered	110 questions	One hour *No*	Prognosis, clinical practice, detection of depression	Attitudes, self-perception and perception of others, intellectual functioning, family relationship, present interests, previous experiences
Social workers	21 items 6 grades	30 minutes *No*	Drug trials, prognosis, clinical practice	Apathy, dissatisfaction, hostility, dependency, health and financial troubles
Physician, psychologist, nurse's aide	64 questions	20-60 minutes *Light*	Drug trials, epidemiological research	Social and family relationship, recent life events
Psychologist, social worker, nurse	6 headings 3 grades	10 minutes *Necessary*	Epidemiological studies	Joy of living, relaxation and rest, family, work and social relationship difficulties
Psychologist, social worker	20 questions	30 minutes *Necessary*	Training of personnel, survey	Attitude, expectations, perception
Psychologist	10 cards	30 minutes *Intensive*	Clinic, research	Perception, adaptation, attitude, personality
Self-administered	67 questions	20 minutes *No*	Survey	Stress and life events
Psychologist	13 themes 21 cards	30-45 minutes *Very intensive* (360 hours)	Prognosis, diagnosis, care planning and therapy	Attitudes toward death, sexuality, communication, loss of work
Social worker, non specialised rater	85 questions	45 minutes *Light*	Psycho-social survey	Social context (needs, resources residence)
Relative	15 items 5 grades	10-15 minutes *No*	Prognosis, therapeutic program, care planning survey	Distress, rejection, disruption

TITLE	YEAR	AUTHOR Country	SPECIFICITY FORM	LANGUAGE	ORIGIN	POPULATION
1. Nursing Load Score	1969	HULTEN Sweden	* * Ordinal rating scale	Swedish, English	Original	Inpatient
2. Instrumental Activities of Daily Living Scale	1969	LAWTON BRODY United States	* * * Nominal rating scale	English, French	Lowenthal, Phillips, Lawton, Barrabee	Out-patient Inpatient
3. Index of A.D.L.	1970	KATZ United States	* * * Ordinal rating scale	English	Original, Dyar, Ford, Steinberg	Inpatient
4. Physical and Mental Health Questionnaire	1972	MILNE Great Britain	* * * Questionnaire and examination	English	Rose, Dyer, Pride and others	Out-patient Inpatient (except demented)
5. Disability Rating Scale	1973	AKHTAR Great Britain	* * * Ordinal rating scale	English	Harris, Bennett, Garrad	Out-patient
6. Geriatric Profile	1973	MISSOURI INSTITUTE United States	* * * Ordinal rating scale	English	Meer, Gurel, Missouri Inpatient Beha- vioral Scale	Inpatient (psychiatric, psychogeriatric)
7. Performance Test of Activities of Daily Living	1976	KURIANSKY United States	* * * Ordinal rating scale	English	Works of Goldfarb	Inpatient (stroke)
8. Ward Function Inventory	1977	NORTON United States	* * * Ordinal rating scale	English	Original	Inpatient
9. Echelle Clinique de Gérontologie	1980	CROCQ France	* * Ordinal rating scale	French	Original	Inpatient Out-patient
10. Evaluation de l'Autonomie	1980	DELOMIER France	* * * Ordinal rating scale	French	Exton-Smith	Inpatient
11. Fischer Symptom Check-List	1981	FISCHER Switzerland	* * Ordinal rating scale	German, French, English, Spanish, Chinese	Original	Out-patient Inpatient (psychiatric)
12. Geriatric Rating Scale	1981	GÖTESTAM Norway	* * * Ordinal rating scale	English	Gottfries, Crichton, Plutchik	Inpatient
13. Bilan Test d'Appréciation de la Perte d'Autonomie	1981	GRAUX France	* * * Questionnaire	French	Original	Out-patient Inpatient
14. G.B.S. Scale	1982	GOTTFRIES Sweden	* * * Ordinal rating scale	Swedish, English	Various works from literature	Inpatient Out-patient
15. Drug Dependency & Overdose Assessment	1982	IDÄNPÄÄN HEIKKILÄ Finland	* * Questionnaire	English, Finnish	Original	Population suffering form drug intoxication
16. Evaluation de la Dépendance en Istitution	1982	KUNTZMANN France	* * * Ordinal rating scale	French	Original Svanborg	Inpatient
17. Rapid Disability Rating Scale 2	1982	LINN United States	* * Ordinal rating scale	English	Various works from literature	Inpatient Out-patient
18. Échelle de Dépendance C.E.N.T.S.	1982	HUGONOT France	* * * Ordinal rating scale	French	Original	Inpatient

ATER	N° OF ITEMS GRADES	TIME REQUIRED *Training*	APPLICATIONS	VARIABLES
urse, hysician	9 items 2-5 grades	Few minutes *No*	Administration, therapy evaluation, program of care	Disturbance, dependency (incontinence dressing, feeding)
ocial worker, urse's aide	14 items 3-5 grades	30 minutes *Light*	Clinical, research, therapy care planning, training of staff	Autonomy, activities of daily living, social life
sychologist, physician, ocial worker	6 items 7 grades	20 minutes *Light*	Prognosis, research, training and teaching, rating of change	Activities of daily living, degree of autonomy and dependency
urse	33 questions examination	30 minutes *Necessary*	Epidemiological research, screening, prevention, program of care	Physical and mental status
hysician, nurse ocial worker	11 items 3, 5, 6 grades	5-10 minutes *No*	Epidemiology, training of personnel	Mobility, continence, mental status, self care, indoor activities
urse's aide	84 items 4 grades	10 minutes *Light*	Clinical, research, prognosis, drug trials	Depression, activities of daily living, physical incapacity, confusion, agitation, sleep disturbances, delusions, hostility, irritability, sociability, physical symptoms
sychiatrist, hysician, nurse, urse's aide	16 items 3 grades	20 minutes *Minimum*	Research, care planning, therapy, administration, diagnosis	Degree of autonomy and dependency, activity of daily living
urse	12 items 5 grades	5 minutes *No*	Research, clinical practice	Cognitive and behavioral deficiency
hysician	87 items	30 minutes *No*	Drug trials, epidemiological studies, therapeutic control	Fatigue, will, cognitive, functions, somatic status, communication, speech existential inventory, mood, appearence
urse	10 items 4 grades	5 minutes *No*	Clinical evaluation of therapy, autonomy and evaluation	Global status, autonomy, sleep, language, activities, feeding, walking, dressing, continence
hysician, psychologist, edical personnel	41 items 4 grades	2-5 minutes after examination *Light*	Clinical differential diagnosis, prognosis, research, drug trials	Psychological and psychiatric symptoms
urse's aide	20 items Different grades	brief *No*	Indications of placement, drug trials, epidemiological studies	Memory, confusion, mood, activities, communication, psychological symptoms, sleep, feeding
hysician, phychologist	20 questions	10 minutes *Light*	Clinical, rating of change, drug trials, diagnosis, epidemiological studies	Mobility, physical and psychiatric stage, continence, hearing, vision
hysician, psychologist, urse	26 items 7 grades	30 minutes *Light*	Clinical, research, drug trials	Motor functioning, emotion, intellect, dementia
hysician	22 questions	30-45 minutes *Necessary*	Epidemiological studies	Drug dependency, aggression, suicidal ideas
sysician, urse's aide	5 indicators	2 minutes per rater *No*	Adaptation to institution, comparison of populations	Self care, bladder and bowel control, physical dependency, need for care, transport and mobility
urse, all personnel cquainted with the atient	1: 16 items 3 grades 2: 18 items 4 grades	5 minutes *Light*	Research, organisation of care, care planning, screening of needs, treatment assessment	Disability, dependency, mental confusion depression, cooperation, etc...
urse's aide	5 items 6 grades	5 minutes *No*	Indications for placement	Level of care, dependency

VALIDATION WORKS – SYNOPTIC TABLES OF SECTION 2

YEARS	AUTHORS	Type of instrument*	VALIDITY					RELIABILITY				SENSITIVITY			
			Face	Construct	Concurrent	External	Predictive	Inter-rater	Test-Retest	Parallel forms / Internal consistency		Inter Individual	Intra Individual	Scoring	Other

MENTAL SOCIAL

YEARS	AUTHORS	Type	Face	Construct	Concurrent	External	Predictive	Inter-rater	Test-Retest	Parallel		Inter Ind.	Intra Ind.	Scoring	Other
1966	PRESTON	Q													
1969	LINN	Ro		X		X		X				X			
1971	PAYKEL	Q.I						X							
1973	KOZAREVIC	Rn													X
1976	ISRAEL	Q	X												
1976	RORSCHACH	T													X
1976	TENNANT	Q													
1977	LAFORESTRIE	T		X											X
1978	ISRAEL	Q	X												
1982	GREENE	Ro		X					X						

PHYSICAL MENTAL

YEARS	AUTHORS	Type	Face	Construct	Concurrent	External	Predictive	Inter-rater	Test-Retest	Parallel		Inter Ind.	Intra Ind.	Scoring	Other
1969	HULTEN	Ro				X						X			X
1969	LAWTON	Ro			X			X							X
1970	KATZ	Ro													
1972	MILNE	Q		X		X		X	X						
1973	AKHTAR	Ro			X			X							
1973	MISSOURI INSTITUTE	Ro		X				X							
1976	KURIANSKY	Ro	X	X	X			X							
1977	NORTON	Ro				X		X				X			
1980	CROCQ	Rmix				X									
1980	DELOMIER	Ro													X
1981	FISCHER	R		X	X	X		X	X				X		X
1981	GOTESTAM	Ro			X			X							
1981	GRAUX	Q				X									
1982	GOTTFRIES	Ro						X							
1982	IDANPAAN	Q													X
1982	KUNTZMANN	Ro				X									X
1982	LINN	Ro		X	X	X	X	X	X				X		

*Type of instrument:

CL	: Check list	R	: Rating scale
Q	: Questionnaire	Ro	: Ordinal rating scale
T	: Test	Rn	: Nominal rating scale
I	: Interview	Rmix	: Mixed rating scale

TITLE	YEAR	AUTHOR Country	SPECIFICITY FORM	LANGUAGE	ORIGIN	POPULATION
1. Stockton Geriatric Rating Scale	1966	MEER United States	* * * Ordinal rating scale	English, French, Dutch	Original Works of Burdock, Ellsworth, Scott, Mc Reynolds	Inpatient
2. Parkside Behaviour Rating Scale	1970	FINE Great Britain	* * * Nominal rating scale	English		Inpatient
3. Geriatric Rating Scale	1970	PLUTCHIK United States	* * * Ordinal rating scale	English	Meer	Inpatient
4. P.A.M.I.E. Scale	1972	GUREL United States	* * * Check list	English	Meer, Plutchik, Watson, Katz, Dobson	Inpatient
5. Functional Life Scale	1973	SARNO United States	* Ordinal rating scale	English	Original	Out-patient
6. Parachek Geriatric Behavior Rating Scale	1974	PARACHEK-MILLER United States	* * * Ordinal rating scale	English	Plutchik	Inpatient
7. Sandoz Clinical Assessment Geriatric	1974	SHADER United States	* * * Ordinal rating scale	English, Swedish, French, German	Original	Out-patient
8. Psychogeriatric Assessment Program	1975	Douglas Hospital Canada	* * * Compound	English	Farina, Plutchik Hamilton, Overall, Doll	Out-patient Inpatient
9. Geriatric Functional Rating Scale	1975	GRAUER United States	* * * Nominal rating scale	English	Original, ADL Katz, Lawton, Lowenthal	Out-patient
10. Echelle d'Appréciation Clinique en Gériatrie	1977	LALLEMAND GEORGES France	* * * Ordinal rating scale	French	S.C.A.G. Shader	Out-patient (with behavioral disorders) Inpatient
11. Comprehensive Assessment & Referral Evaluation	1977	GURLAND United States	* * * Questionnaire	English	Spitzer, Wing	Out-patient
12. Multidimensional Functional Assessment Questionnaire	1978	Center for Aging DUKE UNIVERSITY United States	* * * Questionnaire	English	O.A.R.S. Previous versions	Inpatient Out-patient
13. Geriatric Resident Goals Scale	1978	CORNBLETH United States	* * * Check list	English	Stockton's and Plutchik's rating scales	Inpatient
14. London Psychogeriatric Rating Scale	1978	HERSCH Canada	* * * Ordinal rating scale	English	Various works	Inpatient
15. Origine de la Dépendance	1978	ISRAEL France	* * * Ordinal rating scale	French	Plutchik, Meer Lawton, Linn, Gurel, Crichton	Inpatient
16. Geriatric Rapid Diagnostic Battery	1978	MURKOFSKY United States	* * * Compound instrument	English	Original Zung, Plutchik	Out-patient

ATER	N° OF ITEMS GRADES	TIME REQUIRED *Training*	APPLICATIONS	VARIABLES
urse's aide, urse	Form 1: 30 items Form 2: 33 items 3 grades	10 minutes *No*	Clinical prognosis, drug trials, epidemiological studies	Physical incapacity, apathy, comunication, irritating behavior
urse's aide	6 items 5 grades	15 minutes *No*	Rating of change, longitudinal studies	Self-care, orientation, communication, social interaction, occupation and cooperation during work, psychotic behavior, mood
urse's aide	31 items 3 grades	Brief *No*	Clinical research, rating of treatments, epidemiology	Physical, mental, social (feeding, mobility)
urse	77 items	45 minutes *No*	Clinical, epidemiological studies, program of therapy	Physical disability, mental deteriorations
hysician, psychologist, ecialised nurse's aide	44 items 5 grades	45 minutes *Necessary*	Clinical research, teaching	Cognitive functioning, activities of daily living (indoors and out-doors), social interaction
urse's aide	10 items 5 grades	3 to 5 minutes *No*	Clinical program of therapy, care planning, epidemiological and statistical studies	Physical status, self-care, social behavior
hysician, psychologist, cial worker, nurse	19 items 7 grades	20 minutes *Rating on 5 patients*	Research, drug trials	Estimation of symptoms (physical status, behavior, psychosomatic disorders)
hysician, psychiatrist, cial worker, nurse	Rating scale, clinical examination, laboratory findings	2 days + meetings + interview *Intensive*	Diagnosis, program of therapy, prognosis, prevention,	General health status (neurological, psychological), social problems training of personnel
ocial worker, nurse	30 items	15-20 minutes *No*	Clinical practice, choosing the place of living, indications for placement	Autonomy, physical, mental and social status
hysician	17 items 7 grades (abbreviated form 13 items)	20 minutes *Necessary to familiarize*	Drug trials	Mental (cognitive, mood, social relations) psychosomatic signs, motor and sensory function
ecialist nurse's de	600 items	45-90 minutes *Necessary*	Diagnosis, research, drug trials, epidemiological studies, outcome studies	Medical, social psychiatric imitation activities
hysician, psychiatrist, cial worker, vestigator	101 questions	45 minutes *Special training*	Clinical practice, training, needs assessment, health policy, epidemiological surveys, assessment of services required and of service impact	Physical and mental health activities of daily living, socio-economic resources
urse	86 items 6 headings	1 hour *No*	Clinical practice, defining and evaluating planning	Autonomy, communication
urse	36 items 3 grades	15 minutes *Light*	Drug trials, planning, research, clinic	Degree of general incapacity (mental and physical)
hysician, sychologist, urse's aide	13 items 5 grades	5 minutes *No*	Clinical practice (hospital or institution), impact on dependency	Cause of dependency, sensory functions, intellectual functioning, communication, expression vital functions, self-care
elf-administered cept Plutchik's ting scale	Test, rating-scale questionnaire, inventory	30 minutes *Necessary for interpretation*	Clinical practice, diagnosis, prognosis, etiology, therapy	Depression, activities of daily living, social activities, functioning (cognitive, perceptual, motor) drug medication, and alcohol usage

TITLE	YEAR	AUTHOR Country	SPECIFICITY FORM	LANGUAGE	ORIGIN	POPULATION
17. Batterie de Fiches d'Évaluation	1978	ZAY Canada	* * * Compound	French	Various works	Inpatient Out-patient
18. Disability Assessment Schedule	1979	W.H.O.	* * Rating scale	French, English, numerous others	WHO studies	Out-patient Inpatient (psychiatry)
19. Echelle de Dépendance Autonomie	1980	DELCROS LANOE France	* * * Ordinal rating scale	French	Meer, Crichton, Exton-Smith, Hugonot	Inpatient long stay
20. Comprehensive Health Questionnaire	1980	KOZAREVIĆ Yugoslavia	* * * Questionnaire	Serbo-Croat, English	Authors' works, WHO cooperative study	Out-patient
21. Evaluation Globale de l'Autonomie	1980	PATRON France	* * * Nominal rating scale	French	Original	Residential (dependent)
22. Edinburgh Psychogeriatric Dependency Rating Scale	1980	WILKINSON Great Britain	* * * Ordinal rating scale	English	Stockton Scale Plutchik, Gurel, Grauer, Ferm	Out-patient Inpatient
23. Système d'Information C.T.M.S.P.	1981	E.R.O.S. Canada	* * * Compound Instrument	French	Original	Inpatient Out-patient
24. Échelle d'Expression de l'Autonomie: Geronte	1981	LEROUX-ATTALLI France	* * * Visual rating scale	French	Original	Inpatient Out-patient
25. Clifton Assessment Procedures for Elderly	1981	PATTIE Great Britain	* * * Compound	English, Polish, French	Stockton Scale Clifton	Inpatient Out-patient
26. Questionnaire d'Enquête pour Etudes Épidémiologiques	1981	VIGNAT-ISRAEL France	* * * Questionnaire Rating scale	French	Original	Inpatient Out-patient
27. Self Assessment Scale Geriatric	1981	YESAVAGE United States	* * * Ordinal rating scale	English, French, German	SCAG from Shader	Inpatient Out-patient
28. Multilevel Assessment Instrument	1982	LAWTON United States	* * * Questionnaire	English	O.A.R.S. C.A.R.E.	Inpatient Out.-patient
29. Nürnberger Alters Inventar	1982	OSWALD F.R.G.	* * * Compound	German, English	Wechsler, Chapuis, Cattell, Benton	Inpatient
30. Functional Activities Questionnaire	1982	PFEFFER United States	* * * Ordinal rating scale	English	Original	Out-patient or residential
31. Grille pour l'Evaluation du Degré de Dépendance		C.I.C.P.A. Switzerland	* * * Ordinal rating scale	French	Original	Inpatient (psychiatric and somatic troubles)
32. Grille de Dépendance		CENTRE DE GERIATRIE Switzerland	* * * Ordinal rating scale	French	Dastor, Garrad, Grauer, Williams, Paillard	Out-patient (psychiatrically or physically handicapped)

ATER	Nº OF ITEMS GRADES	TIME REQUIRED *Training*	APPLICATIONS	VARIABLES
hysician, sychologist, urse, social worker, urse's aide	Several rating scales	Different, depending on the format *Light*	Research, planning, administration, care	Health status, sensory status, psychological status, adaptability, social and financial resources, functional capacity
sychologist, hysician, social orker	97 items	30-45 minutes *Light*	Epidemiological longitudinal studies, program of care	Behavior disorders, social role performance
urse's aide	25 items 5 grades	2-3 minutes *Light*	Diagnosis, prognosis for dependency, team work care planning, planning,	Perception, orientation, memory, autonomy, activities of daily living, mental status, social and family relationship, mobility
hysician, nurse	102 questions	50 minutes *Necessary but brief*	Epidemiological longitudinal and cross sectional studies, diagnosis	Socio-cultural historical characteristics of somatic disorders, actual somatic disorders, characteristics of medical care
urse's aide, cial worker, latives	13 items 4 grades	10 minutes *Light*	Research, estimate of likely course	Autonomy, environmental resources, social services
urse	36 items different grades from 2-6	5 minutes *Light*	Clinical, research, administration	Dependency: orientation, behavior, physical condition
ultidisciplinary am	Variable	80 minutes *Necessary*	Indications for placement, planning	Physical characteristic, habits, social and family relationship, impressions and observations of caregiver
hysician, nurse's de, social sistant	27 items 3 grades	2-3 minutes *Light*	Diagnosis, prognosis, epidemiological studies, drug trials, rehabilitation measures	Activities: locomotor, indoor, outdoor, sensory functioning, mental handicap
hysician, sychologist, urse's aide ualified or not	Variable	15-25 minutes *Light*	Clinic, diagnosis, prognosis, epidemiology, experiments	Information, orientation, mental functioning, psychomotor activity, social disturbance, physical incapacity, difficulty in communication, apathy
hysician, sychologist, cial worker	18 principal headings	60 minutes *Intensive*	Epidemiology	Case history, psychological and psychiatric data, personality
elf administered	19 items 7 grades	10-15 minutes *No*	Drug trials, clinical evaluation of treatment, epidemiological studies	Mood, cognitive activities, sociability, autonomy
urse	216 items 5 grades	50 minutes *Necessary*	Research, program of care epidemiological studies	Physical activities, cognitive functioning, activities of daily living, social interaction, psychological well-being, environment
sychologist, urse and elf-adminis-red	Variable	30 minutes *Intensive*	Clinical, drug trials	Dependency, family caregiving, orientation, communication, therapeutic and preventive care
amily, urse, ocial worker	10 items 7 grades	15 minutes *Light*	Diagnosis, prognosis, drug trials, research, epidemiological studies	Activities of daily living
urse's aide, ara-medical ersonnel	14 items 6 grades	15 minutes *Light*	Clinical, rehabilitation	Dependency, family caregiving, orientation, communication, therapeutic and preventive care
urse's aide	11 items different grades	20-45 minutes *Light*	Evaluation of care planning, training, psychological profile	Activities of daily living, communication

PHYSICAL MENTAL SOCIAL

YEARS	AUTHORS	Type of instrument*	VALIDITY					RELIABILITY			SENSITIVITY			Other
			Face	Construct	Concurrent	External	Predictive	Inter-rater	Test-Retest	Parallel forms / Internal consistency	Inter Individual	Intra Individual	Scoring	
1966	MEER	Ro		X		X	X	X		X	X			
1970	FINE	Rn			X									
1970	PLUTCHIK	Ro		X		X	X	X	X		X			
1972	GUREL	CL		X	X	X	X			X				X
1973	SARNO	Ro			X			X	X	X				
1974	PARACHEK	Ro			X	X	X							
1974	SHADER	Ro			X	X		X						
1975	DASTOOR	E		X			X							
1975	GRAUER	Ro					X							
1977	GEORGES	Ro		X	X			X						
1977	GURLAND	Q	X				X	X		X				
1978	CENTER FOR AGING	Q		X	X	X		X	X		X			
1978	CORNBLETH	CL			X			X	X	X	X			
1978	HERSCH	Ro				X	X	X	X		X			
1978	ISRAEL	Ro						X	X					
1978	MURKOFSKY	T.Q								X	X			
1978	ZAY	R.CL												X
1979	O.M.S.	R												
1980	DELCROS	Ro						X	X					
1980	KOZAREVIC	Q												X
1980	PATRON	Rn												
1980	WILKINSON	Ro.a	X		X	X		X						
1981	E.R.O.S.	R.Q.												
1981	LEROUX	R												X
1981	PATTIE	R.Q.T.		X	X				X					X
1981	ISRAEL	Q												
1981	YESAVAGE	Ro		X					X					
1982	LAWTON	Q		X	X	X		X	X					
1982	OSWALD	T.R.CL.		X	X	X		X		X				X
1982	PFEFFER	Ro			X	X								
1982	C.I.C.P.A.	Ro												
1982	CENTRE DE GERIATRIE	Ro												

*Type of instrument:
CL	: Check list	R	: Rating scale
Q	: Questionnaire	Ro	: Ordinal rating scale
T	: Test	Rn	: Nominal rating scale
		Rmix	: Mixed rating scale

III - COMPLEMENTARY INSTRUMENTS

III – COMPLEMENTARY INSTRUMENTS

1. NON INCLUSION CRITERIA

The instruments which were not selected are here analysed and described in a schematic way. They do not include individual bibliographies or detailed identifying information. However, bibliographic details are presented by author in alphabetic order in the fifth chapter reserved for bibliography.

The following characteristics are given for each instrument: *Title, year of publication, author, country, type of instrument, category, language, population, rater, number of items and grades, time required, applications and variables.*

The instruments are presented in the following order:
    Instruments developed before 1965
    Instruments dating from 1965 to 1982

The reason for not including a detailed description is also contained in these tables, according to the following code:

Non-specificity of the *instrument* when it is presented as a simple list of non-measurable *symptoms*. (1)

Non-specificity of the *population concerned* when the instrument is not applicable to the *elderly*. (2)

Inadequacy of content when the instrument is concerned exclusively with the

    Physical aspect (3)
    Social aspect (4)

Instruments whose reference is already presented in the bibliography of the Descriptive Forms in the second chapter of the book. (5)

2. LIST OF COMPLEMENTARY INSTRUMENTS

Instruments dating before 1965 (*)

1. Guilford Schedule	GUILFORD	1939
2. Gardner Behavior Chart	WILCOX	1942
3. Hunt-Minnesota Test	HUNT	1944
4. Psychiatric Rating Scale	MALAMUD	1946
5. Bender-Gestalt Visual Motor Test	BILLINGSLEA	1948
6. L-M Fergus Falls Behavior Rating Sheet	LUCERO	1951
7. Psychiatric Behavior Scale	ROWELL	1951
8. Manifest Anxiety Scale	TAYLOR	1953
9. Normative Social Adjustment Scale	BARRABEE	1955
10. Albany Behavioral Rating Scale	SHATIN	1955
11. Heron Inventory	HERON	1956
12. Clinical Sensorium Test	SHAPIRO	1956
13. Buss-Durkee Hostility Inventory	BUSS	1957
14. Minimal Social Behavior	FARINA	1957
15. Activity-Withdrawal Scale	VENABLES	1957
16. Weyburn Assessment Scale	BLEWETT	1958
17. Activities of Psychiatric Patients	GUERTIN	1959
18. Symptom Rating Scale	JENKINS	1959
19. Ward Behavior Rating Scale	BURDOCK	1960
20. Test d'Apprentissage Psycho-moteur	CLEMENT	1960
21. Adjective Check List	GOUGH	1960
22. Kahn Intelligence Tests	KAHN	1960
23. Psychotic Reaction Profile	LORR	1960
24. Organic Integrity Test	TIEN	1960
25. Multiple Affect Adjective Check-List	ZUCKERMAN	1960
26. Grading Scale for Depressive Reactions	CUTLER	1961
27. Self-Care Inventory	DOBSON	1961
28. Symptom and Adjustment Index	GROSS	1961
29. Life Satisfaction Scale	NEUGARTEN	1961
30. Oberleder Attitude Scale	OBERLEDER	1961
31. Crichton Geriatric Behavioural Rating Scale	ROBINSON	1961
32. Scheier-Cattell Anxiety Battery	SCHEIER	1961
33. Quick Test	AMMONS	1962
34. Associate Learning Test for Elderly Psychiatric Patients	CAIRD	1962
35. Inventaire d'Intérêts pour Personnes Agées	CLEMENT	1962
36. Minimal Social Behavior Scale	DINOFF	1962
37. Twenty-two Item Screening Score	LANGNER	1962
38. Brief Psychiatric Rating Scale	OVERALL	1962
39. Psychiatric Judgment of Depression Scale	OVERALL	1962
40. Longitudinal Observation of Behavior	BUNNEY	1963
41. Epreuve Rapide de Mesure de l'Efficience Intellectuelle	CLEMENT	1963
42. Katz Adjustment Scales	KATZ	1963
43. Dempsey Modification of MMPI	DEMPSEY	1964
44. Evaluation of Levels of Subsistence	GAUGER	1964
45. Measurement of Mental Impairment in Geriatric Practice	ISAACS	1964
46. Senescent Memory Impairment Scale	KRAL	1964
47. Mental Status Schedule	SPITZER	1964

(*) These instruments do not have Descriptive Forms because they do not satisfy the date of publication required. Besides some of them do not fulfil other inclusion criteria.

Instrument dating after 1965 (*)

48. Newcastle Scale	CARNEY	1965
49. Activities of Daily Living Rating Scale	DINNERSTEIN	1965
50. Brief Screening Test of Mental Status	DIXON	1965
51. Quantified Mental Status Scale	ROCKLAND	1965
52. Perceptual Maturity Scale	VAN DE CASTLE	1965
53. Short Form of the WAIS Used with the Aged	BRITTON	1966
54. Middlesex Hospital Questionnaire	CROWN	1966
55. Sad-Glad	SIMPSON	1966
56. Self-Care Inventory	GUREL	1967
57. Mental State Rating Scale	HARRIS	1967
58. Serial Sevens Subtraction Test	SMITH	1967
59. Patient in Nursing Home Schedule	STOTSKY	1967
60. Rapid Approximate Intelligence Test	WILSON	1967
61. Barthel Index	WYLIE	1967
62. Systematic Nursing Observation of Psychopathology	HARGREAVES	1968
63. Verdun Target Rating Scale	SILVER	1968
64. Rating Scales of Psychological Function	TRIER	1968
65. Fourteen-Symptom Behavior and Mood Scale	WYATT	1968
66. Inventory of Psychic and Somatic Complaints	RASKIN	1969
67. Staff and Patient Helping	SIDMAN	1969
68. Psychiatric Screening of the Elderly	SIMON	1969
69. Contentment Index	BLOOM	1970
70. Leyton Obsessional Inventory	COOPER	1970
71. Scales for Nursing Observation of Behavior Syndromes	CRAIG	1970
72. Physician Questionnaire	RICKELS	1970
73. Rating Scale for Extrapyramidal Side Effects	SIMPSON	1970
74. Psychiatric Status Schedule	SPITZER	1970
75. Befindlichkeits-Skala	ZERSSEN	1970
76. Profile of Mood Scale	MacNAIR	1971
77. Current and Past Psychopathology Scales	ENDICOTT	1972
78. Psychiatric Evaluation Form	ENDICOTT	1972
79. Structured and Scaled Interview to Assess Maladjustment	GURLAND	1972
80. Depression Status Inventory	ZUNG	1972
81. Symptom Distress Checklist	DEROGATIS	1973
82. Rating of Mania	PETTERSON	1973
83. Schwab's Depression Scale	SCHWAB	1973
84. Debility Index	SKINNER	1973
85. Hopelessness Scale	BECK	1974
86. Bigot's Life Satisfaction Index	BIGOT	1974
87. Self-Assessment of Anxiety and Depression	SNAITH	1976
88. Comprehensive Psychopathological Rating Scale	ASBERG	1978
89. Schedule for Affective Disorders and Schizophrenia	ENDICOTT	1978
90. WAIS Short Form	HAFNER	1978
91. Pilot Geriatric Arthritis Project	JETTE	1978
92. Category Test	MACK	1978
93. Hand-Held Tachistoscope Perception	PAUKER	1978
94. Ward Behaviour Questionnaire	CLARKE	1979
95. Social Functioning Schedule	REMINGTON	1979
96. Families' Caregiving Capacity	HIRSCHFELD	1980
97. Echelle de Ralentissement Dépressif	WIDLOCHER	1980
98. Echelle d'Autonomie	BERTHAUX	1981
99. Status Physique Fonctionnel	O.M.S.	1981
100. Arbeitsgemeinschaft für Gerontopsychiatrie	FREIE UNIV.	

(*) Specific reasons for not including these instruments are indicated in the last column of descriptive tables.

TITLE	YEAR	AUTHOR Country	FORM	CATEGORY	LANGUAGE	POPULATION
1. Guilford Schedule	1939	GUILFORD United States	Nominal rating scale	Mental behavior	English	Out-patient
2. Gardner Behavior Chart	1942	WILCOX United States	Ordinal rating scale	Mental behavior	English	Out-patient Inpatient
3. Hunt-Minnesota Test	1944	HUNT United States	Test	Mental cognitive	English	Inpatient
4. Psychiatric Rating Scale	1946	MALAMUD United States	Nominal rating scale	Mental behavior	English	Inpatient
5. Bender-Gestalt Visual Motor Test	1948	BILLINGSLEA United States	Test	Mental cognitive	English	Inpatient Out-patient
6. L-M Fergus Falls Behavior Rating Sheet	1951	LUCERO United States	Ordinal rating scale	Mental behavior	English	Inpatient
7. Psychiatric Behavior Scale	1951	ROWELL United States	Ordinal rating scale	Mental behavior	English	Inpatient
8. Manifest Anxiety Scale	1953	TAYLOR United States	Check list	Mental mood	English	Inpatient Out-patient
9. Normative Social Adjustment Scale	1955	BARRABEE United States	Questionnaire	Social	English	Inpatient Out-patient
10. Albany Behavioral Rating Scale	1955	SHATIN United States	Check list	Mental behavior	English	Inpatient
11. Heron Inventory	1956	HERON Great Britain	Check list	Mental Social	English	Inpatient
12. Clinical Sensorium Test	1956	SHAPIRO Sweden	Test	Mental cognitive	Swedish	Inpatient
13. Buss-Durkee Hostility Inventory	1957	BUSS United States	Check list	Mental behavior	English	Inpatient Out-patient
14. Minimal Social Behavior	1957	FARINA United States	Check list	Mental behavior	English	Inpatient
15. Activity- Withdrawal Scale	1957	VENABLES Great Britain	Ordinal rating scale	Mental behavior	English	Inpatient

ATER	N° OF ITEMS GRADES *Time required*	APPLICATIONS	VARIABLES	WHY NOT INCLUDED
elf- administered	89 items 3 grades *30-45 minutes*	Clinical practice	Personality	
urse	50 categories 5 grades *10 minutes*	Rating of changes	Social adjustment and flexibility	
sychologist	*15 minutes*	Programme of care	Organic brain syndrome	
sychiatrist or urse	20 items 5 grades *10-15 minutes*	Rating of changes	Intellectual functions	
elf- administered	9 sub-tests *No time limit*	Clinical practice	Personality perception	
urse or non pecialized ersonnel	11 items 3 grades *10-15 minutes*	Research, care planning	Adaptability	(2)
urse, sychiatrist	20 items 5 points *5 minutes*	Research, rating of changes	Psychotic tendencies	
elf- administered	50 items *20 minutes*	Experimental psychology	Anxiety	
ocial worker, sychiatrist	11 items *One hour*	Research	Professional, family, financial and social life	(4)
urse, ara-medical herapist	100 items *20-30 minutes*	Psychiatric status	Attitudes, adaptability	
elf- administered	110 items *20 minutes*	Research	Social adaptability	(2)
sychologist, hysician	29 items *Two hours*	Clinical research, rating of changes	Memory, perception, intellectual activity	
elf- administered	75 items *30 minutes*	Psychological status	Hostility	
hysician, nurse, ocial worker	32 items *30-45 minutes*	Drug trials, rating of changes	Sociability, attitudes	
urse	10 items 5 grades *20 minutes*	Clinical research, contribution to diagnosis	Activity	(2)

TITLE	YEAR	AUTHOR Country	FORM	CATEGORY	LANGUAGE	POPULATION
16. Weyburn Assessment Scale	1958	BLEWETT Canada	Nominal rating scale	Physical Mental	English	Inpatient
17. Activities of Psychiatric Patients	1959	GUERTIN United States	Nominal rating scale	Mental behavior	English	Inpatient
18. Symptom Rating Scale	1959	JENKINS United States	Ordinal rating scale	Mental	English	Inpatient
19. Ward Behavior Rating Scale	1960	BURDOCK United States	Check list	Mental behavior	English	Inpatient
20. Test d'Apprentissage Psycho-moteur	1960	CLEMENT France	Test	Mental cognitive	French	Out-patient
21. Adjective Check List	1960	GOUGH United States	Check list	Mental Social	English, French, Italian	Out-patient Inpatient
22. Kahn Intelligence Tests: Experimental Form	1960	KAHN F.R.G.	Test	Mental cognitive	German	Inpatient Out-patient
23. Psychotic Reaction Profile	1960	LORR United States	Check list	Mental behavior	English	Inpatient
24. Organic Integrity Test	1960	TIEN United States	Test	Mental cognitive	English	Inpatient Out-patient
25. Multiple Affect Adjective Check List	1960	ZUCKERMAN United States	Check list	Mental mood	English	Out-patient
26. Grading Scale for Depressive Reactions	1961	CUTLER United States	Check list	Mental mood	English	Inpatient
27. Self-Care Inventory	1961	DOBSON United States	Rating scale	Physical mental	English	Inpatient Out-patient
28. Symptom and Adjustment Index	1961	GROSS United States	Ordinal rating scale	Mental behavior	English	Out-patient
29. Life Satisfaction Scale	1961	NEUGARTEN United States	Nominal rating scale	Mental Social	English	Out-patient
30. Oberleder Attitude Scale	1961	OBERLEDER United States	Rating scale	Mental Social	English	Inpatient
31. Crichton Geriatric Behavioural Rating Scale	1961	ROBINSON Great Britain	Rating scale	Mental behavior	English	Inpatient

BLES

RATER	N° OF ITEMS GRADES Time required	APPLICATIONS	VARIABLES	WHY NOT INCLUDED
Psychiatrist	37 items 5 grades 12 minutes	Drug trials	Activities of daily living	(1)
Nurse staff	67 items 6 grades 30 minutes	Drug trials, care planning, research	Psychiatric disorders	(2)
Psychologist, psychiatrist, social worker	80 items 4 grades 40-50 minutes	Prognosis	Psychiatric disorders	
Nurse	150 items 10-15 minutes	Rating of changes, research	Personality	
Not specialised personnel	5 minutes	Contribution to diagnosis	Psychomotor learning	
Psychologist and nurse's aide	300 items 15-20 minutes	Research, care planning	Personality and relationships	(2)
Psychologist	No time limit	Research, diagnosis	Memory, intellectual functioning	
Nurse	85 items 40-45 minutes	Research, diagnosis	Psychiatric disorders	(2)
Self-administered	10 groups of pictures 5 minutes	Differential diagnosis, as between functional and organic illness	Perception	
Self-administered	61 items 5 minutes	Research	Anxiety, depression, hostility	(2)
Physician	27 items 12 minutes	Drug trials, clinical research	Depression	(1)
Nurse, nurse's aide	14 items 5 grades 36 items 4 grades 30 minutes	Research, diagnosis, rating of changes	Self-care, activities of daily living	
Psychiatrist, social worker, psychologist	62 items 5 grades 20-30 minutes	Rating of changes drug trials	Psychiatric symptoms	
Psychologist, self-administered	20 items, 3 grades 30 minutes	Research	Mood, attitudes	(1)
Self-administered	25 items 4 grades 10-15 minutes	Prognosis	Social adjustment	
Physician	10 items 5 grades 10 minutes	Rating of changes, drug trials, care planning	Mood, behavior	

TITLE	YEAR	AUTHOR Country	FORM	CATEGORY	LANGUAGE	POPULATION
32. Scheier-Cattell Anxiety Battery	1961	SCHEIER United States	Nominal rating scale	Mental mood	English	Out-patient
33. Quick Test	1962	AMMONS United States	Test	Mental cognitive	English	Inpatient Out-patient
34. Associate Learning Test for Elderly Psychiatric Patients	1962	CAIRD Canada	Test	Mental cognitive	English	Inpatient Out-patient
35. Inventaire d'Intérêts pour Personnes Agées	1962	CLEMENT France	Questionnaire	Mental Social	French	Out-patient
36. Minimal Social Behavior Scale	1962	DINOFF United States	Check list	Mental behavior	English	Inpatient
37. Twenty-two Item Screening Score	1962	LANGNER United States	Ordinal rating scale	Mental mood	English	Inpatient Out-patient
38. Brief Psychiatric Rating Scale	1962	OVERALL United States	Ordinal rating scale	Mental behavior	English	Inpatient Out-patient
39. Psychiatric Judgment of Depression Scale	1962	OVERALL United States	Ordinal rating scale	Mental behavior	English	Inpatient
40. Longitudinal Observation of Behavior	1963	BUNNEY United States	Check list	Mental mood	English	Inpatient
41. Epreuve Rapide de Mesure de l'Efficience Intellectuelle	1963	CLEMENT France	Test	Mental cognitive	French	Out-patient
42. Katz Adjustment Scales	1963	KATZ United States	Ordinal rating scale	Physical Mental Social	English	Out-patient
43. Dempsey Modification of MMPI	1964	DEMPSEY United States	Check list	Mental mood	English	Out-patient
44. Evaluation of Levels of Subsistence	1964	GAUGER Great Britain	Ordinal rating scale	Physical Mental Social	English	Out-patient
45. Measurement of Mental Impairment in Geriatric Practice	1964	ISAACS Great Britain	Compound	Mental cognitive	English	Inpatient
46. Senescent Memory Impairment Scale	1964	KRAL Canada	Ordinal rating scale	Physical Mental Social	English	Inpatient
47. Mental Status Schedule	1964	SPITZER United States	Questionnaire	Mental mood	English	Inpatient

ATER	N° OF ITEMS GRADES *Time required*	APPLICATIONS	VARIABLES	WHY NOT INCLUDED
elf- administered	95 items 5 grades *15 minutes*	Diagnosis, research	Anxiety	
hysician, ocial worker, sychologist	3 parallel forms *5 minutes*	Research	Intellectual functioning, perception, memory	
sychologist, hysician	*No time limit*	Research, diagnosis, therapeutic studies	Memory	
on specialised staff	59 questions *20 minutes*	Diagnosis, rating of changes	Different interests	
Nurse, non specialised taff	32 items *35-40 minutes*	Diagnosis, therapy, rating of changes	Social behavior	
sychiatrist, sychologist	22 items 4-6 grades *30 minutes*	Screening, diagnosis	Psychiatric disorders	(2)
Physician	16 items 7 grades *20 minutes*	Screening, diagnosis	Psychiatric disorders	
sychiatrist, sychologist, urse, ocial worker	31 items 2 grades *15 minutes*	Drug trials	Depression	
Nurse, hysician, sychologist, ocial worker	24 items *10-15 minutes*	Rating of changes	Depression, anxiety, behavior	(1)
sychologist	*2-5 minutes*	Diagnosis, prognosis	Cognitive processes, memory	
ocial worker	127 items 4 grades *45 minutes*	Screening, care planning	Activities of daily living, adaptability	
Self- administered	30 items *15 minutes*	Diagnosis, screening	Depression	
Physician	20 items 7 grades *20 minutes*	Research, care planning	Activities of daily living, initiative behavior	
Psychologist, psychiatrist	*5-10 minutes*	Prognosis, epidemiological studies	Cognitive functioning, memory, orientation	
Nurse, psychiatrist, social worker, occupational therapist	7 items 4 grades *5-10 minutes*	Diagnosis, prognosis	Memory, physical condition, socialisation	
Psychiatrist	248 items *One hour*	Diagnosis, rating of changes	Anxiety, depression, complaints	(2)

TITLE	YEAR	AUTHOR Country	FORM	CATEGORY	LANGUAGE	POPULATION
48. Newcastle Scale	1965	CARNEY Great Britain	Ordinal rating scale	Mental mood	English	Inpatient
49. Activities of Daily Living Rating Scale	1965	DINNERSTEIN United States	Nominal rating scale	Physical	English	Inpatient
50. Brief Screening Test of Mental Status	1965	DIXON United States	Test	Mental cognitive	English	Inpatient
51. Quantified Mental Status Scale	1965	ROCKLAND United States	Nominal rating scale	Mental behavior	English	Out-patient Inpatient
52. Perceptual Maturity Scale	1965	VAN DE CASTLE United States	Test	Mental cognitive	English	Out-patient Inpatient
53. Short Form of the WAIS Used with the Aged	1966	BRITTON Great Britain	Test	Mental cognitive	English	Out-patient
54. Middlesex Hospital Questionnaire	1966	CROWN Great Britain	Questionnaire	Mental behavior	English	Out-patient
55. Sad-Glad	1966	SIMPSON Canada	Nominal rating scale	Mental mood	English	Out-patient
56. Self-Care Inventory	1967	GUREL United States	Nominal rating scale	Physical dependency	English	Inpatient
57. Mental State Rating Scale	1967	HARRIS Great Britain	Ordinal rating scale	Physical Mental	English	Inpatient
58. Serial Sevens Subtraction Test	1967	SMITH United States	Test	Mental cognitive	English	Out-patient Inpatient
59. Patient in Nursing Home Schedule	1967	STOTSKY United States	Compound	Physical Mental Social	English	Inpatient
60. Rapid Approximate Intelligence Test	1967	WILSON United States	Test	Mental cognitive	English	Inpatient Out-patient
61. Barthel Index	1967	WYLIE United States	Ordinal rating scale	Physical	English	Inpatient
62. Systematic Nursing Observation of Psychopathology	1968	HARGREAVES United States	Ordinal rating scale	Mental behavior	English	Inpatient
63. Verdun Target Rating Scale	1968	SILVER Canada	Test Rating scale	Mental mood	English	Inpatient
64. Rating Scales of Psychological Function	1968	TRIER United States	Ordinal rating scale	Physical Mental Social	English	Inpatient

ATER	N° OF ITEMS GRADES *Time required*	APPLICATIONS	VARIABLES	WHY NOT INCLUDED
sychiatrist	36 items 4 grades *45 minutes*	Diagnosis, prognosis	Depression	(2)
ccupational therapist, irse's aide	11 items 6 classes *40 minutes*	Rating of changes, epidemiological studies	Activities of daily living	(3)
irse	29 items *5 minutes*	Screening, epidemiological studies	Learning	(5)
sychiatrist, ychopharmacologist	16 items 4-8 grades *30-60 minutes*	Research, clinical assessment, rating of changes, drug trials	General status, content of mood, thought, cognitive functions, behavior	(1) - (2)
elf- administered	72 pairs of figures *No time limit*	Clinical research	Perceptual maturity	(2)
sychologist	4 sub tests *30-45 minutes*	Diagnosis, research	Intellectual functioning	(5)
elf-administered	48 items 2-3 grades *5-10 minutes*	Diagnosis, prognosis drug trials, clinical research	Personality	(2)
irse, hysician	9 items 4 grades *5 minutes*	Drug trials, epidemiological studies, rating of changes due to therapy	Depression, fatigue, anxiety	(2)
irse, irse's aide	5 items 5 grades *5 minutes*	Diagnosis, clinical research, rating of changes	Dependency on others for self-care	(3)
sychiatrist, irse	9 items 3-6 grades *5 minutes*	Rating of changes, clinical research	Mood, orientation, learning habits	(2)
elf- administered	*No time limit*	Diagnosis, clinical research, rating of changes	Intellectual functioning, mental deterioration	(2)
irse	101 items 2-7 grades *30 minutes*	Care planning, clinical studies, rating of changes due to therapy	Somatic symptoms, mental status, activities of daily living	(1)
ychiatrist, irse	12 items *2-3 minutes*	Epidemiological studies	Calculation ability	(2)
hysician	10 items 4 grades *5 minutes*	Diagnosis, care planning, rating of changes	Activities of daily living	(3)
irse	24 items 3-6 grades *10-15 minutes*	Epidemiological studies, rating of changes	Depression, behavior, thought disorders	(2)
ychiatrist, hysician	5 items *2-3 minutes*	Prognosis, rating of changes due to therapy	Memory, mood, emotions	(2)
ychiatrist, ychologist, cial worker	12 items 4 grades *5-10 minutes*	Rating of changes	Psychological function, social behavior	(1)

TITLE	YEAR	AUTHOR Country	FORM	CATEGORY	LANGUAGE	POPULATION
65. Fourteen-Symptom Behavior and Mood Scale	1968	WYATT United States	Ordinal rating scale	Mental behavior	English	Inpatient
66. Inventory of Psychic and Somatic Complaints	1969	RASKIN United States	Ordinal rating scale	Mental mood	English	Inpatient
67. Staff and Patient Helping	1969	SIDMAN United States	Questionnaire	Social	English	Hospital nurse assistant
68. Psychiatric Screening of the Elderly	1969	SIMON United States	Check list	Physical Mental	English	Out-patient Inpatient
69. Contentment Index	1970	BLOOM United States	Nominal rating scale	Mental Social	English	Out-patient
70. Leyton Obsessional Inventory	1970	COOPER Great Britain	Questionnaire	Mental behavior	English	Out-patient
71. Scales for Nursing Observation of Behavior Syndromes	1970	CRAIG Canada	Nominal rating scale	Mental behavior	English	Inpatient
72. Physician Questionnaire	1970	RICKELS United States	Questionnaire	Physical Mental	English	Out-patient Inpatient
73. Rating Scale for Extrapyramidal Side Effects	1970	SIMPSON United States	Ordinal rating scale	Physical	English	Inpatient
74. Psychiatric Status Schedule	1970	SPITZER United States	Questionnaire	Mental mood	English	Out-patient Inpatient
75. Befindlichkeits-Skala	1970	ZERSSEN D.R.G.	Nominal rating scale	Mental mood	German	Inpatient
76. Profile of Mood Scale	1971	MAC NAIR United States	Ordinal rating scale	Mental mood	English	Inpatient Out-patient
77. Current and Past Psychopathology Scales	1972	ENDICOTT United States	Nominal rating scale	Mental Social	English	Inpatient Out-patient
78. Psychiatric Evaluation Form	1972	ENDICOTT United States	Ordinal rating scale	Mental Social	English	Inpatient Out-patient
79. Structured and Scaled Interview to Assess Maladjustment	1972	GURLAND United States	Questionnaire	Mental Social	English	Out-patient
80. Depression Status Inventory	1972	ZUNG United States	Ordinal rating scale	Mental mood	English	Inpatient Out-patient
81. Symptom Distress Check-List	1973	DEROGATIS United States	Ordinal rating scale	Mental behavior	English	Out-patient
82. Rating of Mania	1973	PETTERSON Sweden	Ordinal rating scale	Mental behavior	Swedish	Inpatient

BLES

RATER	N° OF ITEMS GRADES *Time required*	APPLICATIONS	VARIABLES	WHY NOT INCLUDED
Nurse, nurse's aide	28 items 8 grades *15 minutes*	Research, rating of changes	Mood, behavior	(2)
Nurse, psychologist, self-administered	50 items 4-7 grades *30-45 minutes*	Therapy assessment, research	Psychosomatic disorders	(2)
Self-administered	140 items 7 grades *30 minutes*	Planning	Possibility of and need for help	(4)
Nurse	30 items *10 minutes*	Screening	Personality depression, memory, physical complaints	(1)
Nurse	10 items 3 grades *5-10 minutes*	Research, planning	Satisfaction	(1)
Self-administered	69 items *30-45 minutes*	Diagnosis, research	Obsessional symptoms, personality	(2)
Nurse	55 items 2-5 grades *15 minutes*	Therapy, diagnosis, care planning	Pessimism, emotion	(2)
Physician	10 items 7 points *5 minutes*	Therapy, rating of changes	Hostility, anxiety, depression, irritability	(2)
Nurse, research worker	10 items 5 grades *10-15 minutes*	Drug trials, diagnosis	Impairment of extrapyramidal system	(3)
Social worker, nurse, psychiatrist, psychologist, research worker	321 items *30-50 minutes*	Clinical research, rating of changes	Anxiety depression, social isolation	(2)
Self-administered	2 x 28 items *10-15 minutes*	Epidemiological studies, rating of changes	Depression, anxiety, mood	(1) (2)
Self-administered, technical and research assistant	65 items 5 grades *3-5 minutes*	Drug trials, clinical research, diagnosis	Feelings, agitation	(2)
Nurse, psychiatrist, psychologist, social worker	171 items 2-7 grades *15-30 minutes*	Diagnosis, prognosis, research	Psychiatric symptoms, social relations	(1)
Psychiatrist, research worker and medical student	19 items 6 grades *20-40 minutes*	Diagnosis, rating of changes	Social relations, behavior disorders, alcoholism	(2)
Psychiatrist	60 items *30 minutes*	Prognosis, diagnosis, research, screening	Behavior disorders, social adjustment	(2)
Nurse, psychiatrist, psychologist	20 items 4 grades *5 minutes*	Drug trials, research, diagnosis, screening	Depression	(5)
Self-administered	90 items 5 grades *20 minutes*	Research, epidemiological studies	Interpersonal relations, anxiety, hostility	(2)
Psychiatrist	9 items 5 grades *30 minutes*	Therapy, drug trials, rating of changes	Manic-depressive, affective disorders	(2)

TITLE	YEAR	AUTHOR Country	FORM	CATEGORY	LANGUAGE	POPULATION
83. Schwab's Depression Scale	1973	SCHWAB United States	Ordinal rating scale	Mental mood	English	Inpatient Out-patient
84. Debility Index	1973	SKINNER United States	Ordinal rating scale	Physical	English	Inpatient Out-patient
85. Hopelessness Scale	1974	BECK United States	Check list	Mental mood	English	Inpatient Out-patient
86. Bigot's Life Satisfaction Index	1974	BIGOT Great Britain	Nominal rating scale	Social	English	Out-patient
87. Self-Assessment of Anxiety and Depression	1976	SNAITH Great Britain	Nominal rating scale	Mental mood	English	Inpatient Out-patient
88. Comprehensive Psychopathological Rating Scale	1978	ASBERG Sweden	Ordinal rating scale	Mental mood	Swedish	Inpatient
89. Schedule for Affective Disorders and Schizophrenia	1978	ENDICOTT United States	Ordinal rating scale	Mental mood	English	Inpatient
90. W.A.I.S. Short Form	1978	HAFNER United States	Test	Mental cognitive	English	Inpatient
91. Pilot Geriatric Arthritis Project	1978	JETTE United States	Ordinal rating scale	Physical	English	Out-patient
92. Category Test	1978	MACK United States	Test	Physical Mental	English	Out-patient
93. Hand-Held Tachistoscope Perception	1978	PAUKER United States	Test	Mental cognitive	English	Out-patient Inpatient
94. Ward Behaviour Questionnaire	1979	CLARKE Great Britain	Check list	Physical	English	Out-patient Inpatient
95. Social Functioning Schedule	1979	REMINGTON Great Britain	Questionnaire	Social	English	Out-patient Inpatient
96. Families' Caregiving Capacity	1980	HIRSCHFELD Israel	Questionnaire	Mental Social	English	Family Care giver
97. Echelle de Ralentissement Dépressif	1980	WIDLÖCHER France	Ordinal rating scale	Mental mood	French	Out-patient
98. Echelle d'Autonomie	1981	BERTHAUX France	Ordinal rating scale	Physical Mental	French	Inpatient
99. Status Physique Fonctionnel	1981	O.M.S. Switzerland	Rating scale	Physical	French	Inpatient
100. Arbeitsgemein- schaft für Gerontopsychiatrie		FREIE UNIV. D.R.G.	Rating scale	Physical	German	Out-patient Inpatient

RATER	N° OF ITEMS GRADES *Time required*	APPLICATIONS	VARIABLES	WHY NOT INCLUDED
Nurse	18 items 5 grades *15 minutes*	Diagnosis, research, epidemiological studies	Depression	(1)
Nurse	5 items 3-5 grades *2-3 minutes*	Care planning	Activities of daily living	(2) (3)
Self- administered or physician	20 items *5 minutes*	Rating of changes, diagnosis, prognosis, clinical research	Depression	(2)
Self- administered	20 items 3 grades *5 minutes*	Research, planning	Life satisfaction	(4)
Self- administered	18 items 4 grades *5 minutes*	Diagnosis, drug trials	Depression, anxiety	(5)
Psychiatrist, psychologist, nurse	65 items 4 grades *1 hour*	Care planning, rating of changes therapy	Memory, mood, depression	(2)
Psychiatrist, psychologist, social worker	88 items 1-7 grades *1-2 hours*	Rating of changes, diagnosis, prognosis	Depression, anxiety, mania	(2)
Psychologist	3 subtests *30 minutes*	Diagnosis, clinical research	Cognitive functions	(2)
Self- administered, physician, nurse	44 items 5 grades *20 minutes*	Prevention, planning	Self-care, level of functional mobility	(3)
Self- administered	5 subtests *30 minutes*	Screening, diagnosis	Intellectual functions, learning	(1)
Physician	*3 minutes*	Diagnosis	Perceptual speed	(2)
Nurse	16 items 2-4 grades *2-3 minutes*	Planning, screening	Activities of daily living, dependency	(3)
Psychiatrist, psychologist	16 items *20-30 minutes*	Planning, therapy, clinical research	Social functioning	(2) (4)
Nurse, physician, social worker	32 items *15-20 minutes*	Planning, research	Family care capacity	(2)
Psychiatrist	14 items 5 grades *8-10 minutes*	Diagnosis, rating of changes, prognosis, drug trials	Slowing of movements, fluency of speech, memory, concentration	(2)
Physician, nurse's aide	8 items *10 minutes*	Diagnosis, prognosis	Mobility, continence, activities of daily living, memory	(1)
Physician	18 items 3-11 grades *15 minutes*	Rating of changes	Instrumental activities of daily living, physical movements	(3)
Physician	343 items *15 minutes*	Epidemiological research, drug trials, diagnosis	Psychosomatic symptoms	(3)

IV - INDEX

IV - INDEX

1 - PRESENTATION

These indices are a new form of classification telling the reader where to find the instruments he wants according to the criteria which may be of particular interest to him. They meet the need to have several ways of classifying the same instrument, allowing rapid location and selection of an instrument according to specification.

They have been designed starting from the content analysis of the 145 instruments establishing the key words identifying the main characteristic features determined by the analytical table. These indices were first compiled by micro-computer then were checked individually by a team of three assessors. The indices were established in accordance with the following classification criteria:

· Author
· Type of instrument
· Categories of classification
· Variables
· Applications
· Translations
· Chronology (year of publication)
· Country
· Degree of specificity
· Population
· Rater (qualifications)

1. INDEX BY AUTHOR

In this alphabetical index, the names of principal authors are given in heavy type, those of co-authors in standard type. The index of the authors of principal instruments is followed by the index of authors of complementary instruments separately presented.

2. INDEX BY TYPE OF INSTRUMENTS

The instruments are listed according to the form they take: scales, check lists, questionnaire, test or composite forms, i.e. those resembling several types.

3. INDEX BY CATEGORY OF CLASSIFICATION

The instruments were first regrouped into sections corresponding to a number of dimensions, and then according to the content of variables.

Section 1: Mental————————→Mood   Cognitive functions   Behavior
                                      (a)   (b)   (c)

Section 2: Mental Social   These three aspects are respectively coded:
           Physical Mental
                                      (a) Mood
                                      (b) Cognitive functions
Section 3: Physical Mental Social   (c) Behavior

- 389 -

4. INDEX BY SUBJECTS

This index is concerned with *variables* and *applications*.

The development of this index passed through two stages of exhaustive enumeration, followed by classification into more reduced categories based on a common logical criterion. The order of presentation retained is the alphabetical order facilitating location.

VARIABLES

The variables retained correspond to the words most often used by authors of the instruments in their answers to the questions contained in the questionnaire.
These variables are presented in the following order:

1. *Activities* of daily living
2. *Anxiety*
3. *Autonomy* – Dependency
4. *Awareness* – Attention
5. *Behavioral* disturbances
6. *Confusion* – Confabulation
7. *Dementia* syndrome
8. *Depressive* symptoms
9. *Economic* aspects
10. *Environment* influences (health and social services)
11. *Family* and social relationships
12. *Instrumental* activities
13. *Intellectual* activities (non-verbal, operational thought, creativity, mental fluency, symbolic processes)
14. *Manic* state
15. *Melancholia*
16. *Memory* (immediate, short-term memory, long-term memory, learning)
17. *Mental* deterioration
18. *Mood*-irritability
19. *Morale* and well-being
20. *Neurological* and sensory status
21. *Organic* pathology
22. *Other psychiatric symptoms* – psychopathology
23. *Perception*
24. *Personality*
25. *Psychomotor* activity
26. *Psychosomatic* disturbances
27. *Self-care*
28. *Sociability* – Adaptability
29. *Spatial* orientation
30. *Stress-Life* events

In using these words, the different authors may not necessarily be applying the same criteria, hence the risk of finding under the same heading instruments which are not measuring the same aspects. This is the reality we have felt obliged to accept in order to stress the urgency of finding a common vocabulary based on a clear definition and well determined criteria that would be a first step towards standardization of the methodology of research on an international level.

The following classification suggests applications that focus on the individual, mixed (individual and group) or group.

Individual	1	Diagnosis
	2	Prognosis
	3	Screening
	4	Care planning.
Mixed	5	Indications for placement
	6	Rating of changes
	7	Review
	8	Experimental or clinical research
Group	9	Drug trials
	10	Epidemiological studies
	11	Administration-management
	12	Teaching – Training of personnel.

5. INDEX BY TRANSLATION

This index indicates for each instrument the different languages in which it has been translated.

6. INDEX CHRONOLOGICAL TABLE

This index is presented in the form of synoptic table with a double entry. In composing this table we were guided by two purposes:

· To give a simultaneous review of several characteristic features of each instrument.
· To enable rapid location of an instrument starting from the point of interest to the user, such as population concerned, rater, etc.

The table is a compilation of information concerned with:

The *country* of the author
The *degree of specificity* (* ** ***)
The *population* to which a particular evaluation can be applied. That population is further distinguished by the place of residence, e.g. institution, out-patient unit or both.
The *rater*. The categories are grouped as below into care giver, non-care giver or the subject himself.

Care giver	**Non-care giver**	**Subject**
1. Physician	4. Social worker	7. Self-evaluation
2. Psychologist	5. Non-medical interviewer	
3. Nurse's aide	6. Immediate family	

2. INDEX

* Main author is indicated by black letters.

Fassio (M.): Ic.17
Feinberg (M.): Ia.17
Ferm (L.): Ic.11
Ferris (S.H.): Ib.32 - Ib.45
Fillenbaum (G.G.): IV.12
Filos (S.): IV.30
Fine (E.W.): IV.2
Fischer-Cornelssen (K.A.): III.11
Fishback (D.B.): Ib.26
Fleischmann (U.M.): IV.29
Fleiss (J.L.): Ic.12
Folstein (M.F.): Ib.22
Folstein (S.E.): Ib.22
Fondarai (J.): Ia.8 - III.9
Fournier (J.): IV.23
Fournier (M.): IV.24
Fowler (R.S.): Ib.10
Fraud (J.P.): III.9
Free (S.M.): Ia.4
Frigard (B.): III.13
Fulcomer (M.): IV.28

Gagne (A.): III.10
Gagnon (G.): IV.23
Gallet (G.): III.9
Gallo (I.): Ic.17
Gardiner (M.): Ic.18 - II.10
Gaucher (J.): Ib.30
Georges (D.): IV.10
Gibson (A.J.): Ib.34
Gilbert (J.G.): Ib.44
Giles (L.): Ic.15
Gilleard (C.J.): IV.25
Girtanner (C.): III.10
Gitz (A.M.): III.16
Goldberg (K.): Ic.12
Goodman (S.P.): II.2
Götestam (K.G.): III.12
Gottfries (C.G.): III.14
Gourlay (A.J.): Ic.12
Graham-White (J.): IV.22
Gram (L.F.): Ia.15
Grauer (H.): IV.9
Graux (P.): III.13
Graziano (C.): Ic.17
Greden (J.F.): Ia.17
Greene (J.G.): Ic.18 - II.10
Grossman (J.): IV.3
Grossman (R.G.): Ib.35
Grotz (R.C.): III.3
Gudiksen (K.S.): II.1
Gurel (L.): IV.4
Gurland (B.J.): IV.11
Gurland (B.J.): Ic.12 - III.7
Guthrie (M.B.): Ia.4

Hachinski (V.C.): Ib.23
Hamilton (M.): Ia.3
Harmatz (J.S.): IV.7
Harrah (C.H.): IV.30
Hasegawa (K.): Ib.19
Heersema (P.H.): Ia.19
Heron (B.): IV.12
Hersch (E.L.): Ib.33 - IV.14
Hodkinson (H.M.): Ib.16
Hodkinson (H.M.): Ib.21
Hogarty (G.E.): Ic.2

Honigfeld (G.): Ic.1
Hugonot (L.): Ic.16 - IV.15
Hugonot (R.): III.18
Hugonot (R.): II.5
Hulten (A.): III.1

Idänpään-Heikkilä (J.): III.15
Iliff (L.D.): Ib.23
Isaacs (B.): Ib.17
Israel (L.): Ib.25 - Ib.39 - Ib.40 - Ib.41 - Ib.42 - Ib.43 - Ib.47 - Ic.16 - II.5 - II.9 - IV.15
Israel (L.): IV.26

Jablensky (A.): IV.18
Jacobs (J.W.): Ib.27
Janakes (C.): Ib.31 - Ic.13
Janin (C.): Ib.30
Jardine (M.Y.): Ia.13
Jasculca (S.): Ic.13
Jefferys (P.M.): Ib.29

Karasu (T.B.): IV.16
Karp (S.A.): Ib.15
Kastenbaum (R.): Ic.6
Katz (S.): III.3
Kelleher (M.J.): Ic.12
Kellett (J.M.): Ic.12
Kendrick (D.C.): Ib.34
Kerstell (J.): III.1
Khan (I.): III.15
Kleban (M.H.): Ic.7
Kleban (M.H.): IV.28
Klett (J.): Ic.1
Kozarević (Dj.): II.4 - IV.20
Kral (V.A.): IV.14
Kramp (P.): Ia.12
Kuntzmann (F.): III.16
Kuriansky (J.): III.7
Kuriansky (J.): IV.11
Kurosaki (T.T.): IV.30

Laboratoire de Gérontologie Sociale.
Université Laval, Québec, Canada: IV.17
Lacava (R.): Ic.17
Laforestrie (R.): II.8
Lallemand (G.): IV.10
Lambert (P.): IV.23
Lanoe (R.): IV.19
Laurie (W.F.): IV.12
Lawton (M.P.): Ia.9 - III.2 - IV.28
Lebeau (A.): IV.23
Lehrman (N.): IV.3
Leroux (R.): IV.24
Lester (D.): Ib.3
Levee (R.F.): Ib.44
Levin (H.S.): Ib.35
Levita (E.): IV.5
Lewis (D.): IV.2
Lieberman (M.): Ib.14 - IV.3
Linn (B.S.): III.17 - IV.4
Linn (M.W.): II.2 - III.17
Linn (M.W.): IV.4
Lipman (A.): Ib.28
Loiseau (P.): Ib.46
Longeot (F.): Ib.20
Loria (Y.): IV.10
Lorr (M.): Ia.5

Walsh (T.J.): IV.12
Wang (R.I.H.): Ia.10
Wechsler (D.): Ib.13
Wells (C.E.): Ib.36
Werner (P.D.): IV.27
Werquin (G.): III.9
White (L.): Ib.11
Whitelem (A.): Ib.46
Wiesen (R.L.): Ia.10
Wilkinson (I.M.): IV.22
Williams (J.R.): Ic.9
Williams (M.): Ib.8

Williamson (J.): III.4
Wing (J.K.): Ic.10
Witkin (H.A.): Ib.15
World Health Organization: Ia.11 – IV.18
World Health Organization: III.15

Yesavage (J.A.): IV.27
Yesavage (J.A.): Ia.19

Zay (N.): IV.17
Zilhka (E.): Ib.23
Zung (W.W.K.): Ia.2 – Ia.16

INDEX BY AUTHORS

COMPLEMENTARY INSTRUMENTS

Ammons (C.H.): 33
Ammons (R.B.): 33
Angus (J.W.S.): 73
Arenberg (D.): 14
Asberg (M.): 88

Ban (T.A.): 63
Barrabee (E.): 9
Barrabee (P.): 9
Beck (A.T.): 85
Berkman (P.L.): 68
Berthaux (P.): 98
Bigot (A.): 86
Billingslea (F.Y.): 5
Blenkner (M.): 69
Blewett (D.B.): 16
Bloom (M.): 69
Brandon (S.): 94
Bridge (G.W.K.): 87
Britton (P.G.): 53
Brownell (W.M.): 44
Bunney (W.E.): 40
Burdock (E.I.): 19
Burdock (E.I.): 47
Buss (A.H.): 13

Cahn (C.): 46
Caird (W.K.): 34
Carlson (N.J.): 92
Carney (M.W.P.): 48
Casey (J.F.): 39
Cattell (R.B.): 32
Clarke (M.): 94
Clement (F.): 20 - 35 - 41
Clyde (D.J.): 28
Cohen (J.): 74
Cooper (J.): 70
Corotto (L.V.): 90
Covi (L.): 81
Craig (W.J.): 71
Crisp (A.H.): 54
Crown (S.): 54
Curnutt (R.H.): 90
Cutler (R.P.): 26

Davis (J.E.): 56
Deboffle (G.): 98
Dempsey (P.): 43
Deniston (O.L.): 91
Derogatis (L.R.): 81
Dexter (M.): 49
Dinnerstein (A.J.): 49
Dinoff (M.): 36
Dixon (J.C.): 50
Dobson (W.R.): 27
Dodd (K.J.): 94
Droppleman (L.F.): 76
Durkee (A.): 13

Endicott (J.): 77 - 78 - 89
Endicott (J.): 74
Epstein (L.J.): 68

Farina (A.): 14
Finesinger (J.): 9
Fleiss (J.L.): 47 - 74 - 79
Folstein (M.F.): 93
Frank (J.D.): 79
Freed (E.X.): 10
Freie Universität. Berlin: 100
Fyrö (B.): 82

Garside (R.F.): 48
Gauger (A.B): 44
Gorham (D.R.): 38
Gough (H.G.): 21
Gross (M.): 28
Guertin (W.H.): 17
Guilford (J.P.): 1
Guilford (R.B.): 1
Gurel (L.): 56
Gurland (B.J.): 79
Guskin (S.): 14

Hackett (E.): 55
Hafner (J.L.): 90
Hakerem (G.): 19
Hamburg (D.A.): 40
Hamilton (M.): 87
Hardesty (A.S.): 19 - 47
Hargreaves (W.A.): 62
Harris (A.D.): 57
Havighurst (R.J.): 29
Heron (A.): 11
Hester (R.): 18
Hirschfeld (M.J.): 96
Hitchman (I.L.): 28
Hoagland (H.): 4
Holden (A.M.): 94
Hollister (L.E.): 39
Holzer (C.E): 83
Hovaguimian (T.): 99
Howard (K.): 72
Hughes (A.O.): 94
Hunt (H.F.): 3

Inglis (J.): 12 - 34
Isaacs (B.): 45

Jenkins (R.L.): 18
Jette (A.M.): 91

Kahn (T.C.): 22
Katz (G.): 39
Katz (M.M.): 42
Kaufman (I.C.): 4
Kline (N.S.): 55

* Indicated numbers correspond to the numbers of the instruments on the summary table pp. 372-373.

Koeller (D.M.): 75
Kral (V.A.): 46
Kral (V.A.): 63
Krüger (H.): 100
Krugman (A.D.): 17
Kupper (D.J.): 65
Kurland (H.D.): 26

Langner (T.S.): 37
Lawrence (J.): 28
Lehmann (H.E.): 63
Lester (D.): 85
Letemendia (F.J.J.): 57
Lipman (R.S.): 81
Löfving (B.): 12
Lorr (M.): 23
Lorr (M.): 76
Lowenthal (M.): 49
Lucero (R.J.): 6
Lyerly (S.B.): 42

Mack (J.L.): 92
Mac Keon (J.J.): 66
Mac Nair (D.M.): 76
Malamud (W.): 4
Meyer (B.T.): 6
Montgomery (S.A.): 88
Moos (R.H.): 67
Moran (T.H.): 93
Morris (J.R.): 36
Moulias (R.): 98
Mueller (H.): 46

Neugarten (B.L.): 29
Newell (P.C.): 28

Oberleder (M.): 30
O'Connor (J.P.): 23
Overall (J.E.): 38 – 39

Palmer (R.L.): 94
Patterson (T.W.): 27
Pauker (N.E.): 93
Pearce (D.): 94
Perris (C.): 88
Petterson (U.): 82
Piette (F.): 98
Pokorny (A.D.): 39
Pollin (W.): 51
Post (F.): 12

Raskin (A.): 66
Raymaker (H.): 36
Reatig (N.): 66
Reeves (W.P.): 28
Remington (M.): 95
Retter (R.W.): 44
Rey (E.R.): 75
Rickels (K.): 72
Robinson (R.A.): 31
Rockland (L.H.): 51
Roth (M.): 48
Rowell (J.T.): 7
Russell (W.W.): 44

Sanderson (R.E.): 34
Savage (R.D.): 53

Schalling (D.): 88
Scheier (I.H.): 32
Schulterbrandt (J.): 66
Schwab (J.J.): 83
Sedvall (G.): 82 – 88
Shapiro (M.B.): 12
Shatin (L.): 10
Sidman (J.): 67
Silver (D.): 63
Simon (A.): 68
Simpson (G.M.): 55 – 73
Skinner (D.E.): 84
Smith (A.): 58
Snaith (R.P.): 87
Spitzer (R.L.): 47 – 74
Spitzer (R.L.): 77 – 78 – 89
Stafford (J.W.): 23
Stauffacher (J.): 18
Stefaniuk (W.B.): 16
Stone (A.R.): 79
Stotsky (B.A.): 59
Sullivan (W.): 32

Taylor (J.): 8
Tien (H.C.): 24
Tobin (S.S.): 29
Trexler (L.): 85
Trier (T.R.): 64
Tyrer (P.): 95

Van De Castle (R.L.): 52
Venables (P.H.): 15

Walkey (F.A.): 45
Warheit (G.J.): 83
Weissman (A.): 85
Widlocher (D.): 97
Wilcox (P.H.): 2
Willems (P.J.A.): 57
Wilson (I.C.): 60
Wolmark (Y.): 98
World Health Organization: 99
Wyatt (R.J.): 65
Wylie (C.M.): 61

Yett (D.E.): 84
Yorkston (N.J.): 79

Zerssen (Von D.V.): 75
Zubin (J.): 19
Zuckerman (M.): 25
Zung (W.W.K.): 80

RATING SCALE

Nurses' Observation Scale for Inpatient Evaluation	Honigfeld	1965	Ic.1
Self Rating Depression Scale	Zung	1965	Ia.2
Discharge Readiness Inventory	Hogarty	1966	Ic.2
Stockton Geriatric Rating Scale	Meer	1966	IV.1
Hamilton Rating Scale for Depression	Hamilton	1967	Ia.3
Dementia Scale	Blessed	1968	Ib.7
New Physician's Rating List	Free	1969	Ia.4
Nursing Load Score	Hulten	1969	III.I
Instrumental Activities of Daily Living Scale	Lawton	1969	III.2
Social Dysfunction Rating Scale	Linn	1969	II.2
Parkside Behaviour Rating Scale	Fine	1970	IV.2
Index of A.D.L.	Katz	1970	III.3
Geriatric Rating Scale	Plutchik	1970	IV.3
VIRO Orientation Scale	Kastenbaum	1972	Ic.6
Adult Personality Rating Schedule	Kleban	1972	Ic.7
Disability Rating Scale	Akhtar	1973	III.5
Personal Habits, Environment & Psychosocial Factors	Kozarević	1973	II.4
Geriatric Profile	Missouri Institute	1973	III.6
Functional Life Scale	Sarno	1973	IV.5
Behavior Rating Scale	Williams	1973	Ic.9
Beck Depression Inventory	Beck	1974	Ia.7
Echelle d'Observation Clinique	Crocq	1974	Ia.8
D. Test	Ferm	1974	Ic.11
Parachek Geriatric Behavior Rating Scale	Parachek	1974	IV.6
Sandoz Clinical Assessment-Geriatric	Shader	1974	IV.7
Geriatric Functional Rating Scale	Grauer	1975	IV.9
Performance Test of Activities of Daily Living	Kuriansky	1976	III.7
Brief Anxiety Rating Scale	Wang	1976	Ia.10
Echelle d'Appréciation Clinique en Gériatrie	Georges	1977	IV.10
Ward Function Inventory	Norton	1977	III.8
Standardized Assessment of Patients with Depressive Disorders	O.M.S.	1977	Ia.11
Mania Rating Scale	Bech	1978	Ia.12
London Psychogeriatric Rating Scale	Hersch	1978	IV.14
Origine de la Dépendance	Israël	1978	IV.15
Irritability-Depression-Anxiety Scale	Snaith	1978	Ia.13
Montgomery & Asberg Depression Rating Scale	Montgomery	1979	Ia.14
Disability Assessment Schedule	O.M.S.	1979	IV.18
W.H.O. Depression Scale	Bech	1980	Ia.15
Echelle Clinique de Gérontologie	Crocq	1980	III.9
Echelle de Dépendance-Autonomie	Delcros	1980	IV.19
Evaluation de l'Autonomie	Delomier	1980	III.10
Evaluation Clinique de la Personnalité	Israël	1980	Ic.16
Echelle Clinique d'Aptitudes Intellectuelles	Israël	1980	Ib.40
Evaluation Globale de l'Autonomie	Patron	1980	IV.21
Self-Rating Anxiety Scale	Zung	1980	Ia.16
Fischer Symptom Checklist	Fischer	1981	III.11
Geriatric Rating Scale	Götestam	1981	III.12
Echelle d'Expression de l'Autonomie: Geronte	Leroux	1981	IV.24
Self Assessment Scale-Geriatric	Yesavage	1981	IV.27
Melancholia Rating Scale	Bech	1982	Ia.18
G.B.S. Scale	Gottfries	1982	III.14
Behavioural & Mood Disturbance Scale	Greene	1982	Ic.18
Relatives' Stress Scale	Greene	1982	II.10
Evaluation de la Dépendance en Institution	Kuntzmann	1982	III.16
Rapid Disability Rating Scale	Linn	1982	III.17
Functional Activities Questionnaire	Pfeffer	1982	IV.30
Grille pour l'Evaluation du Degré de Dépendance	C.I.C.P.A.	1982	IV.31
Grille de Dépendance	Centre de Gériatrie	1982	IV.32
Echelle de Dépendance C.E.N.T.S.	Hugonot	1982	III.18

CHECK LISTS

Depression Adjective Checklist	Lubin	1965	Ia.1
Short Scale for the Assessment of Mental Health	Savage	1967	Ic.4
Patient Activity Checklist	Aumack	1969	Ic.5
Physical & Mental Impairment-of-Function Evaluation in the Aged	Gurel	1972	IV.4
Measurement of Morale in the Elderly	Pierce	1973	Ia.6
Ischemia Score	Hachinski	1975	Ib.23
Philadelphia Geriatric Center Morale Scale	Lawton	1975	Ia.9
Hypochondriasis Scale Institutional Geriatric	Brink	1978	Ic.13
Geriatric Resident Goals Scale	Cornbleth	1978	IV.13
Short Psychiatric Evaluation Schedule	Pfeiffer	1979	Ic.14
Checklist Differentiating Pseudo-Dementia from Dementia	Wells	1979	Ib.36
Carroll Rating Scale	Carroll	1981	Ia.17
Geriatric Depression Scale	Brink-Yesavage	1982	Ia.19

QUESTIONNAIRES

Self Perception Questionnaire	Preston	1966	II.1
Interview for Recent Life Events	Paykel	1971	II.3
Mental Test Score	Hodkinson	1972	Ib.16
Physical & Mental Health Questionnaire	Milne	1972	III.4
Dementia Screening Scale	Hasegawa	1974	Ib.19
Abbreviated Mental Test	Qureshi	1974	Ib.21
Present State Examination	Wing	1974	Ic.10
Short Portable Mental Status Questionnaire	Pfeiffer	1975	Ib.24
Geriatric Mental State Schedule	Copeland	1976	Ic.12
Attitudes et Perceptions Mutuelles des Médecins-Malades-Familles	Israël	1976	II.5
Life Events Inventory	Tennant	1976	II.7
Philadelphia Geriatric Center Mental Status Questionnaire	Fishback	1977	Ib.26
Cognitive Capacity Screening Examination	Jacobs	1977	Ib.27
Comprehensive Assessment & Referral Evaluation	Gurland	1977	IV.11
Confusion Assessment Schedule	Slater	1977	Ib.28
Multidimensional Functional Assessment Questionnaire	Center for Aging	1978	IV.12
Modified Tooting Bec Questionnaire	Denham	1978	Ib.29
Aspects Psychologiques & Sociaux du Vieillissement	Israël	1978	II.9
Galveston Orientation & Amnesia Test	Levin	1979	Ib.35
Orientation Scale for Geriatric Patients	Berg	1980	Ib.37
Comprehensive Health Questionnaire	Kozarević	1980	IV.20
Bilan-Test d'Appréciation de la Perte d'Autonomie	Graux	1981	III.13
Drug Dependency & Overdose Assessment	Idänpään-Heikkilä	1982	III.15
Multilevel Assessment Instrument	Lawton	1982	IV.28

TESTS

Histoire du Lion	Barbizet	1965	Ib.1
Visual Retention Test	Benton	1965	Ib.2
Archétype Test à 9 Eléments	Durand	1967	Ic.3
Shaw Blocks Test	Lester	1967	Ib.3
Memory Battery	Barbizet	1968	Ib.4
Test de Praxie Constructive Tridimensionnelle	Benton	1968	Ib.5
Information-Memory-Concentration Test	Blessed	1968	Ib.6
Scale for the Measurement of Memory	Williams	1968	Ib.8
Praxies Grapho-Motrices	Andrey	1969	Ib.9
Simple Non-Language Test of New Learning	Fowler	1969	Ib.10
Short-Term Memory Test	Dana	1970	Ib.11
Screening Test for Organic Brain Disease	Nahor	1970	Ib.12
Echelle d'Intelligence de Wechsler pour Adultes	Wechsler	1970	Ib.13
Geriatric Interpersonal Evaluation Scale	Plutchik	1971	Ib.14
Embedded Figures Test	Witkin	1971	Ib.15
Set Test	Isaacs	1972	Ib.17
Simple Methods of Testing Ability	Silver	1972	Ib.18
Senior Apperception Technique	Bellak	1973	Ic.8
Echelle de Développement de la Pensée Logique	Longeot	1974	Ib.20
Mini Mental State	Folstein	1975	Ib.22
Batterie de Vigilance en Institution	Israël	1976	Ib.25
Psychodiagnostic de Rorschach	Rorschach	1976	II.6
Test Projectif	Laforestrie	1977	II.8

Echelle d'Efficience Intellectuelle	Janin	1978	Ib.30
Stimulus Recognition Test	Brink	1979	Ib.31
Misplaced Objects Task	Crook	1979	Ib.32
Extended Scale for Dementia	Hersch	1979	Ib.33
Kendrick Battery for the Detection of Dementia in the Elderly	Kendrick	1979	Ib.34
Batterie de Vigilance en Ambulatoire	Israël	1980	Ib.39
Batterie de Fluidité à l'usage des Généralistes	Israël	1980	Ib.41
Batterie de Mémoire en Ambulatoire	Israël	1980	Ib.42
Examen Psychologique pour Personnes Agées Hospitalisées	Israël	1980	Ib.43
Guild Memory Test	Gilbert	1981	Ib.44
Shopping List Task	Mac Carthy	1981	Ib.45
M. Test	Mezzena	1981	Ic.17
Memory Activity Scale	Signoret	1982	Ib.46

COMPOUND INSTRUMENTS

Psychotic Inpatient Profile	Lorr	1969	Ia.5
Psychogeriatric Assessment Program	Douglas Hospital	1975	IV.8
Geriatric Rapid Diagnostic Battery	Murkofsky	1978	IV.16
Batterie de Fiches d'Evaluation	Zay	1978	IV.17
Survey Psychiatric Assessment Schedule	Bond	1980	Ic.15
Hierarchic Dementia Scale	Cole	1980	Ib.38
Edinburgh Psychogeriatric Dependency Rating Scale	Wilkinson	1980	IV.22
Système d'Information C.T.M.S.P.	E.R.O.S.	1981	IV.23
Clifton Assessment Procedures for Elderly	Pattie	1981	IV.25
Questionnaire d'Enquête pour Etude Epidémiologique	Vignat-Israel	1981	IV.26
Nürnberger Alters Inventar	Oswald	1982	IV.29
Bilans de Bel Air 1960-1982	Ecole de Bel Air		IV.33
Bilan d'Evaluation du Syndrome Démentiel	Israël		Ib.47

Hierarchic Dementia Scale	Cole	1980	Ib.38
Batterie de Vigilance en Ambulatoire	Israël	1980	Ib.39
Echelle Clinique d'Aptitudes Intellectuelles	Israël	1980	Ib.40
Batterie de Fluidité à l'usage des Généralistes	Israël	1980	Ib.41
Batterie de Mémoire en Ambulatoirc	Israël	1980	Ib.42
Examen Psychologique pour Personnes Agées Hospitalisées	Israël	1980	Ib.43
Guild Memory Test	Gilbert	1981	Ib.44
Shopping List Task	Mac Carthy	1981	Ib.45
Memory Activity Scale	Signoret	1982	Ib.46
Bilan d'Evaluation de Syndrome Démentiel	Israël		Ib.47

Behavior

Nurses' Observation Scale for Inpatient Evaluation	Honigfeld	1965	Ic.1
Discharge Readiness Inventory (*)	Hogarty	1966	Ic.2
Archétype Test à 9 Elements	Durand	1967	Ic.3
Short Scale for the Assessment of Mental Health	Savage	1967	Ic.4
Patient Activity Checklist (*)	Aumack	1969	Ic.5
VIRO Orientation Scale (*)	Kastenbaum	1972	Ic.6
Adult Personality Rating Schedule (*)	Kleban - Brody	1972	Ic.7
Senior Apperception Technique (*)	Bellak	1973	Ic.8
Behavior Rating Scale	Williams	1973	Ic.9
Present State Examination	Wing-Sartorius	1974	Ic.10
D. Test (*)	Ferm	1974	Ic.11
Geriatric Mental State Schedule	Copeland	1976	Ic.12
Hypochondriasis Scale Institutional Geriatric	Brink	1978	Ic.13
Short Psychiatric Evaluation Schedule	Pfeiffer	1979	Ic.14
Survey Psychiatric Assessment Schedule	Bond	1980	Ic.15
Evaluation Clinique de la Personnalité (*)	Israël	1980	Ic.16
M. Test (*)	Mezzena	1981	Ic.17
Behavioural and Mood Disturbance Scale (*)	Greene	1982	Ic.18

SECTION 2

MENTAL - SOCIAL

Self Perception Questionnaire	Preston	1966	II.1
Social Dysfunction Rating Scale	Linn	1969	II.2
Interview for Recent Life Events	Paykel	1971	II.3
Personal Habits, Environment & Psychosocial Factors	Kozarević	1973	II.4
Attitudes et Perceptions Mutuelles des Médecins-Malades-Familles	Israël	1976	II.5
Psychodiagnostic Test	Rorschach	1976	II.6
Life Events Inventory	Tennant	1976	II.7
Test Projectif	Laforestrie	1977	II.8
Aspects Psychologiques & Sociaux du Vieillissement	Israel	1978	II.9
Relatives' Stress Scale	Greene	1982	II.10

PHYSICAL MENTAL

Nursing Load Score (**) (c)	Hulten	1969	III.1
Instrumental Activities of Daily Living Scale (**) (b)	Lawton-Brody	1969	III.2
Index of A.D.L. (**) (c)	Katz	1970	III.3
Physical & Mental Health Questionnaire (a,b)	Milne	1972	III.4
Disability Rating Scale (**) (c)	Akhtar	1973	III.5
Geriatric Profile (a,b)	Missouri Institute	1973	III.6
Performance Test of Activities of Daily Living (**) (b)	Kuriansky	1976	III.7
Ward Function Inventory (**) (b,c)	Norton	1977	III.8
Echelle Clinique de Gérontologie (a,b)	Crocq	1980	III.9
Evaluation de l'Autonomie (**) (b)	Delomier	1980	III.10
Fischer Symptom Check-list (a)	Fischer	1981	III.11
Geriatric Rating Scale (a,b,c)	Götestam	1981	III.12
Bilan-Test d'Appréciation de la Perte d'Autonomie (**) (b)	Graux	1981	III.13
G.B.S. Scale (**) (a,b)	Gottfries	1982	III.14
Drug Dependency & Overdose Assessment (c)	Idänpään Heikkilä	1982	III.15
Evaluation de la Dépendance en Institution (**) (c)	Kuntzmann	1982	III.16
Rapid Disability Rating Scale (**) (b,c)	Linn	1982	III.17
Echelle de Dépendance C.E.N.T.S. (**) (b)	Hugonot	1982	III.18

PHYSICAL MENTAL SOCIAL

Stockton Geriatric Rating Scale (**) (c)	Meer	1966	IV.1
Parkside Behaviour Rating Scale (c)	Fine	1970	IV.2
Geriatric Rating Scale (**) (c)	Plutchik	1970	IV.3
P.A.M.I.E. Scale (**) (a,c)	Gurel	1972	IV.4
Functional Life Scale (**) (b,c)	Sarno	1973	IV.5
Parachek Geriatric Behavior Rating Scale (c)	Parachek - Miller	1974	IV.6
Sandoz Clinical Assessment-Geriatric (c)	Shader	1974	IV.7
Psychogeriatric Assessment Program (c)	Douglas Hospital	1975	IV.8
Geriatric Functional Rating Scale (**) (c)	Grauer	1975	IV.9
Echelle d'Appréciation Clinique en Gériatrie (c)	Georges-Lallemand	1977	IV.10
Comprehensive Assessment & Referral Evaluation (a,b,c)	Gurland	1977	IV.11
Multidimensional Functional Assessment Quest. (**) (a,b,c,)	Center for Aging	1978	IV.12
Geriatric Resident Goals Scale (**) (c)	Cornbleth	1978	IV.13
London Psychogeriatric Rating Scale (c)	Hersch	1978	IV.14
Origine de la Dépendance (b) (**)	Israël	1978	IV.15
Geriatric Rapid Diagnostic Battery (**) (a,b,c)	Murkofsky	1978	IV.16
Batterie de Fiches d'Evaluation (**) (a,b,c)	Zay	1978	IV.17
Disability Assessment Schedule (**) (c)	W.H.O.	1979	IV.18
Echelle de Dépendance-Autonomie (**) (b,c)	Delcros-Lanoe	1980	IV.19
Comprehensive Health Questionnaire (c)	Kozarević	1980	IV.20
Evaluation Globale de l'Autonomie (**) (a)	Patron	1980	IV.21
Edinburgh Psychogeriatric Dependency Rating Scale (**) (b,c)	Wilkinson	1980	IV.22
Système d'Information C.T.M.S.P. (**) (a,b,c)	E.R.O.S.	1981	IV.23
Echelle d'Expression de l'Autonomie: Geronte (**) (b)	Leroux-Attalli	1981	IV.24
Clifton Assessment Procedures for Elderly (**) (c)	Pattie	1981	IV.25
Questionnaire d'Enquête pour Etude Epidémiologique (a,b,c)	Vignat - Israël	1981	IV.26
Self-Assessment Scale-Geriatric (b,c)	Yesavage	1981	IV.27
Multilevel Assessment Instrument (**) (a,b,c)	Lawton	1982	IV.28
Nurnberger Alters Inventar (b)	Oswald	1982	IV.29
Functional Activities Questionnaire (**) (b)	Pfeffer	1982	IV.30
Grille pour l'Evaluation du Degré de Dépendance (**) (c)	C.I.C.P.A.		IV.31
Grille de Dépendance (**) (c)	Centre de Gériatrie		IV.32
Bilans de Bel Air 1960-1982 (a,b,c)	Ecole de Bel Air		IV.33

(*) Instruments which can be classified as "Mental Social".
(**) Instruments evaluating primarily dependency
(a), (b), (c): Mental components included in instruments dealing with physical status (sections 2 and 3)
        (a): Mood
        (b): Cognitive functions
        (c): Behavior

Gurland (IV 11)
Zay (IV 17)
Lawton (IV 28)

ENVIRONMENTAL INFLUENCES

Kozarević (II 4)
Israël (II 5)
Israël (II 9)
Sarno (IV 5)
Dastoor-Douglas Hospital (IV 8)
Grauer (IV 9)
Gurland (IV 11)
Ctr for Aging. Duke Univ. (IV 12)
Zay (IV 17)
Kozarević (IV 20)
Patron (IV 21)

HEALTH & SOCIAL SERVICES

Gurland (IV 11)
Ctr. for Aging. Duke Univ. (IV 12)
Zay (IV 17)
Kozarević (IV 20)
Patron (IV 21)
Lawton (IV 28)

FAMILY & SOCIAL
RELATIONSHIPS
Kleban (Ic 7)
Bellak (Ic 8)
Ferm (Ic 11)
Mezzena (Ic 17)
Preston (II 1)
Linn (II 2)
Paykel (II 3)
Kozarević (II 4)
Israël (II 5)
Tennant (II 7)
Laforestrie (II 8)
Israël (II 9)
Meer (IV 1)
Plutchik (IV 3)
Sarno (IV 5)
Miller (IV 6)
Grauer (IV 9)
Ctr. for Aging. Duke Univ. (IV 12)
Cornbleth (IV 13)
Jablensky – W.H.O. (IV 18)
Delcros (IV 19)
Patron (IV 21)
E.R.O.S. (IV 23)
Leroux (IV 24)
Pattie (IV 25)
Vignat – Israël (IV 26)
Lawton (IV 28)
C.I.C.P.A. (IV 31)

INSTRUMENTAL ACTIVITIES

Nahor (Ib 12)
Silver (Ib 18)
Folstein (Ib 22)
Hersch (Ib 33)
Cole (Ib 38)
Israël (Ib 47)

Lawton-Brody (III 2)
Kuriansky (III 7)
Pattie (IV 25)
Pfeffer (IV 30)
Bel Air (IV 33)

SPEECH

Barbizet (Ib 1)
Silver (Ib 18)
Folstein (Ib 22)

INTELLECTUAL ACTIVITIES

Barbizet (Ib 1)
Lester (Ib 3)
Wechsler (Ib 13)
Plutchik (Ib 14)
Isaacs (Ib 17)
Hasegawa (Ib 19)
Longeot (Ib 20)
Qureshi (Ib 21)
Folstein (Ib 22)
Pfeiffer (Ib 24)
Israël (Ib 25)
Fishback (Ib 26)
Jacobs (Ib 27)
Janin (Ib 30)
Hersch (Ib 33)
Cole (Ib 38)
Israël (Ib 39)
Israël (Ib 40)
Israël (Ib 41)
Israël (Ib 43)
Durand (Ic 3)
Kastenbaum (Ic 6)
Preston (II 1)
Crocq (III 9)
Graux (III 13)
Gottfries (III 14)
Sarno (IV 5)
Shader (IV 7)
Georges (IV 10)
Delcros (IV 19)
Murkofsky (IV 16)
E.R.O.S. (IV 23)
Pattie (IV 25)
Oswald (IV 29)

NON VERBAL

Benton (Ib 2)
Lester (Ib 3)
Benton (Ib 5)
Andrey (Ib 9)
Fowler (Ib 10)
Nahor (Ib 12)
Witkin (Ib 15)
Longeot (Ib 20)
Brink (Ib 31)
Crook (Ib 32)

OPERATIONAL THOUGHT

Andrey (Ib 9)
Wechsler (Ib 13)
Longeot (Ib 20)
Jacobs (Ib 27)

Hersch (Ib 33)
Cole (Ib 38)
Israël (Ib 47)

CREATIVITY

Lester (Ib 3)

MENTAL FLUENCY

Isaacs (Ib 17)
Pfeiffer (Ib 24)
Israël (Ib 25)
Jacobs (Ib 27)
Israël (Ib 39)
Israël (Ib 41)
Israël (Ib 43)

IMAGINATION

Durand (Ic 3)

MANIC STATE

Bech (Ia 12)

MELANCHOLIA

Hamilton (Ia 3)
Bech (Ia 18)

MEMORY

Barbizet (Ib 1)
Benton (Ib 2)
Barbizet (Ib 4)
Benton (Ib 5)
Blessed (Ib 6)
Williams (Ib 8)
Fowler (Ib 10)
Dana (Ib 11)
Wechsler (Ib 13)
Plutchik (Ib 14)
Hodkinson (Ib 16)
Silver (Ib 18)
Folstein (Ib 22)
Pfeiffer (Ib 24)
Israël (Ib 25)
Fishback (Ib 26)
Jacobs (Ib 27)
Slater (Ib 28)
Denham (Ib 29)
Janin (Ib 30)
Brink (Ib 31)
Crook (Ib 32)
Hersch (Ib 33)
Kendrick (Ib 34)
Levin (Ib 35)
Berg (Ib 37)
Cole (Ib 38)
Israël (Ib 39)
Israël (Ib 41)
Israël (Ib 42)
Israël (Ib 43)
Gilbert (Ib 44)
Mac Carthy (Ib 45)
Signoret (Ib 46)
Ferm (Ic 11)

Norton (III 8)
Götestam (III 12)
Oswald (IV 29)

LEARNING

Barbizet (Ib 4)
Williams (Ib 8)
Fowler (Ib 10)
Israël (Ib 42)
Mac Carthy (Ib 45)
Signoret (Ib 46)

IMMEDIATE MEMORY

Wechsler (Ib 13)
Folstein (Ib 22)
Israël (Ib 25)
Hersch (Ib 33)
Israël (Ib 39)
Israël (Ib 42)
Israël (Ib 43)
Gilbert (Ib 44)
Mac Carhy (Ib 45)
Signoret (Ib 46)

SHORT-TERM MEMORY

Fowler (Ib 10)
Dana (Ib 11)
Folstein (Ib 22)
Pfeiffer (Ib 24)
Israël (Ib 25)
Fishback (Ib 26)
Jacobs (Ib 27)
Janin (Ib 30)
Brink (Ib 31)
Crook (Ib 32)
Hersch (Ib 33)
Kendrick (Ib 34)
Levin (Ib 35)
Cole (Ib 38)
Israël (Ib 39)
Israël (Ib 41)
Israël (Ib 42)
Israël (Ib 43)
Gilbert (Ib 44)
Mac Carthy (Ib 45)
Signoret (Ib 46)

LONG-TERM MEMORY

Pfeiffer (Ib 24)
Fishback (Ib 26)
Janin (Ib 30)
Cole (Ib 38)

MENTAL DETERIORATION

Wechsler (Ib 13)
Israël (Ib 43)
Shader (IV 7)
Georges (IV 10)

MOOD-IRRITABILITY

Wang (Ia 10)
Snaith (Ia 13)

Bond (Ic 15)
Mezzena (Ic 17)
Greene (Ic 18)
Missouri Institute of Psychiatry (III 6)
Crocq (III 9)
Indänpään-Heikkilä (III 15)
Gurel (IV 4)
Dastoor-Douglas Hospital (IV 8)
Georges (IV 10)
Yesavage (IV 27)

MORALE AND WELL-BEING

Pierce (Ia 6)
Lawton (Ia 9)
Pfeiffer (Ic 14)
Israël (Ic 16)
Kozarević (II 4)
Patron (IV 21)
Lawton (IV 28)

NEUROLOGICAL & SENSORY STATUS

Hachinski (Ib 23)
Cole (Ib 38)
Israël (Ib 47)
Gurel (IV 4)
Shader (IV 7)
Dastoor - Douglas Hospital (IV 8)
Kozarevic (IV 20)
Leroux (IV 24)

ORGANIC PATHOLOGY

Zung (Ia 2)
Zung (Ia 16)
Andrey (Ib 9)
Nahor (Ib 12)
Fishback (Ib 26)
Levin (Ib 35)
Savage (Ic 4)
Bond (Ic 15)
Milne (III 4)
Missouri Institute of Psychiatry (III 6)
Crocq (III 9)
Graux (III 13)
Idänpään-Heikkilä (III 15)
Miller (IV 6)
Grauer (IV 9)
Georges (IV 10)
Gurland (IV 11)
Ctr. for Aging. Duke Univ. (IV 12)
Murkofsky (IV 16)
Kozarević (IV 20)
Wilkinson (IV 22)
E.R.O.S. (IV 23)
Lawton (IV 28)

OTHER PSYCHIATRIC SYMPTOMS PSYCHOPATHOLOGY

Lorr (Ia 5)
Crocq (Ia 8)
Honigfeld (Ic 1)
Hogarty (Ic 2)

Durand (Ic 3)
Wing (Ic 10)
Copeland (Ic 12)
Brink (Ic 13)
Pfeiffer (Ic 14)
Bond (Ic 15)
Israël (Ic 16)
Fischer (III 11)
Götestam (III 12)
Dastoor-Douglas Hospital (IV 8)
Grauer (IV 9)
Zay (IV 17)
Vignat - Israël (IV 26)

HALLUCINATIONS

Lorr (Ia 5)

HYPOCHONDRIA

Brink (Ic 13)

NEUROTIC STATES

Bond (Ic 15)

PSYCHOTIC STATES

Lorr (Ia 5)
Honigfeld (Ic 1)
Bond (Ic 15)

PERCEPTION

Andrey (Ib 9)
Plutchik (Ib 14)
Witkin (Ib 15)
Silver (Ib 18)
Israël (Ib 41)
Mezzena (Ic 17)
Israël (II 5)
Rorschach (II 6)
Laforestrie (II 8)
Graux (III 13)
Centre de Gériatrie (IV 32)

PERSONALITY

Kleban (Ic 7)
Williams (Ic 9)
Wing (Ic 10)
Copeland (Ic 12)
Israël (Ic 16)
Mezzena (Ic 17)
Preston (II 1)
Rorschach (II 6)
Vignat - Israël (IV 26)
Oswald (IV 29)

PSYCHOMOTOR ACTIVITY

Andrey (Ib 9)
Nahor (Ib 12)
Folstein (Ib 22)
Israël (Ib 25)
Hersch (Ib 33)
Cole (Ib 38)

Israël (Ib 39)
Israël (Ib 43)

PSYCHOSOMATIC DISTURBANCES

Free (Ia 4)
Wang (Ia 10)
Wing (Ic 10)
Copeland (Ic 12)
Brink (Ic 13)
Milne (III 4)
Missouri Institute of Psychiatry (III 6)
Fischer (III 11)
Yesavage (IV 27)

SELF CARE

Williams (Ic 9)
Lawton-Brody (III 2)
Katz (III 3)
Akhtar (III 5)
Götestam (III 12)
Gottfries (III 14)
Fine (IV 2)
Miller (IV 6)
Cornbleth (IV 13)
Israël (IV 15)
Wilkinson (IV 22)
Oswald (IV 29)
C.I.C.P.A. (IV 31)
Centre de Geriatrie (IV 32)

SOCIABILITY - ADAPTABILITY

Pierce (Ia 6)
Hogarty (Ic 2)
Kastenbaum (Ic 6)
Kleban (Ic 7)
Bellak (Ic 8)
Williams (Ic 9)
Preston (II 1)

Linn (II 2)
Paykel (II 3)
Kozarević (II 4)
Israël (II 5)
Rorschach (II 6)
Laforestrie (II 8)
Israël (II 9)
Greene (II 10)
Missouri Institute of Psychiatry (III 6)
Norton (III 8)
Fischer (III 11)
Meer (IV 1)
Fine (IV 2)
Plutchik (IV 3)
Sarno (IV 5)
Miller (IV 6)
Shader (IV 7)
Georges (IV 10)
Ctr for Aging. Duke Univ. (IV 12)
Cornbleth (IV 13)
Murkofsky (IV 16)
Jablensky-W.H.O. (IV 18)
Kozarević (IV 20)
E.R.O.S. (IV 23)
Pattie (IV 25)
Yesavage (IV 27)
Oswald (IV 29)

ATTITUDES

Bellak (Ic 8)
Preston (II 1)
Linn (II 2)
Israël (II 5)
Rorschach (II 6)
Laforestrie (II 8)
Greene (II 10)

STRESS-LIFE EVENTS

Paykel (II 3)
Kozarević (II 4)

Tennant (II 7)
Israël (II 9)
Greene (II 10)
Vignat - Israël (IV 26)

SPATIAL ORIENTATION

Benton (Ib 2)
Benton (Ib 5)
Blessed (Ib 6)
Wechsler (Ib 13)
Plutchik (Ib 14)
Witkin (Ib 15)
Hodkinson (Ib 16)
Silver (Ib 18)
Pfeiffer (Ib 24)
Fishback (Ib 26)
Slater (Ib 28)
Denham (Ib 29)
Janin (Ib 30)
Hersch (Ib 33)
Kastenbaum (Ic 6)
Fine (IV 2)
Pattie (IV 25)
Oswald (IV 29)
Pfeiffer (IV 30)

Sarno (IV 5)
Miller (IV 6)
Gurland (IV 11)
Ctr for Aging Duke Univ. (IV 12)
Jablensky - W.H.O. (IV 18)
Kozarević (IV 20)
Leroux (IV 24)
Pattie (IV 25)
Vignat - Israël (IV 26)
Yesavage (IV 27)
Lawton (IV 28)
Pfeffer (IV 30)

GENERAL SCHEDULE

Israël (Ib 47)
Savage (Ic 4)
Williams (Ic 9)
Wing (Ic 10)
Copeland (Ic 12)
Pfeiffer (Ic 14)
Israël (Ic 16)
Paykel (II 3)
Milne (III 4)
Missouri Institute of Psychiatry (III 6)
Crocq (III 9)
Fischer (III 11)
Götestam (III 12)
Graux (III 13)
Plutchik (IV 3)
Gurel (IV 4)
Sarno (IV 5)
Dastoor - Douglas Hospital (IV 8)
Grauer (IV 9)
Georges (IV 10)
Gurland (IV 11)
Ctr for Aging. Duke Univ. (IV.12)
Zay (IV 17)
Kozarević (IV 20)
E.R.O.S. (IV 23)
Vignat - Israël (IV 26)
Yesavage (IV 27)
Lawton (IV 20)
C.I.C.P.A. (IV 31)
Bel Air (IV 33)

INDICATION OF PLACEMENT

Silver (Ib 18)
Hogarty (Ic 2)
Ferm (Ic 11)
Greene (Ic 18)
Missuri Institute of Psychiatry (III 6)
Götestam (III 12)
Hugonot (III 18)
Plutchik (IV 3)
Grauer (IV 9)
Israël (IV 15)
Wilkinson (IV 22)
E.R.O.S. (IV 23)
Pattie (IV 25)

PROGNOSIS

Lorr (Ia 5)
Pierce (Ia 6)
Beck (Ia 7)
Carroll (Ia 17)

Brink (Ia 19)
Barbizet (Ib 1)
Wechsler (Ib 13)
Folstein (Ib 22)
Pfeiffer (Ib 24)
Denham (Ib 29)
Crook (Ib 32)
Kendrick (Ib 34)
Levin (Ib 35)
Berg (Ib 37)
Cole (Ib 38)
Durand (Ic 3)
Savage (Ic 4)
Kastenbaum (Ic 6)
Kleban (Ic 7)
Wing (Ic 10)
Copeland (Ic 12)
Pfeiffer (Ic 14)
Greene (Ic 18)
Preston (II 1)
Linn (II 2)
Laforestrie (II 8)
Greene (II 10)
Katz (III 3)
Missouri Institute of Psychiatry (III 6)
Fischer (III 11)
Meer (IV 1)
Dastoor - Douglas Hospital (IV 8)
Gurland (IV 11)
Murkofsky (IV 16)
Jablenksy - W.H.O. (IV 18)
Delcros (IV 19)
Leroux (IV 24)
Pattie (IV 25)
Pfeffer (IV 30)

RATING OF CHANGES

Pierce (Ia 6)
Lawton (Ia 9)
Wang (Ia 10)
Snaith (Ia 13)
Montgomery (Ia 14)
Plutchik (Ib 14)
Longeot (Ib 20)
Israël (Ib 25)
Hersch (Ib 33)
Israël (Ib 39)
Israël (Ib 47)
Honigfeld (Ic 1)
Aumack (Ic 5)
Kleban (Ic 7)
Williams (Ic 9)
Ferm (Ic 11)
Copeland (Ic 12)
Bond (Ic 15)
Israël (Ic 16)
Rorschach (II 6)
Hulten (III 1)
Katz (III 3)
Missouri Institute of Psychiatry (III 6)
Norton (III 8)
Delomier (III 10)
Götestam (III 12)
Graux (III 13)
Linn (III 17)
Fine (IV 2)
Plutchik (IV 3)

Gurel (IV 4)
Sarno (IV 5)
Ctr for Aging. Duke Univ. (IV.12)
Hersch (IV 14)
Israël (IV 16)
Delcros (IV 19)
Leroux (IV 24)
Yesavage (IV 27)
Lawton (IV 28)
Pfeffer (IV 30)

RESEARCH

Zung (Ia 2)
Barbizet (Ib 1)
Benton (Ib 2)
Lester (Ib 3)
Andrey (IB 9)
Wechsler (Ib 13)
Wikin (Ib 15)
Hasegawa (Ib 19)
Folstein (Ib 22)
Janin (Ib 30)
Brink (IB 31)
Hersch (Ib 33)
Gilbert (Ib 44)
Israël (Ib 47)
Durand (Ic 3)
Brink (Ic 13)
Pfeffer (Ic 14)

Greene (Ic 18)
Israël (II 5)
Rorschach (II 6)
Israël (II 9)
Greene (II 10)
Fischer (III 11)
Shader (IV 7)
Cornbleth (IV 13)
Hersch (IV 14)
Murkofsky (IV 16)
Zay (IV 17)
Kozarević (IV 20)
Wilkinson (IV 22)
Bel Air (IV 33)

SCREENING

Lubin (Ia 1)
Zung (Ia 2)
Beck (Ia 7)
Zung (Ia 16)
Carroll (Ia 17)
Brink (Ia 19)
Nahor (Ib 12)
Hodkinson (Ib 16)
Isaacs (Ib 17)
Wells (Ib 36)
Israël (Ib 43)
Gilbert (Ib 44)
Mac (Carthy (Ib 45)
Savage (Ic 4)
Kastenbaum (Ic 6)
Wing (Ic 10)
Ferm (Ic 11)
Copeland (Ic 12)
Pfeiffers (Ic 14)
Milne (III 4)

TEACHING - TRAINING OF PERSONNEL

Kastenbaum (Ic 6)
Israël (II 5)
Lawton - Brody (III 2)
Katz (III 3)
Akhtar (III 5)
Sarno (IV 5)
Dastoor - Douglas Hospital (IV 8)
Ctr. for Aging. Duke Univ. (IV 12)
Cornbleth (IV 13)
Delcros (IV 19)
Centre de Gériatrie (IV 32)

REFERENCE	AUTHOR	ORIGINAL VERSION	TRANSLATIONS

SECTION 1

MENTAL

Mood

Ia.1	Lubin	English	Spanish – Hebrew – Dutch – Chinese.
Ia.2	Zung	English	30 languages
Ia.3	Hamilton	English	All European Languages – Japanese – Corean.
Ia.4	Free	English	
Ia.5	Lorr	English	
Ia.6	Pierce	English	
Ia.7	Beck	English	Indian – Spanish – Polish – Hungarian – Japanese – Dutch – – Finnish – German – French.
Ia.8	Crocq	French	English – Spanish – Arabic
Ia.9	Lawton	English	Japanese.
Ia.10	Wang	English	French.
Ia.11	Sartorius-W.H.O.	English	French – Bulgarian – Polish – German – Hindu – Japanese.
Ia.12	Bech	Danish	English – French – German.
Ia.13	Snaith	English	French – German – Flemish – Italian – Arabic – Swedish – Spanish.
Ia.14	Montgomery	English	French – European languages.
Ia.15	Bech	English	
Ia.16	Zung	English	Chinese – Dutch – French – German – Italian – Thai
Ia.17	Carroll	English	
Ia.18	Bech	Danish	English – French – German – Spanish – Italian – Japanese.
Ia.19	Brink	English	French – Spanish – German.

Cognitive functions

Ib.1	Barbizet	French	English.
Ib.2	Benton	English	French and other European languages.
Ib.3	Lester	English	
Ib.4	Barbizet	English	
Ib.5	Benton	English	French and many other languages.
Ib.6	Blessed	English	
Ib.7	Blessed	English	
Ib.8	Williams	English	
Ib.9	Andrey	French	
Ib.10	Fowler	English	
Ib.11	Dana	English	
Ib.12	Nahor	English	
Ib.13	Wechsler	English	French and many other languages.
Ib.14	Plutchik	English	
Ib.15	Witkin	English	
Ib.16	Hodkinson	English	
Ib.17	Isaacs	English	
Ib.18	Silver	English	
Ib.19	Hasegawa	Japanese	English and French.
Ib.20	Longeot	French	
Ib.21	Qureshi	English	

REFERENCE	AUTHOR	ORIGINAL VERSION	TRANSLATIONS
Ib.22	Folstein	English	Spanish – Portuguese.
Ib.23	Hachinski	English	
Ib.24	Pfeiffer	English	
Ib.25	Israel	French	
Ib.26	Fishback	English	
Ib.27	Jacobs	English	
Ib.28	Slater	English	
Ib.29	Denham	English	French.
Ib.30	Janin	French	
Ib.31	Brink	English	
Ib.32	Crook	English	
Ib.33	Hersch	English	
Ib.34	Kendrick	English	Spanish.
Ib.35	Levin	English	
Ib.36	Wells	English	French.
Ib.37	Berg	Swedish	English.
Ib.38	Cole	English	
Ib.39	Israel	French	
Ib.40	Israel	French	
Ib.41	Israel	French	
Ib.42	Israel	French	
Ib.43	Israel	French	
Ib.44	Gilbert	English	
Ib.45	Mac Carthy	English	
Ib.46	Signoret	French	English.
Ib.47	Israel	French	

Behavior

REFERENCE	AUTHOR	ORIGINAL VERSION	TRANSLATIONS
Ic.1	Honigfeld	English	French – German – Spanish – Italian – Swedish.
Ic.2	Hogarty	English	
Ic.3	Durand	French	Portuguese – English.
Ic.4	Savage	English	
Ic.5	Aumack	English	
Ic.6	Kastenbaum	English	
Ic.7	Kleban	English	
Ic.8	Bellak	English	
Ic.9	Williams	English	French.
Ic.10	Wing	English	Over thirty languages.
Ic.11	Ferm	Finnish	English (abridged version).
Ic.12	Copeland	English	Danish – German – Dutch – French.
Ic.13	Brink	English	Spanish.
Ic.14	Pfeiffer	English	
Ic.15	Bond	English	
Ic.16	Israel	French	English.
Ic.17	Mezzena	Italian	
Ic.18	Greene	English	

REFERENCE	AUTHOR	ORIGINAL VERSION	TRANSLATIONS

SECTION 2

MENTAL - SOCIAL

II.1	Preston	English	
II.2	Linn	English	
II.3	Paykel	English	
II.4	Kozarević	Serbo-Croat	English.
II.5	Israel	French	
II.6	Rorschach	German	French – English – European languages.
II.7	Tennant	English	
II.8	Laforestrie	French	
II.9	Israel	French	
II.10	Greene	English	

PHYSICAL - MENTAL

III.1	Hulten	Swedish	English.
III.2	Lawton	English	French.
III.3	Katz	English	
III.4	Milne	English	
III.5	Akhtar	English	
III.6	Missouri Inst.	English	
III.7	Kuriansky	English	
III.8	Norton	English	
III.9	Crocq	French	
III.10	Delomier	French	
III.11	Fischer	German	English – French – Spanish – Chinese.
III.12	Götestam	English	
III.13	Graux	French	
III.14	Gottfries	Swedish	English.
III.15	Idänpään-Heikkilä	Finnish	English.
III.16	Kuntzmann	French	
III.17	Linn	English	
III.18	Hugonot	French	

SECTION 3

PHYSICAL - MENTAL - SOCIAL

IV.1	aMeer	English	French – Dutch.
IV.2	Fine	English	
IV.3	Plutchik	English	
IV.4	Gurel	English	
IV.5	Sarno	English	
IV.6	Miller	English	
IV.7	Shader	English	French – German – Swedish.
IV.8	Douglas Hospital	English	
IV.9	Grauer	English	
IV.10	Georges	French	
IV.11	Gurland	English	

REFERENCE	AUTHOR	ORIGINAL VERSION	TRANSLATIONS
IV.12	Duke University	English	
IV.13	Cornbleth	English	
IV.14	Hersch	English	
IV.15	Israel	French	
IV.16	Murkofsky	English	
IV.17	Zay	French	
IV.18	Jablensky-W.H.O.	English	Turkish – German – Bulgarian – Arabic – Italian – Chinese – Czechoslowakian – Serbo-Croat – French.
IV.19	Delcros	French	
IV.20	Kozarević	Serbo-Croat	English.
IV.21	Patron	French	
IV.22	Wilkinson	English	
IV.23	E.R.O.S.	French	
IV.24	Leroux	French	
IV.25	Pattie	English	Polish.
IV.26	Vignat-Israel	French	
IV.27	Yesavage	English	Polish-French.
IV.28	Lawton	English	
IV.29	Oswald	German	English.
IV.30	Pfeffer	English	
IV.31	C.I.C.P.A.	French	
IV.32	Centre de Gériatrie	French	
IV.33	Ecole de Bel-Air	French	

YEAR	AUTHOR	COUNTRY – TOWN	SPECIFICITY ***	SPECIFICITY **	SPECIFICITY *	OUT-PATIENT	INPATIENT	PHYSICIAN	PSYCHOLOGIST	NURSES	SOCIAL WORKER	NON SPECIALISED	FAMILY RELATIVES	SELF ADMINISTERED	INDEX
1965	BARBIZET	FRANCE Créteil		X		X	X	X	X						Ib.1
	BENTON	U.S.A. New York		X		X	X		X						Ib.2
	HONIGFELD	U.S.A. East Hannover		X			X			X					Ic.1
	LUBIN	U.S.A. Kansas City		X		X	X							X	Ia.1
	ZUNG	U.S.A. Durham		X		X	X							X	Ia.2
1966	HOGARTY	U.S.A. Chevy Chase		X			X				X				Ic.2
	MEER	U.S.A. Stockton	X				X			X					IV.1
	PRESTON	U.S.A. Seattle	X			X								X	II.1
1967	DURAND	FRANCE Chambéry		X		X	X	X	X						Ic.3
	HAMILTON	G.B. Leeds		X		X	X	X	X	X					Ia.3
	LESTER	U.S.A. Pomona			X	X	X		X						Ib.3
	SAVAGE	AUSTRALIA Murdoch	X			X	X	X	X	X	X				Ic.4
1968	BARBIZET	FRANCE Creteil		X		X	X		X	X					Ib.4
	BENTON	U.S.A. New York		X		X	X			X					Ib.5
	BLESSED - ROTH	G.B. Cambridge	X				X	X	X	X					Ib.6
	BLESSED - ROTH	G.B. Cambridge	X				X	X	X	X					Ib.7
	WILLIAMS	G.B. Cambridge		X		X	X	X	X						Ib.8
1969	ANDREY	FRANCE Grenoble		X		X	X		X						Ib.9
	AUMACK	U.S.A. Danville			X		X	X	X	X					Ic.5
	FOWLER	U.S.A. Seattle		X		X	X	X							Ib.10
	FREE	U.S.A. West Chester		X		X		X							Id.4
	HULTEN	SWEDEN Göteborg		X		X	X	X		X					III.1
	LAWTON - BRODY	U.S.A. Philadelphia	X			X	X			X	X				III.2
	LINN	U.S.A. Miami	X			X	X			X					II.2
	LORR	U.S.A. Washington		X			X	X		X			X		Ia.5
1970	DANA	U.S.A. New York	X				X	X	X	X					Ib.11
	FINE	G.B. Surrey	X				X			X					IV.2
	KATZ	U.S.A. East Lansing	X				X	X		X	X				III.3
	NAHOR	U.S.A. Boston		X		X	X	X	X						Ib.12
	PLUTCHIK	U.S.A. New York (Bronx)	X				X	X	X	X					Ib.13
	WECHSLER	U.S.A. New York		X		X	X			X					Ib.13
1971	PAYKEL	G.B. London			X	X	X	X	X	X					II.3
	PLUTCHIK	U.S.A. New York (Bronx)	X				X			X					Ib.14
	WITKIN	U.S.A. Brooklyn		X		X	X			X					Ib.15

YEAR	AUTHOR	COUNTRY	TOWN	SPEC ***	SPEC **	SPEC *	OUT-PATIENT	INPATIENT	PHYSICIAN	PSYCHOLOGIST	NURSES	SOCIAL WORKER	NON SPECIALISED	FAMILY RELATIVES	SELF ADMINISTERED	INDEX
1972	GUREL	U.S.A.	Arlington	X				X			X					IV.4
	HODKINSON	G.B.	Harrow London	X				X	X	X	X					Ib.16
	ISAACS	G.B.	Birmingham	X			X	X	X	X	X					Ib.17
	KASTENBAUM	U.S.A.	New York	X			X	X	X	X	X	X				Ic.6
	KLEBAN - BRODY	U.S.A.	Philadelphia	X			X	X				X		X		Ic.7
	MILNE	G.B.	Edinburgh	X			X	X			X					III.4
	SILVER	G.B.	London	X			X	X	X	X	X					Ib.18
1973	AKHTAR - BROE	AUSTRALIA	Lidcombe	X			X		X		X	X				III.5
	BELLAK	U.S.A.		X			X	X	X							Ic.8
	KOZAREVIĆ	YUGOSLAVIA	Belgrade		X		X			X	X	X				II.4
	MISSOURI INSTIT.	U.S.A.	Saint Louis	X				X			X					III.6
	PIERCE	U.S.A.	San Rafael	X	X		X	X	X	X						Ia.6
	SARNO	U.S.A.	New York			X	X		X	X	X					IV.5
	WILLIAMS	U.S.A.	Manteno	X				X			X					Ic.9
1974	BECK	U.S.A.	Philadelphia		X		X	X	X	X					X	Ia.7
	CROCQ	FRANCE	Paris			X	X	X	X							Ia.8
	FERM	FINLAND	Helsinski	X			X	X	X	X	X					Ic.11
	HASEGAWA	JAPAN	Kawasaki	X			X	X	X	X						Ib.19
	LONGEOT	FRANCE	Grenoble		X		X	X		X						Ib.20
	PARACHEK-MILLER	U.S.A.	Arizona	X				X			X					IV.6
	QURESHI	G.B.	Harrow London	X				X	X	X	X					Ib.21
	SHADER	U.S.A.	Boston	X			X		X	X	X	X				IV.7
	WING	G.B.	London			X	X	X	X							Ic.10
1975	DASTOOR	CANADA	Verdun	X			X	X	X	X	X	X				IV.8
	FOLSTEIN	U.S.A.	Baltimore	X			X	X	X	X	X	X	X			Ib.22
	GRAUER	CANADA	Montréal	X			X				X	X				IV.9
	HACHINSKI	CANADA	Toronto		X		X	X	X							Ib.23
	LAWTON	U.S.A.	Philadelphia	X			X	X						X		Ia.9
	PFEIFFER	U.S.A.	Tampa	X			X	X	X	X	X	X				Ib.24
1976	COPELAND	G.B.	Liverpool	X			X	X	X	X	X	X				Ic.12
	ISRAEL	FRANCE	Grenoble	X				X	X	X		X				II.5
	ISRAEL	FRANCE	Grenoble	X				X		X						Ib.25
	KURIANSKY	U.S.A.	New York	X				X	X	X	X					III.7
	RORSCHACH	GERMANY			X		X	X		X						II.6
	TENNANT	AUSTRALIA	Little Bay			X	X	X							X	II.7
	WANG	U.S.A.	Milwaukee		X		X	X	X		X					Ia.10

YEAR	AUTHOR	COUNTRY—TOWN	SPECIFICITY ***	SPECIFICITY **	SPECIFICITY *	POPULATION OUT-PATIENT	POPULATION INPATIENT	CAREGIVER PHYSICIAN	CAREGIVER PSYCHOLOGIST	CAREGIVER NURSES	NON CAREGIVER SOCIAL WORKER	NON CAREGIVER NON SPECIALISED	NON CAREGIVER FAMILY RELATIVES	SELF ADMINISTERED	INDEX
1977	FISHBACK	U.S.A. Philadelphia	X			X	X	X		X					Ib.26
	GEORGES	FRANCE Rueil Malmaison	X			X	X	X							IV.10
	GURLAND	U.S.A. New York	X			X	X			X					IV.11
	JACOBS	U.S.A. New York (Bronx)		X		X	X	X	X	X					Ib.27
	LAFORESTRIE	FRANCE Ivry	X			X	X		X						II.8
	NORTON	U.S.A. Lexington	X				X			X					III.8
	W.H.O.	SWITZERLAND Geneva			X	X	X	X	X						Ia.11
	SLATER	G.B. Cardiff	X			X	X						X		Ib.28
1978	BECH	DENMARK Copenhagen			X	X	X	X							Ia.12
	BRINK	U.S.A. San Carlos	X			X	X	X							Ic.13
	CENTER FOR AGING	U.S.A. Durham	X			X	X	X	X		X				IV.12
	CORNBLETH	U.S.A. Pittsburgh	X				X			X					IV.13
	DENHAM	G.B. Harrow London	X				X	X	X	X					Ib.29
	HERSCH	CANADA London	X				X			X					IV.14
	ISRAEL	FRANCE Grenoble	X			X					X	X			II.9
	ISRAEL	FRANCE Grenoble	X			X		X	X	X					IV.15
	JANIN	FRANCE Villeurbanne	X			X	X	X	X						Ib.30
	MURKOFSKY	U.S.A. New York (Bronx)	X			X								X	IV.16
	SNAITH	G.B. Leeds		X		X	X							X	Ia.13
	ZAY	CANADA Québec	X			X	X	X	X	X	X				IV.17
1979	BRINK	U.S.A. Palo Alto	X			X	X			X					Ib.31
	CROOK	U.S.A. Rockville	X			X	X	X	X	X		X			Ib.32
	HERSCH	CANADA London	X			X	X			X					Ib.33
	JABLENSKY. W.H.O.	SWITZERLAND Geneva		X		X	X	X	X		X				IV.18
	KENDRICK	G.B. Hull	X			X	X	X	X	X	X				Ib.34
	LEVIN	U.S.A. Galveston		X		X	X	X	X	X					Ib.35
	MONTGOMERY	G.B. London		X		X	X	X	X	X					Ia.14
	PFEIFFER	U.S.A. Tampa	X			X	X	X	X	X	X				Ic.14
	WELLS	U.S.A. Nashville		X			X	X							Ib.36
1980	BECH	DENMARK Copenhagen			X	X	X	X	X						Ia.15
	BERG	SWEDEN Jönköping	X				X	X	X	X	X				Ib.37
	BOND	G.B. Newcastle Upon Tyne	X			X	X	X	X	X	X				Ic.15
	COLE	CANADA Montréal	X			X	X	X	X	X					Ib.38
	CROCQ	FRANCE Paris		X		X	X	X							III.9
	DELCROS - LANOË	FRANCE Villejuif	X				X					X			IV.19
	DELOMIER	FRANCE Saint Etienne	X				X					X			III.10
	ISRAEL	FRANCE Grenoble	X			X		X	X						Ic.16

YEAR	AUTHOR	COUNTRY	TOWN	SPECIFICITY ***	SPECIFICITY **	SPECIFICITY *	OUT-PATIENT	INPATIENT	PHYSICIAN	PSYCHOLOGIST	NURSES	SOCIAL WORKER	NON SPECIALISED	FAMILY RELATIVES	SELF ADMINISTERED	INDEX
1980	ISRAEL	FRANCE	Grenoble	X			X			X						Ib.39
	ISRAEL	FRANCE	Grenoble	X			X		X	X						Ib.40
	ISRAEL	FRANCE	Grenoble	X				X	X	X	X					Ib.41
	ISRAEL	FRANCE	Grenoble	X				X		X						Ib.42
	ISRAEL	FRANCE	Grenoble	X				X		X						Ib.43
	KOZAREVIĆ	YUGOSLAVIA	Belgrade	X			X		X		X					IV.20
	PATRON	FRANCE	Paris	X			X				X	X		X		IV.21
	WILKINSON	G.B.	Darlington	X			X				X					IV.22
	ZUNG	U.S.A.	Durham			X	X	X							X	Ia.16
1981	CARROLL	U.S.A.	Ann Arbor		X		X	X							X	Ia.17
	E.R.O.S.	CANADA	Montréal	X			X	X	X	X	X	X				IV.23
	FISCHER	SWITZERLAND	Basel		X		X	X	X	X	X					III.11
	GILBERT	U.S.A.	Baltimore		X		X	X		X						Ib.44
	GOTESTAM	NORVEGE	Trondheim	X				X	X	X	X	X				III.12
	GRAUX	FRANCE	Lille	X			X	X	X	X						III.13
	LEROUX-ATTALI	FRANCE	Vierzon	X			X	X	X		X	X				IV.24
	MAC CARTHY	U.S.A.	New York	X			X	X	X	X						Ib.45
	MEZZENA	ITALIA	Turin			X	X	X	X	X						Ic.17
	PATTIE	G.B.	York	X			X	X	X	X	X			X		IV.25
	VIGNAT - ISRAEL	FRANCE	Grenoble	X			X	X	X	X		X				IV.26
	YESAVAGE	U.S.A.	Stanford	X			X	X							X	IV.27
1982	BECH	DENMARK	Copenhagen			X	X	X	X	X	X					Ia.18
	GOTTFRIES	SWEDEN	St. Jörgen	X			X	X	X	X	X					III.14
	GREENE	G.B.	Glasgow	X			X							X		Ic.18
	GREENE	G.B.	Glasgow	X			X							X		II.10
	IDANPAAN	FINLANDIE	Helsinki		X		X	X	X							III.15
	KUNTZMANN	FRANCE	Strasbourg	X				X	X		X					III.16
	LAWTON	U.S.A.	Philadelphia	X			X	X			X					IV.28
	LINN	U.S.A.	Miami		X		X	X			X					III.17
	OSWALD	GERMANY	Nüremberg	X				X		X	X				X	IV.29
	PFEFFER	U.S.A.	Orange	X			X		X	X	X	X		X		IV.30
	YESAVAGE - BRINK	U.S.A.	Palo Alto	X			X	X							X	Ia.19
	SIGNORET	FRANCE	Paris		X		X	X	X	X						Ib.46
	C.I.C.P.A.	SWITZERLAND	Geneva	X				X			X					IV.31
	ECOLE BEL AIR	SWITZERLAND	Geneva	X												IV.33
	CENTRE GERIATRIE	SWITZERLAND	Geneva	X			X				X					IV.32
	HUGONOT	FRANCE	Grenoble	X				X			X					III.18
	ISRAEL	FRANCE	Grenoble	X			X	X	X	X	X					Ib.47

Péguy, interrogeant un jour des tailleurs de pierre sur un chantier au bord de la route, leur avait demandé: "Que faites-vous?"

Le premier interrogé avait répondu:
- "Je casse des cailloux!"

Le second:
- "Je gagne mon pain!"

Le troisième:
- "Je bâtis une maison!"

EPILOGUE

In geriatrics, the diagnostic approach implies more than a mere physical examination. It requires always an adequate estimation of mental function.

It is good and sensible practice to take the patient's mental functioning into account before establishing any therapeutic programme for him. An improvement, or even a recovery, in people over 80 often requires the careful treatment of several chronic conditions, some of which may indeed be mental.

The prognosis is dependant to a considerable degree upon the individual's capacity to adapt to a new psychological situation. Ageing and disease especially if combined are not identical in everyone. The increase in age for example often reinforces the personality or character of each individual and it is unfortunate that it is just when he is more unique than ever that he must fit into the most global of solutions. The functional involution which goes with senescence can undoubtedly bring with it some disorders of the homeostasis which entails a new balance in the biological, psychological or social order which must be recognized and respected.

The traditional clinical approach is insufficient when assessing the elderly person against a background of a complex mixture of physical and psycho-social factors so that not only do we need the tools for our medical examination but also the instruments most appropriate to estimate the patient's psychological capacity.

Every old person should be able to benefit from a comprehensive assessment which is both constructive and reasonable. A constructive approach should consist in making an inventory of all efficient, possible measures, and adapting dynamically the potential efficacy of available resources to the patient's reality.

The resultant profile offers other advantages. In fact, it contributes much towards improving the work of the medical team in that it acknowledges the patient as an adult and authorizes him to choose and formulate the route he intends to take. So long as he is motivated and kept involved and interested in his task of recovery and rehabilitation, an elderly person can master and make use of the abilities at his disposal, at his own pace, despite the handicaps deriving from illness and senescence.

The distinction between mental and physical is extremely arbitrary. The individual is a whole. Geriatrics is, par excellence, a discipline which requires the integration of psychological and biological sciences. However, in order to obtain full knowledge such an integrated approach requires many different inputs.

The authors of this work have performed a necessary task. Primarily, for writing a book of considerable clinical significance. The geriatric specialist, like any other doctor, would like to influence the life-style and hygiene of the patients he is likely to deal with. The doctor who adopts such an action is quickly led to ask himself the following question: "on what criteria of normality should I base the action I intend to perform? What exactly is to be considered as "normal" in geriatric practice and in particular in the area of mental function in the elderly?"

This book makes an important contribution in that it gives us an opportunity

as clinicians to select quickly and easily the instrument suited to our needs and the needs of our patients

as teachers to instruct our students in a significant part of the detailed knowledge for our branch of medicine

as researchers to enable us to study further in the important fields of pharmacological therapeutics by facilitating the provision of comparative data from multicentred trials e.g. the same mental instruments being capable of use in different cities or indeed countries.

We hope that this book, which is clear, well-constructed and well documented, will find the audience it deserves among all those who are interested in the ageing of mental functions. We also hope that other publications of this kind will soon be developed, under the patronage of the World Health Organization.

Docteur J.P. JUNOD
Professeur de Gériatrie
Institutions de Gériatrie
Genève

V - BIBLIOGRAPHIES

Akhtar (A.J.), Broe (G.A.), Crombie (A.), Mc Lean (W.M.R.), Andrews (G.R.), Caird (F.I.): Disability and dependence in the elderly at home. *Age and Ageing*, 1973, 2, 102-111. — III. 5

Andrey (B.): Les praxies grapho-motrices. *Bulletin de Psychologie Scolaire*, 1969, 111-131. — Ib. 9

Aumack (L.): The patient activity checklist: an instrument and an approach for measuring behavior. *Journal of Clinical Psychology*, 1969, 25, 134-137. — Ic. 5

Barbizet (J.), Cany (E.): Clinical and psychometrical study of a patient with memory disturbances. *International Journal of Neurology*, 1968, 7, 44-54. — Ib. 4

Barbizet (J.), Truscelli (D.): L'histoire du lion (considérations sur la fabulation). *La Semaine des Hôpitaux*, 1965, 41, 28, 1688-1694. — Ib. 1

Bech (P.), Gram (L.F.), Reisby (N.), Rafaelsen (O.J.): The WHO depression scale. *Acta Psychiatrica Scandinavica*, 1980, 62, 2, 140-153. — Ia. 15

Bech (P.), Rafaelsen (O.J.): The melancholia scale: development, consistency, validity and utility. In: Sartorius (N.), Ban (T.): "Depression rating scales". 1982. — Ia. 18

Bech (P.), Rafaelsen (O.J.), Kramp (P.), Bolwig (T.G.): The mania rating scale: scale construction and inter-observer agreement. *Neuropharmacology*, 1978, 17, 6, 430-431. — Ia. 12

Beck (A.T.), Beamesderfer (A.): Assessment of depression: the depression inventory. In: Pichot (P.) Ed.: "Psychological measurements in psychopharmacology". Vol. 7. Basel: Karger, 1974, 151-169. — Ia. 7

Bellak (L.), Bellak (S.S.): Manual for the senior apperception technique. Larchmont, New York: C.P.S., 1973. — Ic. 8

Benton (A.L.): Manuel pour l'application du test de rétention visuelle. Applications cliniques et expérimentales. 2ème édition française. Paris: Centre de Psychologie Appliquée, 1965. — Ib. 2

Benton (A.L.): Test de praxie constructive tridimensionnelle. Manuel. Paris: Centre de Psychologie Appliquée, 1968. — Ib. 5

Berg (S.), Svensson (T.): An orientation scale for geriatric patients. *Age and Ageing*, 1980, 9, 215-219. — Ib. 37

Blessed (G.), Tomlinson (B.E.), Roth (M.): The association between quantitative measures of dementia and of senile change in the cerebral grey matter of elderly subjects. *British Journal of Psychiatry*, 1968, 114, 797-811. — Ib. 6, Ib. 7

Bond (J.), Brooks (P.), Carstairs (V.), Giles (L.): The reliability of a survey psychiatric assessment schedule for the elderly. *British Journal of Psychiatry*, 1980, 137, 148-162. — Ic. 15

Brink (T.L.), Belanger (J.), Bryant (J.), Capri (D.), Janakes (C.), Jasculca (S.), Oliveira (C.): Hypochondriasis in an institutional geriatric population: construction of a scale (HSIG). *Journal of the American Geriatrics Society*, 1978, 26, 12, 557-559. — Ic. 13

Brink (T.L.), Bryant (J.), Catalano (M.L.), Janakes (C.), Oliveira (C.): Senile confusion: assessment with a new stimulus recognition test. *Journal of the American Geriatrics Society*, 1979, 27, 3, 126-129. — Ib. 31

Brink (T.L.), Yesavage (J.A.), Lum (O.), Heersema (P.H.), Adey (M.), Rose (T.L.): Screening tests for geriatric depression. *Clinical Gerontologist*, 1982, 1, 1, 37-43. — Ia. 19

Carroll (B.J.), Feinberg (M.), Smouse (P.E.), Rawson (S.G.), Greden (J.F.): The Carroll rating scale for depression. 1: Development, reliability and validation. – 2: Factor analyses of the feature profiles. – 3: Comparison with other rating instruments. *Britsh Journal of Psychiatry*, 1981, 138, 194-200, 201-204, 205-209. — Ia. 17

Center for the Study of Aging and Human Development. Duke University: Multidimensional functional assessment: the OARS methodology. 2nd edition. Duke University: Center for the Study of Aging and Human Development, 1978. Instrument non publié. — IV. 12

Centre d'Information et de Coordination pour Personnes Agées (C.I.C.P.A.). Genève: Grille pour l'évaluation du degré de dépendance des pensionnaires d'une pension de personnes âgées. Instrument non publié. — IV. 31

Centre de Gériatrie. Genève: Appréciation du degré d'autonomie-dépendance dans les activités de la vie quotidienne au Foyer de Jour, à domicile. Instrument non publié. — IV. 32

Cole (M.G.), Dastoor (D.): Development of a dementia rating scale: preliminary communication. *Journal of Clinical and Experimental Gerontology*, 1980, 2, 1, 49-63. — Ib. 38

Copeland (J.R.M.), Kelleher (M.J.), Kellett (J.M.), Gourlay (A.J.), Gurland (B.J.), Fleiss (J.L.), Sharpe (L.): A semi-structured clinical interview for the assessment of diagnosis and mental state in the elderly: the geriatric mental state schedule. 1: Development and reliability – 2: A factor analysis. *Psychological medicine*, 1976, 6, 439-459. — Ic. 12

Cornbleth (T.): Evaluation of goal attainment in geriatric settings. *Journal of the American Geriatrics Society*, 1978, 26, 9, 404-407. — IV. 13

Crocq (L.), Bugard (P.), Fondarai (J.), Boscredon (J.), Bruneaux (J.) Charazac (P.), Clerc (G.), Darondel (A.), Drevet (M.), Fraud (J.P.), Gallet (G.), Louppe (A.), Martin (A.), Meisart (P.), Oules (J.), Patay (M.), Piel (E.), Reverzy (J.P.), Treisser (C.), Werquin (G.): Traitement des états asthéno-dépressifs. Etude multicentrique de 248 cas évalués par l'échelle clinique G.E.F. 4. *Psychologie Médicale*, 1980, 12, 12, 2643-2661. — III. 9

Crocq (L.), Fondarai (J.): Exploitation par ordinaterur des échelles d'appréciation psychiatrique. Extraits du compte rendu du congrès de psychiatrie et de neurologie de langue française, LXXIe session, Monaco, 2-7 juillet 1973. Paris: Masson, 1974, 403-415. — Ia. 8

Crook (T.), Ferris (S.), Mc Carthy (M.): The misplaced-objects task: a brief test for memory dysfunction in the aged. *Journal of the American Geriatrics Society*, 1979, 27, 6, 284-287.   Ib. 32

Dana (L.A.), White (L.), Merlis (S.): A new approach to measuring short-term memory in geriatric ss: a pilot study. *Psychological Reports*, 1970, 27, 8-10.   Ib. 11

Dastoor (D.P.), Norton (S.), Boillat (J.), Minty (J.), Papadopoulou (F.), Muller (H.F.): A psychogeriatric assessment program. 1: Social functioning and ward behavior. *Journal of the American Geriatrics Society*, 1975, 23, 10, 465-471.   IV. 8

Delcros (M.), Lanoe (R.): Une nouvelle échelle d'évaluation de la dépendance des patients dans les établissement de long séjour. *La Revue de Gériatrie*, 1980, 5, 8, 395-400.   IV. 19

Delomier (Y.), Gagne (A.), Girtanner (C.): Evaluation de l'autonomie au centre de jour de Saint-Etienne. *La Revue de Gériatrie*, 1980, 5, 8, 389-392.   III. 10

Denham (M.J.), Jefferys (P.M.): Routine mental testing in the elderly. *Medicine*, 1978, 1, 1.   Ib. 29

Durand (Y.): Eléments d'utilisation pratique et théorique du test A.T. 9. *Annales du Centre d'Enseignement Supérieur de Chambéry*, 1967, 5, 133-172.   Ic. 3

Ecole de Bel-Air. Genève: Bilans d'évaluation du Bel-Air. 1965-1982.   IV. 33

Equipe de Recherche Opérationnelle en Santé (E.R.O.S.). Montréal: C.T.M.S.P.: un système d'information pour un réseau de services prolongés. L'évaluation des services requis et la mesure des ressources requises par le bénéficiaire. Montréal: E.R.O.S., 1981. Instrument non publié.   IV. 23

Ferm (L.): Behavioural activities in demented geriatric patients: study based on evaluations made by nursing staff members and on patients' scores on a simple psychometric test. *Gerontologia Clinica*, 1974, 16, 185-194.   Ic. 11

Fine (E.W.), Lewis (D.), Villa-Landa (I.), Blakemore (C.B.): The effect of cyclandelate on mental function in patients with arteriosclerotic brain disease. *British Journal of Psychiatry*, 1970, 117, 157-161.   IV. 2

Fischer-Cornelssen (K.A.): F.S.C.L.: Fischer symptom check-list. In: Collegium Internationale Psychiatriae Scalarum (C.I.P.S.) Hrsg.: "Internationale Skalen für Psychiatrie". 2nd ed. Weinheim, Germany: Beltz-Test, 1981.   III. 11

Fishback (D.B.): Mental status questionnaire for organic brain syndrome, with a new visual counting test. *Journal of the American Geriatrics Society*, 1977, 25, 4, 167-170.   Ib. 26

Folstein (M.F.), Folstein (S.E.), Mc Hugh (P.R.): "Mini-mental state": a practical method for grading the cognitive state of patients for the clinician. *Journal of Psychiatric Research*, 1975, 12, 189-198.   Ib. 22

Fowler (R.S.): A simple non-language test of new learning. *Perceptual and Motor Skills*, 1969, 29, 895-901.   Ib. 10

Free (S.M.), Guthrie (M.B.): A new rating scale for evaluating clinical response in psychoneurotic outpatients. *Journal of Clinical Pharmacology*, 1969, 9, 187-194.   Ia. 4

Georges (D.), Lallemand (A.), Coustenoble (J.), Loria (Y.): Validation par l'analyse factorielle d'une échelle d'évaluation clinique des troubles de la sénescence cérébrale. Application à l'essai thérapeutique. *Thérapie*, 1977, 32, 173-180.   IV. 10

Gilbert (J.G.), Levee (R.F.), Catalano (F.L.): Guild memory test manual. Bloomfield: Unico National Mental Health Research Foundation, 1981.   Ib. 44

Götestam (K.G.): A geriatric rating scale empirically derived from three rating scales for geriatric behaviour. *Acta Psychiatrica Scandinavica. Supplementa*, 1981, 294, 54-63.   III. 12

Gottfries (C.G.), Brane (G.), Steen (G.): A new rating scale for dementia syndromes. *Gerontology*, 1982, 28, Suppl. 2, 20-31.   III. 14

Grauer (H.), Birnbom (F.): A geriatric functional rating scale to determine the need for institutional care. *Journal of the American Geriatrics Society*, 1975, 23, 10, 472-476.   IV. 9

Graux (P.), Frigard (B.): Bilan-test-permettant d'apprécier la perte d'autonomie. In: "Accidents vasculaires cérébraux. Recherche épidémiologique". Premier congrès francophone de gérontologie, Paris, 17-18 septembre 1979. Paris: Masson, 1981, 548-552.   III. 13

Greene (J.G.), Smith (R.), Gardiner (M.), Timbury (G.C.): Measuring behavioural disturbance of elderly demented patients in the community and its effects on relatives: a factor analytic study. *Age and Ageing*, 1982, 11, 121-126.   Ic. 18 / II. 10

Gurel (L.), Linn (M.W.), Linn (B.S.): Physical and mental impairment – of – function evaluation in the aged: the PAMIE scale. *Journal of Gerontology*, 1972, 27, 1, 83-90.   IV. 4

Gurland (B.), Kuriansky (J.), Sharpe (L.), Simon (R.), Stiller (P.): The comprehensive assessment and referral evaluation (CARE): rationale, development, and reliability. *International Journal of Aging and Human Development*, 1977-1978, 8, 1, 9-41.   IV. 11

Hachinski (V.C.), Iliff (L.D.), Zilhka (E.), Du Boulay (G.H.), Mc Allister (V.L.), Marshall (J.), Russell (R.W.R.), Symon (L.): Cerebral blood flow in dementia. *Archives of Neurology*, 1975, 32, 632-637.   Ib. 23

Hamilton (M.): Development of a rating scale for primary depressive illness. *British Journal of social and clinical Psychology*, 1967, 6, 278-296.   Ia. 3

Hasegawa (K.): Validity and reliability of rating scales for psychogeriatric assessment. The study on Hasegawa's dementia scale. Kawasaki: Dpt of Psychiatriy, St Marianna University, 1974. Instrument non publié.   Ib. 19

Hersch (E.L.): Development and application of the extended scale for dementia. *Journal of the American Geriatrics Society*, 1979, 27, 8, 348-354.   Ib. 33

Hersch (E.L.), Kral (V.A.), Palmer (R.B.): Clinical value of the London psychogeriatric rating scale. *Journal of the American Geriatrics Society*, 1978, 26, 8, 348-354.   IV. 14

Hodkinson (H.M.): Evaluation of a mental test score for assessment of mental impairment in the elderly. *Age and Ageing*, 1972, 1, 233-238. — Ib. 16

Hogarty (G.E.): Discharge readiness: the components of casework judgment. *Social Casework*, 1966, 47, 165-171. — Ic. 2

Honigfeld (G.), Klett (C.J.): The nurses'observation scale for inpatient evaluation: a new scale for a measuring improvement in chronic schizophrenia. *Journal of Clinical Psychology*, 1965, 21, 65-71. — Ic. 1

Hugonot (R.): Evaluation de la dépendance des personnes âgées: C.E.N.T.S. Instrument non publié. — III. 18

Hulten (A.), Kerstell (J.), Olsson (R.), Svanborg (A.): A method to calculate nursing load. *Scandinavian Journal of Rehabilitation Medicine*, 1969, 1, 117-125. — III. 1

Idänpään-Heikkilä (J.), Khan (I.): Psychotropic substances and public health problems: report of a seminar convened by the World Health Organization with the collaboration of the Government of Finland and the United Nations Fund for Drug Abuse Control. Helsinki: Government of Finland, 1982. — III. 15

Isaacs (B.), Akhtar (A.J.): The set test: a rapid test of mental function in old people. *Age and Ageing*, 1972, 1, 222-226. — Ib. 17

Israel (L.): Questionnaire d'enquête sur les aspects psychologiques et sociaux du vieillissement. 1978. Instrument non publié. — II. 9

Israel (L.), Hugonot (R.): Relations malades – médecins – familles en milieu gériatrique. *Médecine et Hygiène*, 1976, 34, 1196, 846-848. — II. 5

Israel (L.), Ohlmann (T.): Mise au point et étalonnage d'une batterie d'épreuves psychométriques pour l'examen des personnes âgées. *Gerontology*, 1976, 22, 3, 141-156. — Ib. 25

Israel (L.), Ohlmann (T.): Structure factorielle de la mémoire appréciée à travers une batterie d'épreuves psychologiques chez des personnes âgées ambulatoires: son application aux essais cliniques contrôlés. *Encéphale*, 1980, 6, 181-195. — Ib. 42

Israel (L.), Ohlmann (T.): Tests psychométriques pour malades très détériorés. 1980. Manuscrit non publié. — Ib. 43

Israel (L.), Ohlmann (T.), Chappaz (M.): Batterie d'épreuves psychométriques pour personnes âgées ambulatoires. *Psychologie Médicale*, 1980, 12, 3, 669-678. — Ib. 39

Israel (L.), Ohlmann (T.), Chappaz (M.): Batterie psychométrique à l'usage du médecin généraliste pour apprécier les conduites intellectuelles des personnes âgées. *Psychologie Médicale*, 1980, 12, 4, 921-938. — Ib. 40 / Ib. 41

Israel (L.), Ohlmann (T.), Hugonot (L.): Techniques psychométriques particulières adaptées aux personnes âgées: application aux essais cliniques contrôlés. In: "Recherche expérimentale et investigations cliniques dans la sénescence cérébrale". Symposium, Bâle, 5-6 juin 1978. Paris: Sandoz, 1978, 185-199. — IV. 15

Israel (L.), Ohlmann (T.), Hugonot (L.), Drouet d'Aubigny (G.): Echelle clinique d'évaluation de la personnalité. La validation par analyse factorielle en gériatrie. *Encéphale*, 1980, 6, 81-91. — Ic. 16

Jacobs (J.W.), Bernhard (M.R.), Delgado (A.), Strain (J.J.): Screening for organic mental syndromes in the medically ill. *Annals of Internal Medicine*, 1977, 86, 40-46. — Ib. 27

Janin (C.), Gaucher (J.), Chapuy (P.): Echelle d'efficience intellectuelle de la personne âgée. *La Revue de Gériatrie*, 1978, 3, 5, 245-251. — Ib. 30

Kastenbaum (R.), Sherwood (S.): VIRO: a scale for assessing the interview behavior of elderly people. In: Kent (D.P.), Kastenbaum (R.), Sherwood (S.) Eds.: "Research planning and action for the elderly: the power and potential of social science". New York: Behavioral publications, 1972, 166-200. — Ic. 6

Katz (S.), Downs (T.D.), Cash (H.R.), Grotz (R.C.): Progress in development of the index of ADL. *Gerontologist*, 1970, Part. I, 20-30. — III. 3

Kendrick (D.C.), Gibson (A.J.), Moyes (I.C.A.): The revised Kendrick battery: clinical studies. *British Journal of social and clinical Psychology*, 1979, 18, 329-340. — Ib. 34

Kleban (M.H.), Brody (E.M.): Prediction of improvement in mentally impaired aged: personality ratings by social workers. *Journal of Gerontology*, 1972, 27, 1, 69-76. — Ic. 7

Kozarević (Dj.), Milicevic (L.J.), Vojvodic (N.): Health status and health care system of war veterans in Yougoslavia. Beograd: 1980. — IV. 20

Kozarević (Dj.), Roberts (A.): Personal habits, environment and psycho-social factors (P.H.E.P.S.F.). In: "Respiratory diseases". Beograd: Postgraduate Medical Institute, 1973. — II. 4

Kuntzmann (F.), Rudloff (H.), Etheve (M.), Berthel (M.), Gitz (A.M.), Strubel (D.), Artzner (M.): Evaluation des besoins des pensionnaires des établissements gériatriques. *La Revue de Gériatrie*, 1982, 7, 6, 263-271. — III. 16

Kuriansky (J.), Gurland (B.): The performance test of activities of daily living. *International Journal of Aging and Human Development*, 1976, 7, 4, 343-352. — III. 7

Laforestrie (R.), Missoum (G.): Un test projectif pour personnes âgées. *La Revue de Gériatrie*, 1977, 2, 5, 351-356. — II. 8

Lawton (M.P.): The Philadelphia geriatric center morale scale: a revision. *Journal of Gerontology*, 1975, 30, 85-89. — Ia. 9

Lawton (M.P.), Brody (E.M.): Assessment of older people: self maintaining and instrumental activities of daily living. *Gerontologist*, 1969, 9, 179-186. — III. 2

Lawton (M.P.), Moss (M.), Fulcomer (M.). Kleban (M.H.): A research and service oriented multilevel assessment instrument. *Journal of Gerontology*, 1982, 37, 1, 91-99. — IV. 28

Leroux (R.), Viau (G.), Fournier (M.), Bergeot (R.), Attalli (G.): Visualisation d'une échelle simple d'autonomie: Géronte. *La Revue de Gériatrie*, 1981, 6, 9, 433-436. — IV. 24

Lester (D.): The shaw blocks test: a description. *Journal of Clinical Psychology*, 1967, 23, 1, 88-89. Ib. 3

Levin (H.S.), O'Donnell (V.M.), Grossman (R.G.): The Galveston orientation and amnesia test: a practical scale to assess cognition after head injury. *Journal of Nervous and Mental Disease*, 1979, 167, 11, 675-684. Ib. 35

Linn (M.W.), Linn (B.S.): The rapid disability rating scale - 2. *Journal of the American Geriatrics Society*, 1982, 30, 6, 378-382. III. 17

Linn (M.W.), Sculthorpe (W.B.), Evje (M.), Slater (P.H.), Goodman (S.P.): A social dysfunction rating scale. *Journal of Psychiatric Research*, 1969, 6, 299-306. II. 2

Longeot (F.): L'échelle de développement de la pensée logique. Issy-Les-Moulineaux: Editions Scientifiques et Psychotechniques, 1974. Ib. 20

Lorr (M.), Vestre (N.D.): The psychotic inpatient profile: a nurse's observation scale. *Journal of Clinical Psychology*, 1969, 25, 137-140. Ia. 5

Lubin (B.): Adjective checklists for measurement of depression. *Archives of General Psychiatry*, 1965, 12, 57-62. Ia. 1

Mac Carthy (M.), Ferris (S.H.), Clark (E.), Crook (T.): Acquisition and retention of categorized material in normal aging and senile dementia. *Experimental Aging Research*, 1981, 7, 2, 127-135. Ib. 45

Meer (B.), Baker (J.A.): The Stockton geriatric rating scale. *Journal of Gerontology*, 1966, 21, 392-403. IV. 1

Mezzena (G.), Fassio (M.), Gallo (I.), Graziano (C.), Lacava (R.), Mazzone (M.), Panero (A.), Veronese-Morosini (M.): M test: un contributo all'esplorazione dello stile di vita. *Quaderno della Rivista di Psicologia Individuale*, 1981, 5. Ic. 17

Miller (E.R.), Parachek (J.F.): Validation and standardization of a goal-oriented, quick-screening geriatric scale. *Journal of the American Geriatrics Society*, 1974, 22, 6, 278-283. IV. 6

Milne (J.S.), Maule (M.M.), Cormack (S.), Williamson (J.): The design and testing of a questionnaire and examination to assess physical and mental health in older people using a staff nurse as the observer. *Journal of Chronic Diseases*, 1972, 25, 385-405. III. 4

Missouri Institute of Psychiatry: Geriatric profile. Missouri Institute of Psychiatry, 1973. Instrument non publié. III. 6

Montgomery (S.A.), Asberg (M.): A new depression scale designed to be sensitive to change. *British Journal of Psychiatry*, 1979, 134, 382-389 Ia. 14

Murkofsky (C.), Conte (H.R.), Plutchik (R.), Karasu (T.B.): Clinical utility of a rapid diagnostic test series for elderly psychiatric outpatients. *Journal of the American Geriatrics Society*, 1978, 26, 1, 22-26. IV. 16

Nahor (A.), Benson (D.F.): A screening test for organic brain disease in emergency psychiatric evaluation. *Behavioral Neuropsychiatry*, 1970, 2, 1/2, 23-26. Ib. 12

Norton (J.C.), Romano (P.O.), Sandifer (M.G.): The ward function inventory (WFI): a scale for use with geriatric and demented inpatients. *Diseases of the Nervous System*, 1977, 38, 1, 20-23. III. 8

Oswald (W.D.), Fleischmann (U.M.): Nürnberger-Alters-Inventar: NAI (the Nuremberg gerontopsychological inventory). 1982. Instrument non publié. IV. 29

Patron (C.): L'évaluation de l'autonomie dans le cadre du maintien à domicile de la personne âgée. *La Revue de Gériatrie*, 1980, 5, 8, 381-386. IV. 21

Pattie (A.H.), Gilleard (C.J.): Manual of the Clifton assessment procedures for the elderly (C.A.P.E.). Kent: Hodder and Stoughton, 1979. IV. 25

Paykel (E.S.), Prusoff (B.A.), Uhlenhuth (E.H.): Scaling of life events *Archives of General Psychiatry*, 1971, 25, 340-347. II. 3

Pfeffer (R.I.), Kurosaki (T.T.), Harrah (C.H.), Chance (J.M.), Filos (S.): Measurement of functional activities in older adults in the community. *Journal of Gerontology*, 1982, 37, 3, 323-329. IV. 30

Pfeiffer (E.): A short portable mental status questionnaire for the assessment of organic brain deficit in elderly patients. *Journal of the American Geriatrics Society*, 1975, 23, 10, 433-441. Ib. 24

Pfeiffer (E.): A short psychiatric evaluation schedule: a new 15-item monotonic scale indicative of functional psychiatric disorder. In: "Brain function in old age": Bayer-Symposium VII, 1979. Springer-Verlag, 1979, 228-236. Ic. 14

Pierce (R.C.), Clark (M.M.): Measurement of morale in the elderly. *International Journal of Aging and Human Development*, 1973, 4, 2, 83-101. Ia. 6

Plutchik (R.), Conte (H.), Lieberman (M.): Development of a scale (GIES) for assessment of cognitive and perceptual functioning in geriatric patients. *Journal of the American Geriatrics Society*, 1971, 19, 7, 614-623. Ib. 14

Plutchik (R.), Conte (H.), Lieberman (M.), Bakur (M.), Grossman (J.), Lehrman (N.): Reliability and validity of a scale for assessing the functioning of geriatric patients. *Journal of the American Geriatrics Society*, 1970, 18, 6, 491-500. IV. 3

Preston (C.E.), Gudiksen (K.S.): A measure of self-perception among older people. *Journal of Gerontology*, 1966, 21, 63-71. II. 1

Qureshi (K.N.), Hodkinson (H.M.): Evaluation of a ten-question mental test in the institutionalized elderly. *Age and Ageing*, 1974, 3, 152-157. Ib. 21

Rorschach (H.): Psychodiagnostic. Méthode et résultats d'une expérience diagnostique de perception. Interprétation libre de formes fortuites. 5e édition française. Paris: Presses Universitaires de France, 1976. II. 6

Sarno (J.E.), Sarno (M.T.), Levita (E.): The functional life scale. *Archives of Physical Medicine and Rehabilitation*, 1973, 54, 214-220. IV. 5

Savage (R.D.), Britton (P.G.): A short scale for the assessment of mental health in the community aged. *British Journal of Psychiatry*, 1967, 113, 521-523. Ic. 4

Shader (R.I.), Harmatz (J.S.), Salzman (C.): A new scale for clinical assessment in geriatric population: Sandoz clinical assessment – geriatric (SCAG). *Journal of the American Geriatrics Society*, 1974, 22, 3, 107-113. — IV. 7

Signoret (J.L.), Whitelem (A.): Memory battery scale. *I.N.S. Bulletin*, 1979, 2, 26. — Ib. 46

Silver (C.P.): Simple methods of testing ability in geriatric patients. *Gerontologia Clinica*, 1972, 110-122. — Ib. 18

Slater (R.), Lipman (A.): Staff assessments of confusion and the situation of confused residents in homes for old pecple. *Gerontologist*, 1977, 17, 6, 523-530. — Ib. 28

Snaith (R.P.), Constantopoulos (A.A.), Jardine (M.Y.), Mc Guffin (P.): A clinical scale for the self-assessment of irritability. *British Journal of Psychiatry*, 1978, 132, 164-171. — Ia. 13

Tennant (C.), Andrews (G.): A scale to measure the stress of life events. *Australian and New Zealand Journal of Psychiatry*, 1976, 10, 27-32. — II. 7

Vignat (J.P.), Israel (L.), Broutchoux (F.): Recueil des données psychologiques et psychiatriques dans les enquêtes épidémiologiques chez les personnes âgées. In: «Accidents vasculaires cérébraux. Recherche épidémiologique». Premier congrès francophone de gérontologie, Paris, 17-18 septembre 1979. Paris: Masson, 1981, 421-441. — IV. 26

Wang (R.I.H.), Wiesen (R.L.), Treul (S.), Stockdale (S.): A brief anxiety rating scale in evaluation anxiolytics. *Journal of Clinical Pharmacology*, 1976, 16 2/3, 99-105. — Ia. 10

Wechsler (D.): Echelle d'intelligence de Wechsler pour adultes: WAIS. 2e édition. Paris: Centre de Psychologie Appliquée, 1970. — Ib. 13

Wells (C.E.): Pseudodementia. *American Journal of Psychiatry*, 1979, 136, 7, 895-900. — Ib. 36

Wilkinson (I.M.), Graham-White (J.): Psychogeriatric dependency rating scales (PGDRS): a method of assessment for use by nurses. *British Journal of Psychiatry*, 1980, 137, 558-565. — IV. 22

Williams (J.R.): Preliminary studies aimed at increasing the reliability of a behavior rating scale for use with geriatric and infirm patients. *Journal of Gerontology*, 1973, 28, 4, 510-515. — Ic. 9

Williams (M.): The measurement of memory in clinical practice. *British Journal of social and clinical Psychology*, 1968, 7, 19-34. — Ib. 8

Wing (J.K.), Cooper (J.E.), Sartorius (N.): Measurement and classification of psychiatric symptoms: an instruction manual for the P.S.E. and CATEGO program. London: Cambridge University Press, 1974. — Ic. 10

Witkin (H.A.), Oltman (P.K.), Raskin (E.), Karp (S.A.): Manual for embedded figures test, children embedded figures test, and group embedded figures test. Palo Alto, CA: Consulting Psychologists Press, 1971. — Ib. 15

World Health Organization: Schedule for a standardized assessment of patients with depressive disorders. Geneva: World Health Organization, March 1977. Instrument non publié. — Ia. 11

World Health Organization: Disability assessment schedule (DAS). Geneva: World Health Organization, 1979. — IV. 18

Yesavage (J.A.), Adey (M.), Werner (P.D.): Development of a geriatric behavioral self-assessment scale. *Journal of the American Geriatrics Society*, 1981, 29, 6, 285-288. — IV. 27

Zay (N.), Boily-Sirois (H.): Indicateurs sociaux et système statistique pour les services aux personnes âgées. III: Le système d'information. Université Laval, Québec: Laboratoire de Gérontologie sociale, 1978. Instrument non publié. — IV. 17

Zung (W.W.K.): A self rating depression scale. *Archives of General Psychiatry*, 1965, 12, 63-70. — Ia. 2

Zung (W.W.K.): How normal is anxiety? (Current concepts). Upjohn Company, 1980. — Ia. 16

REFERENCES OF 100 COMPLEMENTARY INSTRUMENTS

Ammons (R.B.), Ammons (C.H.): The Quick test (QT): provisional manual. *Psychological Reports*, 1962, 11, 111-161.

Asberg (M.), Montgomery (S.A.), Perris (C.), Schalling (D.), Sedvall (G.): A comprehensive psychopathological rating scale. *Acta Psychiat. Scand.*, 1978, Suppl. 271, 5-27.

Barrabee (P.), Barrabee (E.), Finesinger (J.): A normative social adjustment scale. *Amer. J. Psychiat.*, 1955, 112, 252-259.

Beck (A.T.), Weissman (A.), Lester (D.), Trexler (L.): The measurement of pessimism: the hopelessness scale. *Journal of Consulting and Clinical Psychology*, 1974, vol. 42, n°. 6, 861-865.

Berthaux (P.), Piette (F.), Wolmark (Y.), Deboffle (G.), Moulias (R.): Echelle d'autonomie et efficacité des services de moyen séjour. Hambourg, 1981. Instrument non publié.

Bigot (A.): The relevance of american life satisfaction indices for research on british subjects before and after retirement. *Age and Ageing*, 1974, 3, 113-121.

Billingslea (F.Y.): The Bender-Gestalt: an objective scoring method and validating data. *Journal of Clinical Psychology*, 1948, 4, 1, 1-27.

Blewett (D.B.), Stefaniuk (W.B.): Weyburn assessment scale. *J. Ment. Sci.*, 1958, 104, 359-371.

Bloom (M.), Blenkner (M.): Assessing functioning of older persons living in the community. *Gerontologist*, 1970, 31-37.

Britton (P.G.), Savage (R.D.): A short form of the WAIS for use with aged. *Brit. J. Psychiat.*, 1966, 112, 417-418.

Bunney (W.E.), Hamburg (D.A.): Methods for reliable longitudinal observation of behavior. *Arch. Gen. Psychiat.*, 1963, 9, 280-294.

Burdock (E.I.), Hardesty (A.S.), Hakerem (G.), Zubin (J.): A ward behavior rating scale for mental hospital patients. *J. Clin. Psychol.*, 1960, 16, 246-247.

Buss (A.H.), Durkee (A.): An inventory for assessing different kinds of hostility. *J. of Consulting Psychology*, 1957, 21, 343-349.

Caird (W.K.), Sanderson (R.E.), Inglis (J.): Cross-validation of a learning test for use with elderly psychiatric patients. *J. Ment. Sci.*, 1962, 108, 368-370.

Carney (M.W.P.), Roth (M.), Garside (R.F.): The diagnosis of depressive syndromes and the prediction of E.C.T. response. *Brit. J. Psychiat.*, 1965, 111, 659-674.

Clarke (M.), Hughes (A.O.), Dodd (K.J.), Palmer (R.L.), Brandon (S.), Holden (A.M.), Pearce (D.): The elderly in residential care: patterns of disability. *Health Trends*, 1979, vol. 11, 17-20.

Clément (F.): Un test d'apprentissage psycho-moteur: influence de l'âge et de divers facteurs sur ces résultats. *Gerontologia*, 1960, 4, 120-139.

Clément (F.): Un inventaire d'intérêts pour personnes âgées: élaboration et résultats. *Revue de Psychologie Appliquée*, 1962, vol. 12, n°. 1, 1-13.

Clément (F.): Une épreuve rapide de mesure de l'efficience intellectuelle. *Revue de Psychologie Appliquée*, 1963, vol. 13, n° 1, 1-15.

Cooper (J.): The Leyton obsessional inventory. *Psychological Medicine*, 1970, 1, 48-64.

Craig (W.J.): Scales for nursing observation of behavior syndromes. *J. Clin. Psychol.*, 1970, 26, 91-97.

Crown (S.), Crisp (A.H.): A short clinical diagnostic self-rating scale for psychoneurotic patients. *Brit. J. Psychiat.*, 1966, 112, 917-923.

Cutler (R.P.), Kurland (H.D.): Clinical quantification of depressive reactions. *Arch. Gen. Psychiat.*, 1961, 5, 280-285.

Dempsey (P.): An unidimensional depression scale for the MMPI. *Journal of Consulting Psychology*, 1964, vol. 28, n°. 4, 364-370.

Derogatis (L.R.), Lipman (R.S.), Covi (L.): SCL-90: an outpatient psychiatric rating scale: preliminary report. *Psychopharm. Bull.*, 1973, 9, 13-28.

Dinnerstein (A.J.), Lowenthal (M.), Dexter (M.): Evaluation of a rating scale of ability in activities of daily living. *Arch. of Physical Med. & Rehab.*, 1965, 579-584.

Dinoff (M.), Raymaker (H.), Morris (J.R.): The reliability and validity of the minimal social behavior scale and its use as a selection device. *J. Clin. Psychol.*, 1962, 18, 441-444.

Dixon (J.C.): Cognitive structure in senile conditions with some suggestions for developing a brief screening test of mental status. *J. Gerontol.*, 1965, 20, 41-49.

Dobson (W.R.), Patterson (T.W.): A behavioral evaluation of geriatric patients living in nursing homes as compared to a hospitalized group. *Gerontologist*, 1961, vol. 1, 135-139.

Endicott (J.), Spitzer (R.L.): Current and past psychopathology scales (CAPPS). *Arch. Gen. Psychiat.*, 1972, vol. 27, 678-687.

Endicott (J.), Spitzer (R.L.): What! Another rating scale? The psychiatric evaluation form. *The Journal of Nervous and Mental Disease*, 1972, vol. 154, n° 2, 88-104.

Endicott (J.), Spitzer (R.L.): A diagnostic interview: the schedule for affective disorders and schizophrenia. *Arch. Gen. Psychiat.*, 1978, vol. 35, 837-844.

Farina (A.), Arenberg (D.), Guskin (S.): A scale for measuring minimal social behavior. *Journal of Consulting Psychology*, 1957, 21, 3, 265-268.

Freie Universität. Berlin: AGP: Dokumentetionssystem der Arbeitsgemeinschaft für Gerontopsychiatrie. Instrument non publié.

Gauger (A.B.), Brownell (W.M.), Russell (W.W.), Retter (R.W.): Evaluation of levels of subsistence. *Archives of Physical Medicine and Rehabilitation*, 1964, 286-292.

Gough (H.G.): The adjective check list as a personality assessment research technique. *Psychological Reports*, 1960, 6, 107-122.

Gross (M.), Hitchman (I.L.), Reeves (W.P.), Lawrence (J.), Newell (P.C.), Clyde (D.J.): Objective evaluation of psychotic patients under drug therapy: a symptom and adjustment index. *The Journal of Nervous and Mental Disease*, 1961, vol. 133, 399-409.

Guertin (W.H.), Krugman (A.D.): A factor analytically derived scale for rating activities of psychiatric patients. *J. Clin. Psychol.*, 1959, 15, 32-36.

Guilford (J.P.), Guilford (R.B.): Personality factors D.R.T, and A. *Journ. Abnorm. Soc. Psychol.*, 1939, 34, 21-36.

Gurel (L.), Davis (J.E.): A survey of self-care dependency in psychiatric patients. *Hospital and Community Psychiatry*, May 1967, 135-138.

Gurland (B.J.), Yorkston (N.J.), Stone (A.R.), Frank (J.D.), Fleiss (J.L.): The structured and scaled interview to assess maladjustment (SSIAM). *Arch. Gen. Psychiat.*, Aug. 1972, vol. 27, 259-267.

Hafner (J.L.), Corotto (L.V.), Curnutt (R.H.): The development of a WAIS short form for clinical populations. *J. Clin. Psychol.*, 1978, vol. 34, n. 4, 935-937.

Hargreaves (W.A): Systematic nursing observation of psychopatholgy. *Arch. Gen. Psychiat.*, 1968, 18, 518-531.

Harris (A.D), Letemendia (F.J.J.), Willems (P.J.A.): A rating scale of the mental state: for use in the chronic population of the psychiatric hospital. *Brit. J. Psychiat.*, 1967, 113, 941-949.

Heron (A.): A two-part personality measure for use as a research criterion. *Brit. J. Psychol.*, Nov. 1956, vol. 47, n. 4, 243-251.

Hirschfeld (M.J.): The use of a formula predictive of families'caregiving capacity. In: International Association of Gerontology: "Psychological and sociological aspects of the health care of the aged: research, methods and results": proceedings for the XXth Symposium of social gerontology, Prage, Czechoslovakia, August 18-22 1980.

Hunt (H.F.): A note on the clinical use of the Hunt-Minnesota test for organic brain damage. *J. Appl. Psychol.*, 1944, 28, 175-178.

Isaacs (B.), Walkey (F.A.): Measurement of mental impairment in geriatric practice. *Geront. Clin.*, 1964, 6, 114-123.

Jenkins (R.L.), Stauffacher (J.), Hester (R.): A symptom rating scale for use with psychotic patients. *Arch. Gen. Psychiat.*, Aug. 1959, vol. 1, 197-204.

Jette (A.M.), Deniston (O.L.): Inter-observer reliability of a functional status assessment instrument. *J. Chron. Dis.*, 1978, vol. 31, 573-580.

Kahn (T.C.): A new "culture-free" intelligence test. *Psychological Reports*, 1960, 6, 239-242.

Katz (M.M.), Lyerly (S.B.): Methods for measuring adjustment and social behavior in the community. I: Rationale, description, discriminative validity and scale development. *Psychological Reports*, 1963, 13, 503-535.

Kral (V.A.), Cahn (C.), Mueller (H.): Senescent memory impairment and its relation to the general health of the aging individual. *Journal of the American Geriatrics Society*, 1964, vol. 12, n°. 2, 101-113.

Langner (T.S.): A twenty-two item screening score of psychiatric symptoms indicating impairment. *J. of Health and Human Behavior*, 1962, 3, 269-276.

Lorr (M.), O'Connor (J.P.), Stafford (J.W.): The psychotic reaction profile. *J. Clin. Psychol.*, 1960, 16, 241-245.

Lucero (R.J.), Meyer (B.T.): A behavior rating scale suitable for use in mental hospitals. *J. Clin. Psychol.*, 1951, 7, 250-254.

Mack (J.L.), Carlson (N.J.): Conceptual deficits and aging: the category test. *Perceptual and Motor Skills*, 1978, 46, 123-128.

Mac Nair (D.M.), Lorr (M.), Droppleman (L.F.): Profile of mood states. San Diego: Educational and industrial testing service, 1971.

Malamud (W.), Hoagland (H.), Kaufman (I.C.): A new psychiatric rating scale. *Psychosom. Med.*, 1946, 8, 243-245.

Neugarten (B.L.), Havighurst (R.J.), Tobin (S.S.): The measurement of life satisfaction. *J. Geront.*, 1961, 16, 134-143.

Oberleder (M.): An attitude scale to determine adjustment in institutions for the aged. *J. Chron. Dis.*, 1961, vol. 15, 915-923.

Overall (J.E.), Gorham (D.R.): The brief psychiatric rating scale. *Psychological Reports*, 1962, 10, 799-812.

Overall (J.E.), Hollister (L.E.), Pokorny (A.D.), Casey (J.F.), Katz (G.): Drug therapy in depressions: controlled evaluation of imipramine, isocarboxazide, dextroamphetamine-amobarbital, and placebo. *Clinical Pharmacology and Therapeutics*, 1962, vol. 3, n° 1, 16-22.

Pauker (N.E.), Folstein (M.F.), Moran (T.H.): The clinical utility of the hand-held tachistoscope. *The Journal of Nervous and Mental Disease*, 1978, vol. 166, n° 2, 126-129.

Petterson (U.), Fyrö (B.), Sedvall (G.): A new scale for the longitudinal rating of manic states. *Acta Psychiat. Scand.*, 1973, 49, 248-256.

Raskin (A.), Schulterbrandt (J.), Reatig (N.), Mc Keon (J.J.): Replication of factors of psychopathology in interview, ward behavior and self-report ratings of hospitalized depressives. *The Journal of Nervous and Mental Disease*, 1969, vol. 148, n°. 1, 87-98.

Remington (M.), Tyrer (P.): The social functioning schedule. A brief semi-structured interview. *Social Psychiatry*, 1979, 14, 151-157.

Rickels (K.), Howard (K.): The physician questionnaire: a useful tool in psychiatric drug research. *Psychopharmacologia*, 1970, 17, 338-344.

Robinson (R.A.): Some problems of clinical trials in elderly people. *Geront. Clin.*, 1961, 3, 247-257.

Rockland (L.H.), Pollin (W.): Quantification of psychiatric mental status. *Archives of General Psychiatry*, Jan. 1965, vol. 12, 23-28.

Rowell (J. T.): An objective method of evaluating mental status. *J. Clin. Psychol.*, 1951, 7, 255-259.

Scheier (I.H.), Cattell (R.B.), Sullivan (W.): Predicting anxiety from clinical symptoms of anxiety. I: Background, and measurements employed. *Psychiat. Quart. Suppl.*, 1961, 35, 114-126.

Schwab (J.J.), Holzer (C.E.), Warheit (G.J.): Depressive symptomatology and age. *Psychosomatics*, May-June 1973, vol. 14, 135-141.

Shapiro (M.B.), Post (F.), Löfving (B.), Inglis (J.): "Memory function" in psychiatric patients over sixty, some methodological and diagnostic implications. *J. Ment. Sci.*, 1956, 102, 233-246.

Shatin (L.), Freed (E.X.): A behavioural rating scale for mental patients. *J. Ment. Sci.*, 1955, 101, 644-653.

Sidman (J.), Moos (R.H.): Staff and patient helping questionnaire. 1969. Instrument non publié.

Silver (D.), Lehmann (H.E.), Kral (V.A.), Ban (T.A.): Experimental geriatrics: selection and prediction of therapeutic responsiveness in geriatric patients. *Canad. Psychiat. Assoc. J.*, Dec. 1968, vol. 13, n°. 6, 561-563.

Simon (A.), Berkman (P.L.), Epstein (L.J.): Psychiatric screening of the elderly. *California Mental Health Research Digest*, 1969, 7, 2, 62-63.

Simpson (G.M.), Angus (J.W.S.): A rating scale for extrapyramidal side effects. *Acta Psychiatrica Scandinavica*, 1970, Suppl. 212, 11-19.

Simpson (G.M.), Hackett (E.), Kline (N.S.): Difficulties in systematic rating of depression during out-patient drug treatment. *Canad. Psychiat. Assoc. J.*, 1966, Suppl. I, 116-122.

Skinner (D.E.), Yett (D.E.): Debility index for long-term-care patients. In: Berg (R.L.): "Health status indexes": proceedings of a conference conducted by Health Service Research, Tucson, Arizona, October 1-4 1972. Chicago: Hospital Research and Educational Trust, 1973, 69-89.

Smith (A.): The serial sevens subtraction test. *Arch. neurol.*, July 1967, vol. 17, 78-80.

Snaith (R.P.), Bridge (G.W.K.), Hamilton (M.): The Leeds scales for the self-assessment of anxiety and depression. *Brit. J. Psychiat.*, 1976, 128, 156-165.

Spitzer (R.L.), Endicott (J.), Fleiss (J.L.), Cohen (J.): The psychiatric status schedule: a technique for evaluating psychopathology and impairment in role functioning. *Arch. Gen. Psychiat.*, July 1970, vol. 23, 41-55.

Spitzer (R.L.), Fleiss (J.L.), Burdock (E.I.), Hardesty (A.S.): The mental status schedule: rationale, reliability and validity. *Comprehensive Psychiatry*, Dec. 1964, vol. 5, n° 6, 384-395.

Stotsky (B.A.): A systematic study of therapeutic interventions in nursing homes. *Genetic Psychology Monographs*, 1967, 76, 257-320.

Taylor (J.): A personality scale of manifest anxiety. *The Journal of Abnormal and Social Psychology*, 1953, vol. 48, n° 2, 285-290.

Tien (H.C.): Organic Integrity Test (O.I.T.): a quick diagnostic aid to rule in organic brain diseases. *Archives of General Psychiatry*, July 1960, vol. 3, 67/43-76/52.

Trier (T.R.): A study of change among elderly psychiatric inpatients during their first year of hospitalization. *Journal of Gerontology*, 1968, 23, 354-362.

Van De Castle (R.L.): Development and validation of a perceptual maturity scale using figure preferences. *Journal of Consulting Psychology*, 1965, vol. 29, n° 4, 314-319.

Venables (P.H.): A short scale for rating "activity-withdrawal" in schizophrenics. *J. Ment. Sci.*, 1957, 103, 197-199.

Widlocher (D.): L'évaluation quantitative du ralentissement psychomoteur dans les états dépressifs. *Psychologie Médicale*, 1980, 12, 13, 2725-2729.

Wilcox (P.H.): The Gardner behavior chart. *Amer. J. Psychiatry*, 1942, 98, 874-880.

Wilson (I.C.): Rapid approximate intelligence test. *Amer. J. Psychiatry*, Apr. 1967, 123, 10, 1289-1290.

World Health Organization: Status physique fonctionnel: étude concertée sur la comparaison des soins hospitaliers à la population âgée en service général ou spécialisé. Sept. 1981. Instrument non publié.

Wyatt (R.J.), Kupper (D.J.): A fourteen-symptom behavior and mood rating scale for longitudinal patient evaluation by nurses. *Psychological Reports*, 1968, 23, 1331-1334.

Wylie (C.M.): Gauging the response of stroke patients to rehabilitation. *Journal of the American Geriatrics Society*, 1967, vol. 15, n° 9, 797-805.

Zerssen (Von D.V.), Koeller (D.M.), Rey (E.R.): Die Befindlichkeits-Skala (B-S), ein einfaches Instrument zur Objektivierung von Befindlichkeitsstörungen, insbesondere im Rahmen von Längsschnittuntersuchungen. *Arzneim. Forsch.*, 1970, vol. 20, n° 7, 915-918.

Zuckerman (M.): The development of an affect adjective check list for the measurement of anxiety. *Journal of Consulting Psychology*, 1960, vol. 24, n° 5, 457-462.

Zung (W.W.K.): The depression status inventory: an adjunct to the self-rating depression scale. *Journ. Clin. Psychol.*, 1972, 28, 539-543.

BALINSKY (W.), BERGER (R.): A review of the research on general health status indexes. *Medical Care*, 1975, 13, 283-293.

BANOUB (S.N.): Methodology of social and health surveys of the elderly in developing countries: problems and alternative approaches. Paper submitted to the Scientific Group Meeting on the Epidemiology of Aging, Geneva, 11-17 January 1983.

BECH (P.): Rating scales for affective disorders: their validity and consistency. *Acta Psychiatrica Scandinavica*, 1981 Suppl. 295.

BELLOC (N.B.), Breslow (L.), Hochstim (J.R.): Measurement of physical health in a general population survey. *American Journal of Epidemiology*, 1971, vol. 93, n° 5, 328-336.

BERG (R.L.) ED.: Health status indexes: proceedings of a conference conducted by Health Service Research, Tucson, Arizona, October 1-4, 1972. Chicago: Hospital Research and Educational Trust, 1973.

BIRREN (J.E.), SCHAIE (K.W.) EDS.: Handbook of the psychology of aging. New York: Van Nostrand Reinhold Company, 1977.

BIRREN (J.E.), SLOANE (R.B.) Eds.: Handbook of mental health and aging. Englewood Cliffs, N.J.: Prentice-Hall, 1980.

BLAHA (L.): Psychopathometry in elderly patients. In: "Drugs and methods in C.V.D.": proceedings of the international symposium on Experimental and Cinical Methodologies for Study of Acute and Chronic Cerebrovascular Diseases, Paris, March 24-26 1980. New York: Pergamon Press, 1981.

BLOOM (M.): Evaluation instruments: tests and measurements in long-term care. In: Sherwood (S.): "Long-term care: a handbook for researchers, planners and providers". New York: Spectrum, 1975, 573-638.

BRODY (J.): Research priorities in the epidemiology of aging. Paper submitted to the Scientific Group Meeting on the Epidemiology of Aging, 11-17 January 1983.

BROOK (R.H.), WARE (J.E.), DAVIES-AVERY (A.), STEWART (A.), DONALD (C.A.), ROGERS (W.H.), WILLIAMS (K.N.), JOHNSTON (S.A.): Conceptualization and measurement of health for adults in the health insurance study. Vol. VIII: overview. *Medical Care*, July 1979, vol. 17, n° 7, 1-131.

BRUETT (T.L.), OVERS (R.P.): A critical review of 12 ADL scales. *Physical Therapy*, 1969, vol. 49, n° 8, 857-862.

CHUN (K.T.), COBB (S.), FRENCH (J.R.P.): Measures for psychological assessment: a guide to 3000 original sources and their applications. Ann Arbor, Michigan: Survey Research Center, Institute for Social Research, 1975.

COHEN (J.), BRODY (J.): The epidemiologic importance of psychological factors in longevity. *American Journal of Epidemiology*, 1981, 114, 4, 451-461.

COLE (J.O.), BARRETT (J.E.) Eds.: Psychopathology in the aged. New York: Raven Press, 1980.

COMREY (A.), BACKER (T.), GLASER (E.): A sourcebook for mental health measures. Los Angeles, California: Human Interaction Research Institute, 1973.

DENTON (C.F.): The design of health and social surveys of the elderly. Paper submitted to the Scientific Group Meeting on the Epidemiology of Aging, Geneva 11-17 January 1983.

DONALD (C.A.) ET AL.: Social health. In: "Conceptualization and measurement of health for adults in the health insurance study". Santa Monica: Rand Corporation, 1979, vol. 4.

DONALDSON (S.W.), WAGNER (C.C.), GRESHAM (G.E.): A unified ADL evaluation form. *Arch. Phys. Med. Rehabil.*, April 1973, vol. 54, 175-179.

EISDORFER (C.), FRIEDEL (R.O.) EDS.: Cognitive and emotional disturbance in the elderly. Chicago: Year Book Medical Publishers, 1977.

ERICKSON (R.C.), SCOTT (M.L.): Clinical memory testing: a review. *Psychological Bulletin*, 1977, vol. 84, n° 6, 1130-1149.

FAVERGE (J.M.): Méthodes statistiques en psychologie appliquée. 7e éd. Paris: Presses Universitaires de France, 1975.

FILLENBAUM (G.G.): Comparison of two brief tests of organic brain impairment, the MSQ and the Short Portable MSQ. *Journal of the American Geriatrics Society*, 1980, 28, 381-384.

FILLENBAUM (G.G.): The wellbeing of the elderly: approaches to multidimensional assessment. Copenhagen: World Health Organization, 1982.

GALLAGHER (D.), THOMPSON (L.W.), LEVY (S.M.): Clinical psychological assessment of older adults. In: Poon (L.) Ed. "Aging in the 1980's: selected contemporary issues in the psychology of aging". Washington: American Psychological Association, 1980.

GEORGE (L.K.): Developing measures of functional status and service utilization for program evaluation of services for the elderly. Proposal funded by NRTA-AARP Andrus Foundation, 1981.

GEORGE (L.K.), BEARON (L.B.): Quality of life in older persons: meaning and measurement. New York: Human Sciences Press, 1980.

GILMORE (A.J.J.): Rating scales and their value. *Geront. Clin.*, 1974, 16, 137-142.

GILMORE (A.J.J.), SVANBORG (A.), MAROIS (M.), BEATTIE (W.M.), PIOTROWSKI (J.): Ageing: a challenge to science and society. Oxford: Oxford University Press, 1981.

GOGA (J.A.), HAMBACHER (W.O.): Psychologic and behavioral assessment of geriatric patients: a review. *Journal of the American Geriatrics Society*, 1977, vol. 25, n° 5, 232-237.

GRANEY (M.J.), GRANEY (E.E.): Scaling adjustment in older people. *Intern. J. of Aging and Human Development*, 1973, vol. 4, n° 4, 351-359.

GRANEY (M.J.), GRANEY (E.E.): Communication activity substitutions on aging. *Journal of Communication*, 1974, 24, 88-96.

GRAWITZ (M.): Méthode des sciences sociales. 5e éd. Paris: Dalloz, 1981.

GRINBLAT (J.): Aging in the world: demographic determinants, past trends and long-term perspective to 2075. Geneva: World Health Organization, 1982.

GUY (W.) ED.: ECDEU assessment manual for psychopharmacology. Revised. Rockville, Maryland: U.S. Department of Health, Education, and Welfare, 1976.

HABERMAN (P.W.): Appendix. The reliability and validity of the data. In: Kosa (J.) et al. Eds.: "Poverty and health". Cambridge: Harvard University Press, 1969.

HALL (J.N.): Assessment procedures used in studies on long-stay patients. *Brit. J. Psychiat.*, 1979, 135, 330-335.

HALL (J.N.): Ward rating scales for long-stay patients: a review. *Psychological Medicine*, 1980, 10, 277-288.

HÉBERT (R.): L'autonomie fonctionnelle des personnes âgées: pour une prévention des dépendances pathologiques. Mémoire non publié. Grenoble: Centre Pluridisciplinaire de Gérontologie, Université des Sciences Sociales, 1981.

HEIKKINEN (E.), WATERS (W.) BREZEZINSKI: The elderly in eleven countries: a sociomedical survey. Copenhagen: WHO Regional Office for Europe, 1982.

HENNES (J.D.): The measurement of health. *Medical Care Review*, 1972, 29, 1268-1288.

HONIGFELD (G.): The evaluation of ward behavior rating scales for psychogeriatric use. *Psychopharmacology Bulletin*, October 1981, vol. 17, n° 4, 82-95.

HUGONOT (L.): Contribution à l'étude des échelles de dépendance en gériatrie. Thèse Méd., Grenoble, 1977.

Institut National de la Santé et de la Recherche Médicale (I.N.S.E.R.M.). Paris: Santé publique et vieillissement: colloque, Paris, 18-19 Juin 1981. Paris: Editions de l'INSERM, 1982.

ISAACS (B.), NEVILLE (Y.): The measurement of need in old people. Scottish Home and Health Department, 1976. (Scottish Health Service Studies, n° 34).

ISAACS (B.), NEVILLE (Y.): The needs of old people: the "interval" as a method of measurement. *British Journal of preventive and social Medicine*, 1976, 30, 79-85.

ISRAEL (L.): Memory disorders as a criteria of dependency in old people: evaluation and measurement. In: Munnichs (J.M.A.), Van den Heuvel (W.J.A.) Eds.: "Dependency or interdependency in old age". The Hague: Martinus Nijhoff, 1976.

ISRAEL (L.): Application de techniques psychométriques à l'étude des thérapeutiques à visée cérébrale en milieu gériatrique. Thèse Psychol., Doctorat 3e cycle, Grenoble, 1977.

ISRAEL (L.): Means of prevention of mental disability in the elderly through memory stimulation. Paper submitted to Working Group to Define Means of Prevention of Disability in the Elderly, Cologne, 16-19 November 1981.

ISRAEL (L.): Application of psychometric techniques to the study of treatment affecting brain functioning. In: "Drugs studies in CVD and PVD": proceedings of the international symposium, Geneva, May 25-26 1981. New York, Paris: Pergamon Press, 1982.

ISRAEL (L.), Kozarevic (D.): Multidimensions of health in assessing the elderly: WHO informal meeting on Measuring Cognitive Improvement, Health and Functioning in the Elderly, Geneva, 22-24 Sept. 1982.

KAHN (R.L.), ZARIT (S.H.), NIEDEREHE (G.): Memory complaint and impairment in the aged. *Arch. Gen. Psychiat.*, December 1975, vol. 32, 1569-1573.

KANE (R.L.), KANE (R.A.): Assessing the elderly: a practical guide to measurement. Lexington, Mass.: Lexington Books, 1981.

KATZ (M.M.), COLE (J.O.), BARTON (W.E.) EDS: The role and methodology of classification in psychiatry and psychopathology: proceedings of a conference held in Washington, November 1965. Chevy Chase, Md: U.S. Department of Health, Education and Welfare, Public Health Service, National Institute of Mental Health.

KATZ (S.), AKPOM (C.A.): A measure of primary sociobiological functions. *International Journal of Health Services*, 1976, 6, 493-507

KATZ (S.), HEDRICK (S.C.), HENDERSON (N.S.): The measurement of long-term care needs and impact. *Health and Medical Care Services Review*, Spring 1979, vol. 2, n° 1, 1-21.

KENT (D.P.), KASTENBAUM (R.), SHERWOOD (S.) EDS.: Research planning and action for the elderly: the power and potential of social science. New York: Behavioral Publications, 1972.

KNOX (E.G.): Epidemiology in health care planning. Oxford: Oxford University Press, 1979.

KOZAREVIĆ (Dj.): Health status and performance in activities of daily living in old age. Paper submitted to Working Group to Define Means of Prevention of Disability in the Elderly, Cologne, 16-19 November 1981.

KOZAREVIĆ (Dj.): Performance in activities of daily living and clinical data. Presented at Working Group on the Organization of services to prevent disability among the elderly, Sokobanja, 1982.

KOZAREVIĆ (Dj.): The design of health and social surveys of the elderly. Paper submitted to Scientific Group on the Epidemiology of Aging, Geneva, 11-17 January 1983.

LARSON (R.): Thirty years of research on the subjective well-being of older americans. *Journal of Gerontology*, 1978, vol. 33, n° 1, 109-125.

LEAVEL (H.R.), CLARK (E.G.): Preventive medicine for the doctor in the community. 2nd ed. New York: Mc Graw-Hill, 1958.

LEROY (M.), SALAUN (P.), CHOVELON (R.), BOUILLOUX (E.): Approche clinique et psychométrique en gériatrie. Méthodes d'études et choix d'une thérapeutique. *La Vie Médicale*, 28 novembre 1978, 2513-2519.

LINN (M.W.): Studies in rating the physical, mental, and social dysfunction of the chronically ill aged. *Medical Care*, May 1976, vol. 14, n° 5 (Suppl.), 119-125.

LOEB (C.): Clinical diagnosis of multi-infarct dementia. In: Amaducci (L.) et al.: "Aging of the brain and dementia" – Aging, vol. 13. New York: Raven Press, 1980.

LORR (M.): Rating scales, behavior inventories, and drugs. In: Uhr (L.), Miller (J.G.): "Drugs and behavior". New York, London: John Wiley and sons, 1960, 519-538.

LYERLY (S.B.) ED.: Handbook of psychiatric rating scales. Second edition. Rockville, Maryland: National Institute of Mental Health, 1978.

MAC MAHON (M.), PUGH (T.), IPSEN (J.): Epidemiologic methods. Little Brown and Comp., 1960.

MADDOX (G.): Sociology, aging, and guided social change: relating alternative organization of helping resources to well-being. In: Yinger (M.), Cutler (S.) Eds.: "Major social issues: a multidisciplinary view". New York: The Free Press, 1978.

MADDOX (G.L.) ET AL.: Extending the use of the LRHS data set. *Review of public data use*, 1979, 7, 57-62.

MADDOX (G.L.), DELLINGER (D.C.): Assessment of functional status in a program evaluation and resource allocation model *Annals of the American Academy of Political and Social Science*, 1978, 438, 59-70.

MADDOX (G.L.), MANTON (K.): Purposive data archiving as a component of information systems for planning policy and research in aging. Paper submitted to the Scientific Group Meeting on the Epidemiology of Aging, 11-17 January 1983.

MALCOLM (L.): A health information system for service planning for the aging. Paper submitted to the Scientific Group Meeting on the Epidemiology of Aging, 11-17 January 1983.

MANGEN (D.J.), PETERSON (W.A.) EDS.: Research instruments in social gerontology. Minneapolis: University of Minnesota, 1982 and forthcoming, vol. 1-3.

MECHANIC (D.): Readings in medical sociology. New York: The Free Press, 1980.

MEEGAMA (S.A.): Aging in developing countries. Geneva: World Health Organization, 1982.

MIGDAL (S.), ABELES (R.), SHERROD (L.) EDS.: An inventory of longitudinal studies of middle and old age. New York: Social Science Research Council, 1981.

MUNNICHS (J.M.A.), VAN DEN HEUVEL (W.J.A.) EDS.: Dependency or interdependency in old age. The Hague: Martinus Nijhoff, 1976.

NATIONAL INSTITUTE ON AGING. U.S.: Federal demographic and health research data: resources and needs. Bethesda, Maryland, unpublished conference proceedings, June 25-27 1979.

PERSE (M.J.), PELICIER (Y.), HUBER (J.P.), BENICHOU (S.): Les tests d'intelligence. *Psychologie Médicale*, 1978, 10, 1, 129-134.

PICHOT (P.): Le problème de quantification dans la recherche psychiatrique. *Bulletin de L'Académie Suisse des Sciences Médicales*, 1970, 25, 147-159.

POITRENAUD (J.), MOREAUX (C.): Normes psychométriques pour sujets âgés. *Revue de Psychologie Appliquée*, 1974, 24, 3.

POWELL (C.), CROMBIE (A.): The Kilsyth questionnaire: a method of screening elderly people at home. *Age and Ageing*, 1974, 3, 23-28.

Preventing disability in the elderly: report on a WHO Working Group. Copenhagen: WHO Regional Office for Europe, 1982. (EURO Reports and Studies, n° 65).

RASKIN (A.), JARVIK (L.F.): Psychiatric symptoms and cognitive loss in the elderly: evaluation and assessment techniques. Washingtom: Hemisphere Publishing Corporation, 1979.

REISBERG (B.), FERRIS (S.H.): Diagnosis and assessment of the older patients. *Hospital and Community Psychiatry*, February 1982, 33, 2, 104-110.

REUCHLIN (M.): Précis de statistique. 2e édition. Paris: Presses Universitaires de France, 1979.

REUCHLIN (M.): La psychologie différentielle. 3e édition. Paris: Presses Universitaires de France, 1980.

SACHUK: The value of early detection of high risk cases in maintaining independence of the elderly. Paper submitted to the Scientific Group Meeting on the Epidemiology of Aging, Geneva, 11-17 January 1983.

SAINSBURY (S.): Measuring disability. London: Bell and sons, 1973.

SALZMAN (C.), KOCHANSKY (G.E.), SHADER (R.I.): Rating scales for geriatric psychopharmacology: a review. *Psychopharmacology Bullettin*, 1972, 8, 3, 3-50.

SALZMAN (C.), SHADER (R.I.), KOCHANSKY (G.E.), CRONIN (D.M.): Rating scales for psychotropic drug research with geriatric patients. 1: Behavior ratings. *Journal of the American Geriatrics Society*, 1972, 20, 5.

SARTORIUS (N.): The research component of the WHO mental health program. *Psychological Medicine*, 1980, 10, 175-185.

SAVAGE (R.D.): Intellectual assessment. In: Mittler (P.) Ed.: "The psychological assessment of mental and physical handicaps". London: Methuen and co., 1970.

Science Citation Index (Annual): an international interdisciplinary index to the literature of science, medicine, agriculture, technology, and the behavioral sciences. Philadelphia, Pennsylvania: Institute for Scientific Information.

SHERWOOD (S.) ED.: Long-term care: a handbook for researchers, planners and providers. New York: Spectrum, 1975.

SIEGEL (J.S.): Demographic aspects of the health of the elderly to the year 2000 and beyond. Copenhagen: World Health Organization, 1982.

SNAITH (R.P.): Rating scales. *Brit. J. Psychiat.*, 1981, 138, 512-514.

SPRIET (A.), Fermanian (J.), Simon (P.): L'utilisation des échelles d'évaluation en psycho-pharmacologie. *L'Encéphale*, 1978, 4, 119-129.

SPRIET (A.), SIMON (P.): Méthodologie des essais cliniques des médicaments. Paris. Editions de la Prospective Médicale, 1980.

SVANBORG (A.), BERGSTRÖM (G.), MELLSTRÖM (D.): Epidemiological studies on social and medical conditions of the elderly. Copenhagen: WHO Regional Office for Europe, 1982. (EURO Reports and Studies, n° 62).

WORLD HEALTH ORGANIZATION: International classification of impairments, disabilities, and handicaps. A manual of classification relating to the consequences of disease. Geneva: World Health Organization, 1980.